# Pediatric Brain Tumors Update

*Editor*

LARA A. BRANDÃO

# NEUROIMAGING CLINICS
# OF NORTH AMERICA

www.neuroimaging.theclinics.com

*Consulting Editor*
SURESH K. MUKHERJI

February 2017 • Volume 27 • Number 1

**ELSEVIER**

1600 John F. Kennedy Boulevard • Suite 1800 • Philadelphia, Pennsylvania, 19103-2899

http://www.neuroimaging.theclinics.com

**NEUROIMAGING CLINICS OF NORTH AMERICA Volume 27, Number 1**
**February 2017 ISSN 1052-5149, ISBN 13: 978-0-323-49654-4**

Editor: John Vassallo (j.vassallo@elsevier.com)
Developmental Editor: Casey Potter

*Neuroimaging Clinics of North America* (ISSN 1052-5149) is published quarterly by Elsevier Inc., 360 Park Avenue South, New York, NY 10010-1710. Months of issue are February, May, August, and November. Business and editorial offices: 1600 John F. Kennedy Blvd., Suite 1800, Philadelphia, PA 19103-2899. Business and editorial offices: 6277 Sea Harbor Drive, Orlando, FL 32887-4800. Periodicals postage paid at New York, NY, and additional mailing offices. Subscription prices are USD 365 per year for US individuals, USD 581 per year for US institutions, USD 100 per year for US students and residents, USD 415 per year for Canadian individuals, USD 740 per year for Canadian institutions, USD 525 per year for international individuals, USD 740 per year for international institutions and USD 260 per year for Canadian and foreign students and residents. To receive student/resident rate, orders must be accompanied by name of affiliated institution, date of term, and the *signature* of program/residency coordinator on institution letterhead. Orders will be billed at individual rate until proof of status is received. Foreign air speed delivery is included in all *Clinics* subscription prices. All prices are subject to change without notice. POSTMASTER: Send address changes to *Neuroimaging Clinics of North America*, Elsevier Health Sciences Division, Subscription **Customer Service, 3251 Riverport Lane, Maryland Heights, MO 63043. Telephone: 1-800-654-2452 (U.S. and Canada); 314-447-8871 (outside U.S. and Canada). Fax: 314-447-8029. E-mail: journalscustomer service-usa@elsevier.com (for print support); journalsonlinesupport-usa@elsevier.com (for online support).**

*Reprints.* For copies of 100 or more of articles in this publication, please contact the Commercial Reprints Department, Elsevier Inc., 360 Park Avenue South, New York, NY 10010-1710. Tel.: 212-633-3874; Fax: 212-633-3820; E-mail: reprints@elsevier.com.

*Neuroimaging Clinics of North America* is covered by *Excerpta Medical/EMBASE,* the RSNA Index of Imaging Literature, *MEDLINE/PubMed (Index Medicus),* MEDLINE/MEDLARS, SciSearch, Research Alert, and Neuroscience Citation Index.

## PROGRAM OBJECTIVE
The goal of *Neuroimaging Clinics of North America* is to keep practicing radiologists and radiology residents up to date with current clinical practice in radiology by providing timely articles reviewing the state of the art in patient care.

## TARGET AUDIENCE
Practicing radiologists, radiology residents, and other healthcare professionals who utilize neuroimaging findings to provide patient care.

## LEARNING OBJECTIVES
Upon completion of this activity, participants will be able to:
1. Review imaging techniques in pediatric brain tumors.
2. Discuss clinical applications for advanced MRI in pediatric brain tumors.
3. Recognize neuroimaging techniques for brain tumors in the neonate.

## ACCREDITATION
The Elsevier Office of Continuing Medical Education (EOCME) is accredited by the Accreditation Council for Continuing Medical Education (ACCME) to provide continuing medical education for physicians.

The EOCME designates this enduring material for a maximum of 15 *AMA PRA Category 1 Credit*(s)™. Physicians should claim only the credit commensurate with the extent of their participation in the activity.

All other health care professionals requesting continuing education credit for this enduring material will be issued a certificate of participation.

## DISCLOSURE OF CONFLICTS OF INTEREST
The EOCME assesses conflict of interest with its instructors, faculty, planners, and other individuals who are in a position to control the content of CME activities. All relevant conflicts of interest that are identified are thoroughly vetted by EOCME for fair balance, scientific objectivity, and patient care recommendations. EOCME is committed to providing its learners with CME activities that promote improvements or quality in healthcare and not a specific proprietary business or a commercial interest.

**The planning committee, staff, authors and editors listed below have identified no financial relationships or relationships to products or devices they or their spouse/life partner have with commercial interest related to the content of this CME activity:**
Stefan Blüml, PhD; Thangamadhan Bosemani, MD; Lara A. Brandão, MD; Rafael Ceschin, BS; Marjolein H.G. Dremmen, MD; Anjali Fortna; Andre D. Furtado, MD; Jeroen Hendrikse, MD, PhD; Thierry A.G.M. Huisman, MD; Izlem Izbudak, MD; Regina I. Jakacki, MD; Maarten Lequin, MD, PhD; Gary Mason, MD; Suresh K. Mukherji, MD, MBA, FACR; Marvin Nelson, MD, MBA; Ashok Panigrahy, MD; Ian F. Pollack, MD; Andrea Poretti, MD; Tina Young Poussaint, MD, FACR; Erin Simon Schwartz, MD; Daniel P. Seeburg, MD, PhD; Karuna V. Shekdar, MD; Karthik Subramaniam; Megan Suermann; Benita Tamrazi, MD; Mary Tenenbaum, MD; John Vassallo; Carlos Zamora, MD, PhD.

**The planning committee, staff, authors and editors listed below have identified financial relationships or relationships to products or devices they or their spouse/life partner have with commercial interest related to the content of this CME activity:**
**Hideho Okada, MD** is an inventor in a patent with Stemline Therapeutics, Inc.

## UNAPPROVED/OFF-LABEL USE DISCLOSURE
The EOCME requires CME faculty to disclose to the participants:
1. When products or procedures being discussed are off-label, unlabelled, experimental, and/or investigational (not US Food and Drug Administration [FDA] approved); and
2. Any limitations on the information presented, such as data that are preliminary or that represent ongoing research, interim analyses, and/or unsupported opinions. Faculty may discuss information about pharmaceutical agents that is outside of FDA-approved labelling. This information is intended solely for CME and is not intended to promote off-label use of these medications. If you have any questions, contact the medical affairs department of the manufacturer for the most recent prescribing information.

## TO ENROLL
To enroll in the *Neuroimaging Clinics of North America* Continuing Medical Education program, call customer service at 1-800-654-2452 or sign up online at http://www.theclinics.com/home/cme. The CME program is available to subscribers for an additional annual fee of USD 235.

## METHOD OF PARTICIPATION
In order to claim credit, participants must complete the following:
1. Complete enrolment as indicated above.

2. Read the activity.
3. Complete the CME Test and Evaluation. Participants must achieve a score of 70% on the test. All CME Tests and Evaluations must be completed online.

**CME INQUIRIES/SPECIAL NEEDS**

For all CME inquiries or special needs, please contact elsevierCME@elsevier.com.

# NEUROIMAGING CLINICS OF NORTH AMERICA

**THE CLINICS ARE AVAILABLE ONLINE!**
Access your subscription at:
www.theclinics.com

# Contributors

## CONSULTING EDITOR

**SURESH K. MUKHERJI, MD, MBA, FACR**
Professor and Chairman, Walter F. Patenge
Endowed Chair, Department of Radiology,
Michigan State University, Chief Medical
Officer & Director of Health Care Delivery,
Michigan State University Health Team, East
Lansing, Michigan

## EDITOR

**LARA A. BRANDÃO, MD**
Chief of Neuroradiology, Radiologic
Department, Clínica Felippe Mattoso, Fleury
Medicina Diagnóstica, Neuroradiologist,
Radiologic Department, Clínica IRM-
Ressonância Magnética, Rio De Janeiro, Rio
De Janeiro, Brazil

## AUTHORS

**STEFAN BLÜML, PhD**
Department of Radiology, Children's Hospital
of Los Angeles, Keck School of Medicine,
University of Southern California, Los Angeles,
California

**THANGAMADHAN BOSEMANI, MD**
Section of Pediatric Neuroradiology, Division of
Pediatric Radiology, The Russell H. Morgan
Department of Radiology and Radiological
Science, Charlotte R. Bloomberg Children's
Center, The Johns Hopkins School of
Medicine, Baltimore, Maryland

**LARA A. BRANDÃO, MD**
Chief of Neuroradiology, Radiologic
Department, Clínica Felippe Mattoso, Fleury
Medicina Diagnóstica, Neuroradiologist,
Radiologic Department, Clínica IRM-
Ressonância Magnética, Rio De Janeiro, Rio
De Janeiro, Brazil

**RAFAEL CESCHIN, BS**
Departments of Radiology and Bioinformatics,
University of Pittsburgh, Pittsburgh,
Pennsylvania

**MARJOLEIN H.G. DREMMEN, MD**
Division of Pediatric Radiology,
Department of Radiology, Erasmus
MC – University Medical Center, Rotterdam,
The Netherlands

**ANDRE D. FURTADO, MD**
Assistant Professor, Department of Radiology,
University of Pittsburgh, Pittsburgh,
Pennsylvania

**JEROEN HENDRIKSE, MD, PhD**
Neuroradiology, Department of Radiology and
Nuclear Medicine, University Medical Center
Utrecht, Utrecht, Netherlands

**THIERRY A.G.M. HUISMAN, MD**
Professor, Director of Pediatric
Radiology and Pediatric Neuroradiology,
The Russell H. Morgan Department of
Radiology and Radiological Science,
The Johns Hopkins School of Medicine,
Baltimore, Maryland

**IZLEM IZBUDAK, MD**
Associate Professor, Division of
Neuroradiology, Section of Pediatric
Neuroradiology, The Russell H. Morgan
Department of Radiology and Radiological
Science, The Johns Hopkins School of
Medicine, Baltimore, Maryland

**REGINA I. JAKACKI, MD**
Department of Pediatrics, University of
Pittsburgh, Pittsburgh, Pennsylvania

**MAARTEN LEQUIN, MD, PhD**
Neuroradiology, Department of Radiology and
Nuclear Medicine, University Medical Center
Utrecht, Utrecht, Netherlands

**GARY MASON, MD**
Department of Pediatrics, University of
Pittsburgh, Pittsburgh, Pennsylvania

**MARVIN NELSON, MD, MBA**
Department of Radiology, Children's Hospital
Los Angeles, Los Angeles, California

**HIDEHO OKADA, MD**
Professor of Neurological Surgery, Department
of Neurosurgery, University of California,
San Francisco, San Francisco, California

**ASHOK PANIGRAHY, MD**
Associate Professor, Department of Radiology,
University of Pittsburgh, Pittsburgh,
Pennsylvania

**IAN F. POLLACK, MD**
Professor, Department of Neurosurgery,
Children's Hospital of Pittsburgh,
University of Pittsburgh Cancer Institute,
University of Pittsburgh School of Medicine,
University of Pittsburgh, Pittsburgh,
Pennsylvania

**ANDREA PORETTI, MD**
Section of Pediatric Neuroradiology, Division of
Pediatric Radiology, The Russell H. Morgan
Department of Radiology and Radiological
Science, Charlotte R. Bloomberg Children's
Center, The Johns Hopkins School of
Medicine, Baltimore, Maryland

**ERIN SIMON SCHWARTZ, MD**
Associate Professor of Radiology;
Neuro-Radiologist, The Children's Hospital of
Philadelphia, Perelman School of Medicine at
University of Pennsylvania, Philadelphia,
Pennsylvania

**DANIEL P. SEEBURG, MD, PhD**
Divisions of Pediatric Radiology and
Neuroradiology, The Russell H. Morgan
Department of Radiology and Radiological
Science, The Johns Hopkins Hospital, The
Johns Hopkins Medical Institutions, Baltimore,
Maryland

**KARUNA V. SHEKDAR, MD**
Assistant Professor of Clinical Radiology;
Neuro-Radiologist, The Children's Hospital of
Philadelphia, Perelman School of Medicine at
University of Pennsylvania, Philadelphia,
Pennsylvania

**BENITA TAMRAZI, MD**
Department of Radiology, Children's Hospital
Los Angeles, Los Angeles, California

**MARY TENENBAUM, MD**
Department of Radiology, Baystate Medical
Center, Springfield, Massachusetts

**TINA YOUNG POUSSAINT, MD, FACR**
Division of Neuroradiology, Department of
Radiology, Boston Children's Hospital,
Harvard Medical School, Boston,
Massachusetts

**CARLOS ZAMORA, MD, PhD**
Clinical Fellow, Division of Neuroradiology, The
Russell H. Morgan Department of Radiology
and Radiological Science, The Johns Hopkins
School of Medicine, Baltimore, Maryland;
Assistant Professor, Division of
Neuroradiology, Department of Radiology,
University of North Carolina School of
Medicine, Chapel Hill, North Carolina

# Contents

Pediatric brain tumors are the leading cause of death from solid tumors in childhood. The most common posterior fossa tumors in children are medulloblastoma, atypical teratoid/rhabdoid tumor, cerebellar pilocytic astrocytoma, ependymoma, and brainstem glioma. Location, and imaging findings on computed tomography (CT) and conventional MR (cMR) imaging may provide important clues to the most likely diagnosis. Moreover, information obtained from advanced MR imaging techniques increase diagnostic confidence and help distinguish between different histologic tumor types. Here we discuss the most common posterior fossa tumors in children, including typical imaging findings on CT, cMR imaging, and advanced MR imaging studies.

The breadth of tumors that can arise in the supratentorial brain in children is extensive. With the exception of those that result in seizures and the highly malignant histologies, supratentorial tumors may come to medical attention later compared with infratentorial tumors, as they are less commonly associated with ventricular obstruction. This article presents an overview of the neuroimaging characteristics of these entities, with particular attention to relevant features that may aid in narrowing the differential diagnosis, including correlation with demographics and clinical presentation.

Brain tumors can develop in the prenatal and neonatal time periods. Neuroimaging studies are crucial for the early detection of prenatal and neonatal brain tumors. Imaging allows for characterization of morphology, as well as the detection of hydrocephalus, local invasion, and distant spread. The imaging features of the more common neonatal brain tumors, including teratomas, choroid plexus tumors, ATRTs, and neoplasm mimics are described.

A review of pediatric pineal region tumors is provided with emphasis on advanced imaging techniques. The 3 major categories of pineal region tumors include germ cell tumors, pineal parenchymal tumors, and tumors arising from adjacent structures such as tectal astrocytomas. The clinical presentation, biochemical markers, and imaging of these types of tumors are reviewed.

Daniel P. Seeburg, Marjolein H.G. Dremmen, and Thierry A.G.M. Huisman

Masses in the sella and parasellar region comprise about 10% of all pediatric brain tumors but type and frequency differ from those in adults. Imaging is critical for diagnosis and characterization of these lesions. By assessing the site of origin and the signal and contrast enhancement characteristics, the differential diagnostic considerations can be narrowed. The clinical presentation is often suggestive of a specific disease entity and should be considered. This article summarizes the characteristic imaging features of the most frequent pediatric tumors and tumor-mimicking lesions in children in this region.

Mary Tenenbaum

Extraparenchymal lesions of childhood include neoplastic and nonneoplastic entities. Lesions affecting children are different from the most common entities affecting adults. Although there are imaging features that are highly suggestive of extraparenchymal origin, it can be difficult to distinguish extraparenchymal from intraparenchymal lesions. MR imaging is the examination of choice for the evaluation of extraparenchymal lesions given greater sensitivity and anatomic detail. Syndromic associations should be considered, especially for unusual lesions in the pediatric age group such as meningioma and schwannoma.

Thangamadhan Bosemani and Andrea Poretti

There are several tumors and tumorlike masses involving multiple spaces in the pediatric brain. Accurate diagnosis of tumors and distinguishing them from tumorlike masses is an important aspect in the diagnostic workup and plays a key role for management and prognosis. Neuroimaging plays an important role in (1) identification of a brain mass, (2) determining its location, (3) demonstrating involvement of a single space versus multiple spaces, and (4) distinguishing a tumor from tumorlike masses.

Andre D. Furtado, Rafael Ceschin, Stefan Blüml, Gary Mason, Regina I. Jakacki, Hideho Okada, Ian F. Pollack, and Ashok Panigrahy

The potential benefits of peptide-based immunotherapy for pediatric brain tumors are under investigation. Treatment-related heterogeneity has resulted in radiographic challenges, including pseudoprogression. Conventional MR imaging has limitations in assessment of different forms of treatment-related heterogeneity, particularly regarding distinguishing true tumor progression from efficacious treatment responses. Advanced neuroimaging techniques, including diffusion magnetic resonance (MR), perfusion MR, and MR spectroscopy, may add value in the assessment of treatment-related heterogeneity. Observations suggest that recent delineation of specific response criteria for immunotherapy of adult brain tumors is likely relevant to the pediatric population and further validation in multicenter pediatric brain tumor peptide-based vaccine studies is warranted.

Maarten Lequin and Jeroen Hendrikse

Advanced MR imaging techniques, such as spectroscopy, perfusion, diffusion, and functional imaging, have improved the diagnosis of brain tumors in children and also play an important role in defining surgical as well as therapeutic responses in these patients. In addition to the anatomic or structural information gained with conventional MR imaging sequences, advanced MR imaging techniques also provide physiologic information about tumor morphology, metabolism, and hemodynamics. This article reviews the physiology, techniques, and clinical applications of diffusion-weighted and diffusion tensor imaging, MR spectroscopy, perfusion MR imaging, susceptibility-weighted imaging, and functional MR imaging in the setting of neuro-oncology.

# Foreword
# Pediatric Brain Tumors

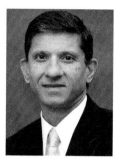

Suresh K. Mukherji, MD, MBA, FACR
*Consulting Editor*

This issue is the second part to Dr Brandao's two-part series on advanced imaging of brain tumors. The prior issue focused on adult brain tumors, while this issue focuses on pediatric brain neoplasms. This issue provides a superb review for neuroradiologists and radiologists who routinely interpret neuroimaging studies. Equally important, this issue also integrates the latest information from the updated World Health Organization classification. The updated classification makes substantive and important changes by integrating imaging and molecular and genetic markers into brain tumor classification and staging. The new classification especially impacts medulloblastomas.

I want to both thank and congratulate all of these world-class authors for making the effort to integrate the latest information into their superbly written articles. This issue will be a "ready" reference for years to come.

Finally, once again, I want to thank "Superwoman"! Lara, you are a wonderful friend and colleague! Thank you again for your unparalleled contributions to our scientific and educational community.

Suresh K. Mukherji, MD, MBA, FACR
Department of Radiology
Michigan State University
Michigan State University Health Team
846 Service Road
East Lansing, MI 48824, USA

E-mail address:
mukherji@rad.msu.edu

Neuroimag Clin N Am 27 (2017) xiii
http://dx.doi.org/10.1016/j.nic.2016.10.002
1052-5149/17/© 2016 Published by Elsevier Inc.

# Preface

# Pediatric Brain Tumors Update: Imaging Characterization of Pediatric Brain Tumors in the Central Nervous System Including Findings on Advanced MR Imaging Techniques

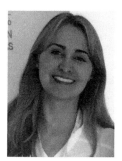

Lara A. Brandão, MD

*Editor*

This issue of *Neuroimaging Clinics* focuses on pediatric and neonatal brain tumors.

The first article, "Posterior fossa tumors," offers a detailed overview of the most common brain tumors in the posterior fossa in children.

Findings on conventional MR imaging as well as on diffusion-weighted imaging, MR spectroscopy, perfusion-weighted imaging, and permeability in medulloblastomas and other embryonal tumors, as well as in cerebellar astrocytomas, ependymomas, and brainstem gliomas, are discussed in detail.

The four molecular subgroups of medulloblastomas are also addressed, due to their prognostic significance.

The article by Zamora and colleagues addresses supratentorial tumors in the pediatric population, offering a fairly complete review of the extensive list of differential diagnosis in the supratentorial compartment.

While there is overlap in the imaging appearance of some of these entities, many have relatively characteristic features that in combination with the patient's demographics and clinical presentation may aid in narrowing the differential diagnosis.

Neuroimaging features play an important role in the early detection and characterization of antenatal and neonatal brain tumors. In the article by Shekdar and Schwartz, we find a vey nice discussion of the most common neonatal brain tumors.

A review of pediatric pineal region tumors is provided in the article, "Pineal region masses in pediatric patients," with an emphasis on advanced imaging techniques. The three major categories of pineal region tumors, germ cell tumors, pineal parenchymal tumors, and tumors arising from adjacent structures such as tectal astrocytomas, are discussed.

The clinical presentation, biochemical markers, and imaging of these types of tumors are reviewed.

In the article, "Imaging of the sella and parasellar region in the pediatric population," the authors summarize the characteristic imaging features of the most frequent pediatric tumors and tumor-mimicking lesions in children in these regions. The differential of extraparenchymal lesions in the pediatric age group differs from that in adults.

The article, "Extraparenchymal lesions in pediatric patients," offers a very nice review of the

Neuroimag Clin N Am 27 (2017) xv–xvi
http://dx.doi.org/10.1016/j.nic.2016.10.001
1052-5149/17/© 2016 Published by Elsevier Inc.

most common extraparenchymal lesions in children.

There are several tumors and tumorlike masses involving multiple spaces in the pediatric brain. Accurate diagnosis of tumors and the capability of distinguishing them from tumorlike masses is an important aspect in the diagnostic workup and plays a key role in management and prognosis. A very nice and organized approach of tumor and tumorlike masses in pediatric patients that involve multiple spaces is offered in the article by Bosemani and Poretti entitled, "Tumor and tumorlike masses in pediatric patients that involve multiple spaces."

The article, "Neuroimaging of peptide-based vaccine therapy in pediatric brain tumors: initial experience," discusses peptide-based immunotherapy for pediatric brain tumors and its association with the presence of treatment-related heterogeneity, including that of pseudoprogression. Advanced neuroimaging techniques, including diffusion MR, perfusion MR, and MR spectroscopy, may add value in the assessment of treatment-related heterogeneity.

In the last article, "Advanced MR imaging in pediatric brain tumors: clinical applications," the authors review the physiology, techniques, and clinical applications of diffusion-weighted and diffusion-tensor imaging, MR spectroscopy, perfusion MR imaging, susceptibility-weighted imaging, and functional MR imaging, in the setting of neuro-oncology. Advanced MR imaging techniques not only have improved the diagnosis of brain tumors in children but also play an important role in defining surgical approach as well as therapeutic response in these patients.

This issue of *Neuroimaging Clinics* provides the reader with a nice and organized review of the most common pediatric brain tumors, including information on advanced MR imaging techniques.

I would like to sincerely thank all of the authors of this issue for their invaluable contributions. I wish to express my gratitude to the consulting editor, Dr Suresh K. Mukherji, for the opportunity to lead this project. I would also like to thank the series editor, John Vassallo, developmental editor, Casey Potter, and editorial assistant, Nicole Congleton, for their guidance and support during the preparation of this issue.

Lara A. Brandão, MD
Radiologic Department
Clínica Felippe Mattoso
Fleury Medicina Diagnóstica
Avenida das Américas 700sala 320, Barra Da
Tijuca, Rio de Janeiro
Rio de Janeiro CEP 22640-100, Brazil

Radiologic Department
Clínica IRM-Ressonância Magnética
Rua Capitão Salomão
Humaitá, Rio de Janeiro
Rio de Janeiro CEP 22271-040, Brazil

E-mail address:
larabrandao.rad@terra.com.br

# Posterior Fossa Tumors

Lara A. Brandão, MD[a,b],*, Tina Young Poussaint, MD[c]

## KEYWORDS

- Posterior fossa tumor • Medulloblastoma • Atypical teratoid/rhabdoid tumor
- Cerebellar astrocytoma • Ependymoma • Brainstem glioma

## KEY POINTS

- Medulloblastoma is the most common posterior fossa tumor in children.
- Due to high cell density and high nuclear-to-cytoplasmic ratio, medulloblastomas are typically hyperdense on computed tomography, isointense to the cerebellar cortex on T2 and present with restricted diffusion, as well as a very high choline peak and a taurine peak on magnetic resonance spectroscopy.
- Cerebellar pilocytic astrocytoma is a World Health Organization grade I tumor with a solid portion that is typically hyperintense to the cerebellar cortex on T2 due to high water content along with low cell density.
- Extension through the fourth ventricular outflow foramina, although typical, is not entirely pathognomonic of ependymoma.
- Brainstem gliomas are usually located in the pons, with diffuse midline glioma H3 K27-mutant the most common.

## INTRODUCTION

Pediatric brain tumors are the leading cause of death from solid tumors in childhood.[1,2] The most common posterior fossa tumors in children are medulloblastoma (MB), atypical teratoid/rhabdoid tumor (ATRT), cerebellar pilocytic astrocytoma (CPA), ependymoma, and brainstem glioma (BG). Location, as well as imaging findings on computed tomography (CT) and conventional magnetic resonance (cMR) imaging may provide important clues to the most likely diagnosis. Moreover, information obtained from advanced MR imaging techniques, such as diffusion-weighted imaging (DWI), MR spectroscopy (MRS), perfusion-weighted imaging, and dynamic contrast-enhanced (DCE) studies, increase diagnostic confidence and help distinguish between different histologic tumor types.

Here we discuss the most common posterior fossa tumors in children, including typical imaging findings on CT, cMR imaging, and advanced MR imaging studies.

## MEDULLOBLASTOMA

Medulloblastoma (MB), a highly malignant neoplasm, is the most common posterior fossa

Funding Sources: None.
Conflict of Interest: None.
[a] Radiologic Department, Clínica Felippe Mattoso, Fleury Medicina Diagnóstica, Avenida das Américas 700, sala 320, Barra Da Tijuca, Rio De Janeiro, Rio De Janeiro CEP 22640-100, Brazil; [b] Department of Radiology, Clínica IRM- Ressonância Magnética, Rua Capitão Salomão, Humaitá, Rio De Janeiro, Rio De Janeiro CEP 22271-040, Brazil; [c] Division of Neuroradiology, Department of Radiology, Boston Children's Hospital, Harvard Medical School, 300 Longwood Avenue, Boston, MA 02115, USA
* Corresponding author. Clínica Felippe Mattoso, Fleury Medicina Diagnóstica, Avenida das Américas 700, sala 320, Barra Da Tijuca, Rio De Janeiro, Rio De Janeiro CEP 22640-100, Brazil.
*E-mail address:* larabrandao.rad@terra.com.br

neoplasm in children, representing 15% to 20% of all pediatric brain tumors and 30% to 40% of posterior fossa neoplasms.[3–8] Medulloblastomas are classified as embryonal tumors, the largest group of malignant tumors in the pediatric population.[3]

This highly malignant neoplasm occurs more frequently in boys, usually before 10 years of age.[3,9] Although less common, the disease may also occur in adults, usually in the third and fourth decades of life.[9]

### Clinical Picture and Treatment

Clinical symptoms and signs are generally brief, typically less than 3 months in duration, and reflect the strong predilection of this tumor to arise within the cerebellum, most often in the vermis. Symptoms may include headache, general malaise, failure to thrive, vomiting, and clumsiness, among other presentations that mimic common and benign childhood pathologies seen in primary care.[10,11]

Typically, the treatment strategies for MB are threefold: maximal safe resection (which may include cerebrospinal fluid [CSF] diversion), neuraxis radiotherapy, and chemotherapy.[11]

### Location

The tumor usually arises at the midline within the vermis and exhibits growth into the fourth ventricle (Fig. 1).[12–17]

Less typical locations include nonventricular superior or inferior vermian tumor, cerebellar hemispheric lesions, and extension into the foramina of Magendie and foramina of Luschka to the cerebellopontine angle (CPA).[18]

### Computed Tomography and Conventional MR Imaging

On unenhanced CT, the tumor is usually characterized as hyperdense (Fig. 2), and on T2 images, as isointense to hypointense compared with gray matter (Fig. 3).[14] These imaging findings are likely secondary to high cell density and high nuclear-to-cytoplasmic ratio.[2]

The tumor typically may appear heterogeneous on imaging, with findings related to cyst formation and hemorrhage on MR, and calcification seen on CT (see Fig. 3A–C). Intratumoral cyst or necrosis is observed in 40% to 50% of cases.[19]

MBs typically enhance.[4]

Atypical imaging findings, such as high signal intensity compared with the cerebellar cortex on T2, as well as no enhancement may be demonstrated (Fig. 4).[18]

Sometimes the tumor presents with an infiltrative pattern instead of a solid solitary mass (Fig. 5).

Evidence of leptomeningeal metastatic spread is present in 33% of all cases at the time of diagnosis and is well evaluated with contrast-enhanced MR imaging of the brain and the spine.[20] MR imaging is more sensitive than CSF studies for the detection of CSF spread of primary brain tumors.[2,4]

Metastases may be leptomeningeal, dural-based, intraventricular, adherent to the spinal roots, or even to the liver (Fig. 6).

Metastasis to the brain parenchyma may bleed, resembling cavernoma (Fig. 7).

### Diffusion-Weighted MR Imaging

Apparent diffusion coefficient (ADC) values are significantly lower in MBs than in all other posterior

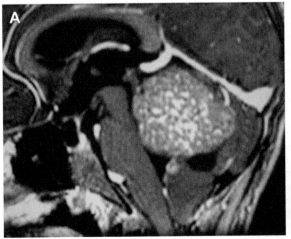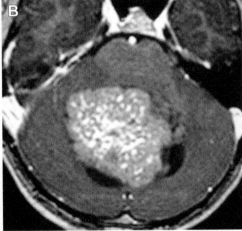

Fig. 1. MB: location. (A, B) Contrast-enhanced MR T1 images from a 6-year-old girl presenting with MB in the midline vermis, with growth into the fourth ventricle and hydrocephalus.

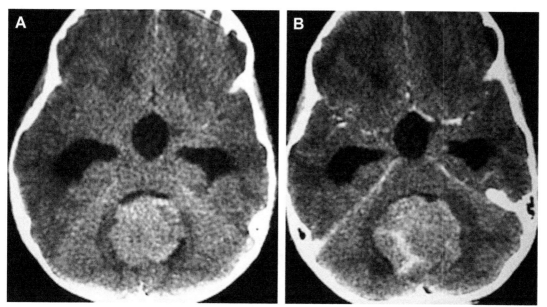

Fig. 2. MB: CT. A 9-year old boy presenting with headache and vomiting. There is a well-circumscribed solid lesion in the midline vermis, that occupies the fourth ventricle with hydrocephalus. The lesion is hyperdense on the non-contrast CT (A) and enhances after contrast injection (B).

fossa tumors (P<.001) related to high cell density (Fig. 8, see also Figs. 3D, E and 5E).[21–23]

A study by Jaremko and colleagues[21] confirmed that diffusion imaging is the single most useful sequence for differentiating pediatric posterior fossa tumors and that, as expected, diffusion restriction is rare in grade 1 tumors and common in grade 4 tumors. The optimal threshold for distinguishing MB and juvenile pilocytic astrocytomas (JPAs), ADC minimum = $800 \times 10^{-6}$ mm²/s, was lower than the threshold of $900 \times 10^{-6}$ mm²/s used by Rumboldt and colleagues,[22] likely because they used ADC mean rather than ADC minimum.

Desmoplastic medulloblastoma, a histologically less aggressive subtype with better prognosis than the classic type, is expected to have less highly restricted diffusion than the classic type. Some of these tumors present with no restricted diffusion at all (Fig. 9).[21]

### Proton Magnetic Resonance Spectroscopy

#### Choline

On MRS, MBs usually demonstrate a significant elevation of the choline (Cho) peak related to high cell density and elevated Cho/Cr and Cho/N-acetyl-aspartate (NAA) ratios, reflecting its malignant nature (Fig. 10, see also Figs. 3F and 5F).[2,24–26]

High Cho has been previously reported as a characteristic finding of embryonal tumors.[12,27]

Elevation of the Cho peak is useful in distinguishing between MB and L'Hermitte-Duclos disease (LDD), as MBs occasionally may present with a laminated appearance, and with no contrast enhancement, mimicking LDD. The Cho peak is typically elevated in patients with MB when compared with patients with LDD.[8]

Desmoplastic MBs may present with no elevation of the choline in the spectra. In these tumors, a huge myo-inositol peak may be seen related to the desmoplastic nature (Lara A. Brandão, MD, personal communication, 2013) (Fig. 11).

#### Taurine

Spectra with a short echo time (TE) show a significantly elevated taurine (Tau) concentration at 3.3 ppm in patients with MB when compared with other tumors (see Fig. 10).[24,28–32] Furthermore, at a TE of 30 ms, the Tau peak projects above the baseline; whereas, at a TE of 144 ms, the Tau peak occurs below the baseline.[28]

Tau has been established as an important biomarker in distinguishing MBs from other common pediatric brain tumors, such as cerebellar astrocytomas.[24,28,31,33,34] Higher Tau levels are associated with increased cellular proliferation and tumoral aggressiveness.[23,24,28,29,35]

#### Glutamine and glutamate and alanine

In a study of 60 children with untreated brain tumors, Panigrahy and colleagues[24] measured the highest glutamate (Glu) concentrations in pineal germinoma

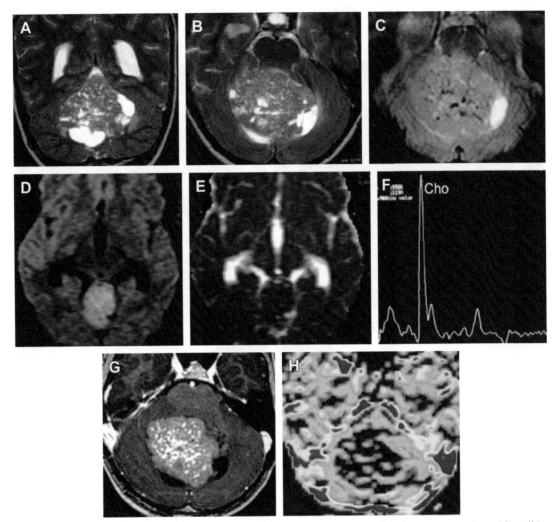

Fig. 3. MB: MR imaging. Same patient as Fig. 1. A 6-year old girl complaining of neck pain, presenting with walking difficulty and ataxia. There is a well-circumscribed lesion in the midline vermis, with growth into the fourth ventricle. Some cysts with high signal intensity on T2 (*A*: coronal and *B*: axial) as well as some foci of low signal intensity on the gradient echo (*C*) that may be related to calcification or blood are demonstrated within the lesion. The solid portion is isointense to the cerebellar cortex on T2, due to high cell density along with high nuclear-cytoplasmic ratio, also responsible for the restricted diffusion (*D*: DWI, *E*: ADC map) and high Cho peak (*F*) demonstrated in the lesion. There is significant enhancement (*G*: axial T1 with contrast) and no elevation of the blood volume (*H*: rCBV map) in the perfusion study.

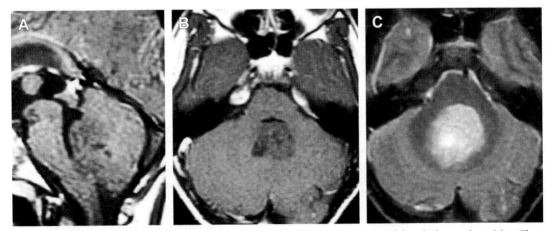

Fig. 4. MB: high signal on T2 and no enhancement. An 8-year old boy presenting with headaches and vomiting. There is a solid MB within the inferior vermis growing into the fourth ventricle, with no enhancement (*A*: sagittal, *B*: axial T1 with contrast) presenting with high signal intensity compared with the cerebellar cortex on T2 (*C*: axial T2).

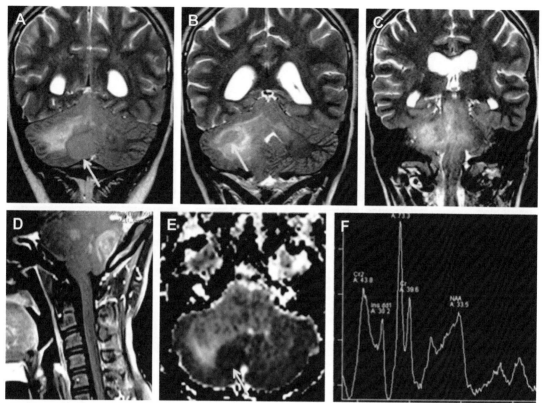

**Fig. 5.** MB: infiltrative pattern. A 12-year old girl presenting with ataxia, headache, and vomiting. There is a diffuse infiltrative lesion (*A–C*: coronal T2), involving the right greater than left cerebellum, infiltrating into the brainstem. Most of the lesion is hyperintense on T2, with some hypointense areas (*arrows* in *A* and *B*), probably related to high cell density. The neurosurgeon suspected ADEM (acute disseminated encephalomyelitis). Pathology was consistent with classic MB. There is heterogeneous enhancement (*D*: sagittal T1 with contrast) as well as evidence of high cell density and high nuclear-cytoplasmic ratio characterized by restricted diffusion (*arrow* in *E*: ADC map) and high choline on spectra (*F*).

and in MB (see **Fig. 10**B). Specifically, the MB, pineal germinoma, and astrocytoma showed mean glutamine and glutamate (Glx) concentrations above the mean in all tumors; whereas, Glx concentration was low in both the choroid plexus papilloma and carcinoma. The quantitation of these metabolites proved useful in separating either MB or astrocytoma from choroid plexus papilloma. Panigrahy and colleagues[24] have also reported the highest mean alanine (Ala) concentration among posterior fossa tumors in MBs.

### Lipids and lactate
Prominent lipid (Lip) resonances can be observed in some, but not all, spectra of malignant MB (see **Fig. 11**B).[24,28]

High lactate (Lac) values are usually found in the spectra of MB.[36]

### Magnetic resonance spectroscopy in metastatic versus localized medulloblastomas
Metastatic MBs are characterized by higher total Cho (tCho), which is consistent with increased

cell turnover and tumor growth, a finding substantiated by a significant positive correlation between tCho and the Ki67 index.[37] Tau is present in both metastatic and localized tumors, although higher levels are typically found in metastatic tumors, which is consistent with previous findings in neuroblastoma (ie, Tau is a reliable biomarker for more aggressive subtypes of neural tumors).[37–39] The fact that higher mobile Lip levels are observed in localized tumors may also reflect a higher proportion of necrotic tumor in these cases.

### Dynamic Susceptibility Contrast and Dynamic Contrast-Enhanced MR Imaging

There can be variable perfusion and permeability characteristics in MB, with some lesions showing elevated perfusion and permeability and others not (**Fig. 12**, see also **Fig. 3**H).

### Important considerations
**Radiologic-pathologic correlation** The World Health Organization (WHO) classification system

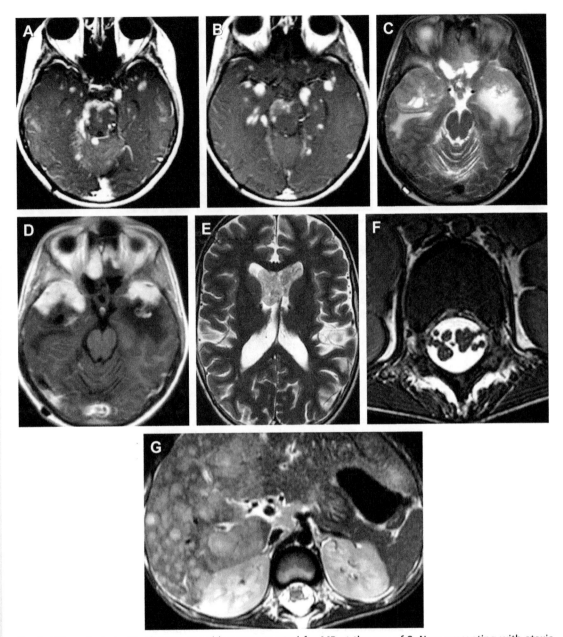

Fig. 6. MB: metastasis. (*A, B*) A 26-year-old woman treated for MB at the age of 8. Now presenting with ataxia and incoordination. Enhancing leptomeningeal metastases are demonstrated surrounding the brainstem, basal cisterns, temporal lobes, and occipital lobes (*A, B*: axial T1 with contrast). (*C, D*) A 20-year-old man treated for MB 2 years ago. MR imaging shows dural-based metastasis in the temporal and frontal basal regions, isointense to the cortex on T2 (*C*: axial) with solid enhancement (*D*: axial T1 with contrast). Metastasis also may compromise the ventricular system (*E*), the spinal roots, which may look thickened (*F*), as well as the liver (*G*).

2007 uses histology to classify MBs into 4 major groups, including classic, desmoplastic, MB with extensive nodularity (MBEN), and large cell/anaplastic MB subtypes[3,40]:

*Classic* Classic MB represents the most common histologic subtype and is composed of sheets of densely packed small round blue cells (basophilic) with a high nuclear-to-cytoplasmic ratio, mitotic and apoptotic activity, and may occur in the midline.[3]

Elevation of Tau is seen specifically in this histologic subtype.

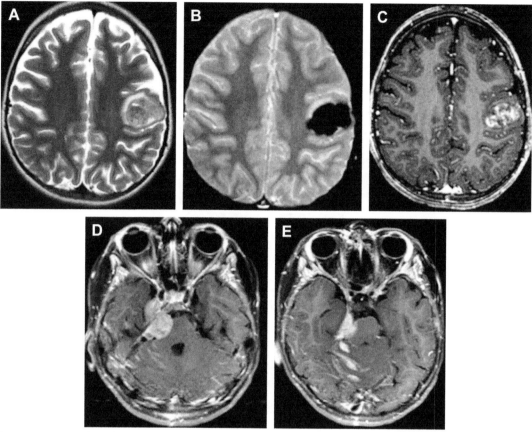

**Fig. 7.** MB: parenchymal metastasis resembling cavernoma. A 7-year-old girl presenting with headaches and paresthesia on the right. A solid lesion is demonstrated in the left frontal region, which is heterogeneous, hypo-intense on T2 (*A*: axial T2), has significant low signal on the gradient echo image (*B*: axial gradient echo [GRE]) and some enhancement (*C*: axial T1 with contrast). Lesion was diagnosed as cavernoma. Two months later (*D, E*: axial T1 with contrast) dural-based, as well as leptomeningeal metastasis are demonstrated with final diagnosis of metastatic MB.

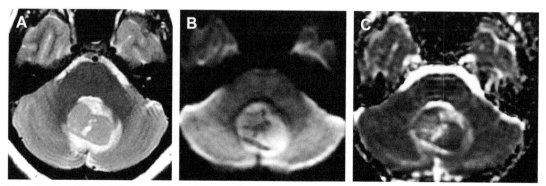

**Fig. 8.** MB-restricted diffusion. Patient diagnosed with MB, presenting with dizziness and nausea in the previous 2 months. There is a solid lesion in the midline vermis, mostly isointense to the cerebellar cortex on T2 (*A*: axial T2), presenting with restricted diffusion (*B*: DWI, *C*: ADC map).

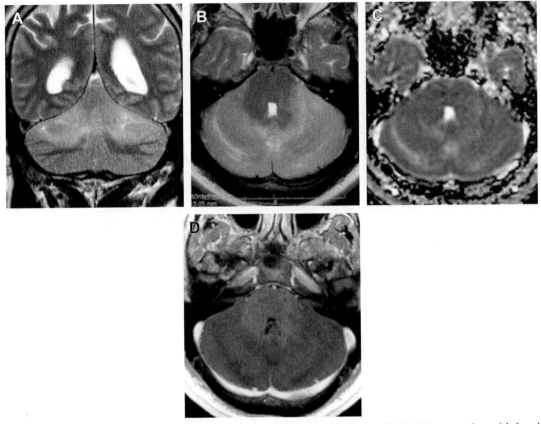

Fig. 9. MB: no restricted diffusion. A 51-year-old man diagnosed with desmoplastic MB, presenting with headaches and nausea in the preceding 3 months. There is an infiltrative lesion compromising most of the cerebellar parenchyma, presenting with mild high signal intensity on T2 (*A*: coronal, *B*: axial T2), and no restricted diffusion (*C*: ADC map). The lesion does not enhance (*D*: axial T1 with contrast).

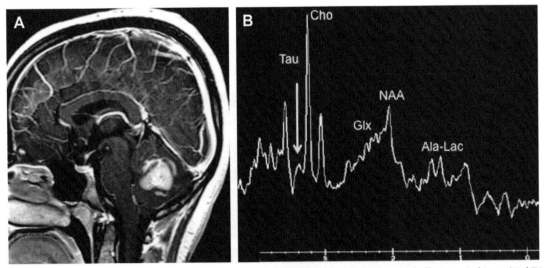

Fig. 10. MB: MRS. Same patient as in Fig. 8. There is a solid enhancing MB in the cerebellar vermis (*A*: sagittal T1 with contrast), presenting with very high Cho as well as Tau peak in the spectra (*B*: MRS). NAA is very low and there is elevation of Glx as well as presence of Ala and lactate.

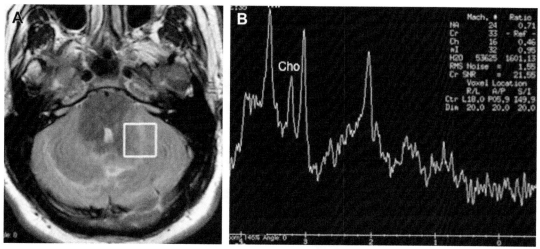

Fig. 11. MB: no elevation of Cho. Patient diagnosed with desmoplastic MB. MRS (*A*: voxel placement-axial T2) demonstrates no elevation of the Cho peak (*B-curve*). The most striking finding is elevation of the myo-inositol peak (mI).

*Desmoplastic* This subtype is hypocellular, presents with lower Tau concentration compared with the classic subtype and carries a favorable prognosis.[3,41]

This histologic subtype is often found in adult patients with MB, demonstrating a cerebellar hemispheric mass extending to the overlying meninges, with desmoplastic reaction evoked by prominent leptomeningeal involvement (Fig. 13).[19]

*Anaplastic* Anaplastic MBs (15%) are characterized by marked nuclear pleomorphism, nuclear molding, and cell–cell wrapping, and the large cell variant (2%–4%) displays a monomorphous population of large cells whose nuclei exhibit prominent nucleoli.[3,42] Both variants are characterized by a very high proliferative activity, abundant apoptosis, and a much poorer prognosis.[3,43,44]

This is the most aggressive subtype, characterized by presence of necrosis.

*Extensively nodular* MBENs tend to develop in the vermis in children younger than 3 years in most cases and is frequently represented as a nodular enhancing appearance on CT scans or MR images. Prognosis is better than for the classic MB.[19,41]

Molecular subgroups More recently there has been the development of a classification of 4 main subgroups of MBs based on molecular profiling.[42,45–51]

The WNT and SHH groups were named after the predominant signaling pathways thought to be

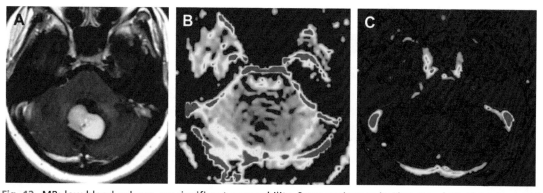

Fig. 12. MB: low blood volume, no significant permeability. Same patient as in Figs. 8 and 10. There is a solid enhancing MB in the cerebellar vermis (*A*: axial T1 with contrast), showing no elevation of the blood volume (*B*: rCBV map), as well as no significant elevation of the permeability (*C*: maximum slope of increase map).

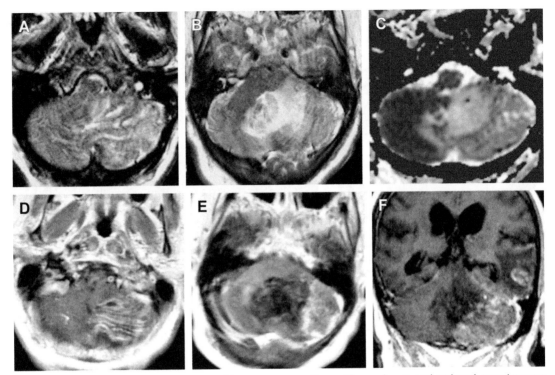

**Fig. 13.** MB: desmoplastic type. A 64-year-old woman presenting with numbness and reduced consciousness. There is an infiltrative cerebellar lesion in the left cerebellar hemisphere, extending laterally to the cerebellopontine angle, hyperintense on T2 (*A, B*: axial T2) with a laminated appearance. There is no restricted diffusion, which may be demonstrated in desmoplastic MBs (*C*: ADC map). There is nonhomogeneous enhancement in the lesion, associated with thickening of the adjacent meninges due to desmoplastic reaction (*D, E*: axial, *F*: coronal T1 with contrast).

affected in their pathogenesis. Less is known currently regarding the pathogenesis of groups 3 (tending to harbor MYC amplification) and 4 (tending to have isochromosome 17q) and therefore generic names were chosen until they are better understood.[45]

The SHH group has become of increasing interest because of the availability and

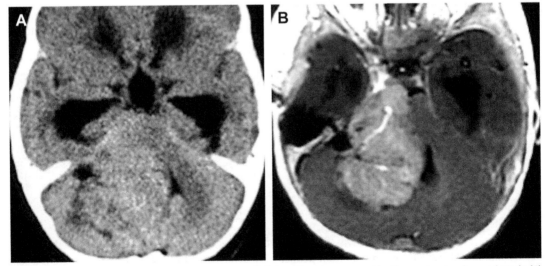

**Fig. 14.** ATRT: CT. ATRT hyperdense on noncontrast CT (*A*), with enhancement in the contrast-enhanced study (*B*). (*Courtesy of* A. James Barkovich, MD, San Francisco, CA.)

temporary success of small molecule inhibitors to smoothened (SMO), which is part of the SHH pathway.

For a detailed comprehensive review on the molecular subgroups of MB, see the consensus article by Taylor and colleagues.[52]

MB is the most common malignant brain tumor in children and, as such, has been the focus of tremendous efforts to genomically characterize it.[53]

What was once thought to be a single disease has been divided into multiple, molecularly unique subgroups through gene expression profiling. Each subgroup is not only unique in its origin and pathogenesis, but also in the prognosis and potential therapeutic options. The molecular

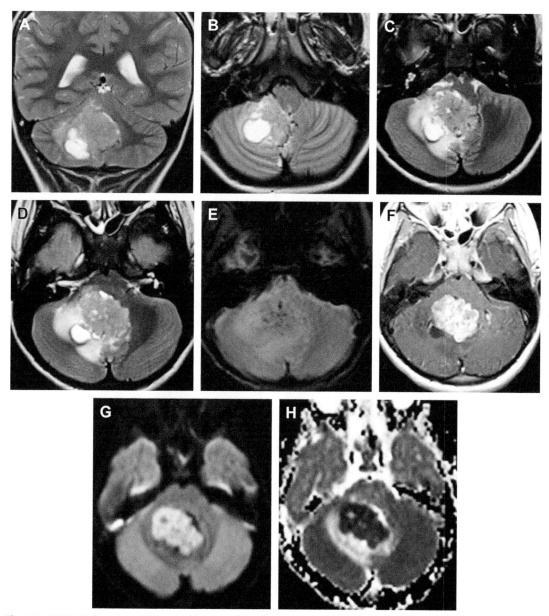

**Fig. 15.** ATRT: MR imaging. A 5-year-old girl with irritability and hypersexuality, sent to a psychiatrist. There is a nonhomogeneous lesion presenting with a solid component isointense to the cerebellar cortex on T2 (*A*: coronal and *B–D*: axial). Cysts are demonstrated within and adjacent to the solid component. The lesion is located off midline and extends to the CPA on the right, which favors ATRT instead of MB. Some low signal intensity foci are demonstrated within the solid portion, which may be related to blood products (*E*: axial GRE). There is heterogeneous enhancement (*F*: axial T1 with contrast) and significant restricted diffusion (*G*: DWI, *H*: ADC map).

classification system has a potential use in developing prognostic models as well as for the advancement of targeted therapeutic interventions.

MB is currently stratified into 4 molecular variants through the advances in transcriptional profiling.[54,55]

They include sonic hedgehog (SHH), wingless (WNT), Group III, and Group IV.

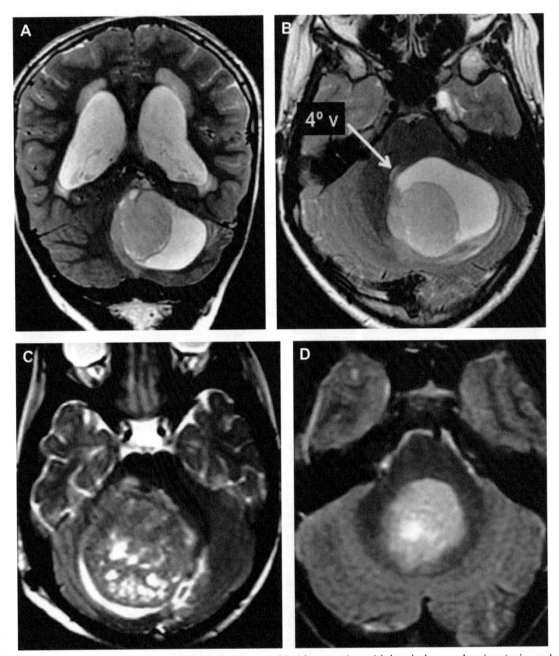

**Fig. 16.** PA: location and signal on T2. (*A, B*) A 9-year-old girl presenting with headaches, neck pain, ataxia, and vomiting. There is a PA in the left cerebellar hemisphere, compressing and displacing the fourth ventricle (*A*: coronal and *B*: axial T2). The solid component is hyperintense to the cerebellar cortex on T2. (*C, D*) Children diagnosed with MB. The lesion is located in the midline vermis, filling the fourth ventricle. The solid component of MB is usually isointense to the cerebellar cortex on T2 (*C*). Some MBs may present with high signal intensity on T2 (*D*), resembling a PA.

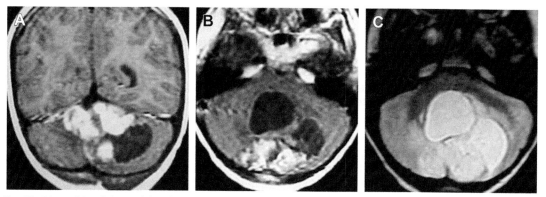

Fig. 17. PA: multinodular/multicystic appearance. PA presenting with multiple enhancing nodules (*A*: coronal, *B*: axial T1 with contrast) hyperintense on T2 (*C*: axial T2), as well as multiple cystic nonenhancing components.

*SHH (sonic hedgehog) medulloblastomas* SHH tumors are thought to account for 28% of all medulloblastomas.[42]

They have an intermediate prognosis between good prognosis WNT tumors and poor prognosis group 3 tumors, and may be similar in prognosis to group 4.[52,53] SHH MBs show a dichotomous age distribution being more common in both infants (<4 years) and adults (>16 years).[56–58]

Most tumors in this group are of the desmoplastic subtype, located in the cerebellar hemisphere more often than in the midline.

*WNT (wingless) medulloblastomas (∼10%)* WNT tumors are thought to be the rarest subgroup of medulloblastoma, accounting for 11% of these tumors,[58] but they have probably been the most studied and have a very good long-term prognosis with overall survivals reaching 90%.[51,59,60]

WNT tumors also show a specific age distribution being almost absent in infants (aged <4 years) but predominantly affecting children with a peak incidence of 10 to 12 years.[59]

Most (97%) WNT MBs show classic histology; however, rarely, they are phenotypically large cell/anaplastic[3] and may remarkably retain their relatively good prognosis with this phenotype.[47] They tend to occur in the middle cerebellar peduncle/cerebellopontine angle.[55]

*Group 3* Group 3 tumors account for 28% of all MBs.

They are associated with the worst prognosis of all the subgroups and are frequently

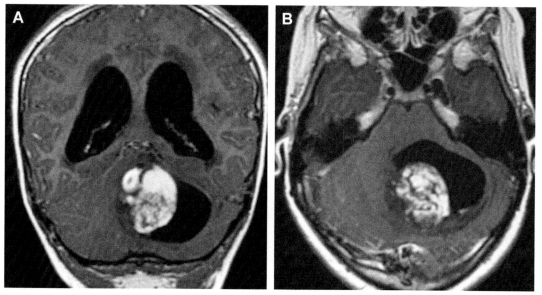

Fig. 18. PA: striking solid enhancement. Same patient as in Fig. 16A, B. The solid portion of the PA presents with striking enhancement. (*A*) Coronal and (*B*) axial T1 with contrast.

metastatic.[45,51] Group 3 tumors are found in infants and children but very rarely in adults.[52] Group 3 MBs are mostly classic or large cell/anaplastic morphology.[51,52] MYC amplification appears to be highly associated with group 3 tumors and is associated with a worse prognosis.[47] The tumors in this subgroup tend to be ill-defined on imaging.[55]

*Group 4* Group 4 MBs are thought to be the most common "typical" subgroup of MB, accounting for approximately 34%,[52] and can be thought of conceptually as being associated with isochromosome 17q.[52] Group 4 medulloblastomas rarely affect infants (0–3 years) and mainly affect children, with a peak age of 10 years.[52]

Although they frequently metastasize, they still have an intermediate prognosis compared with the poor prognosis of group 3.[11,46,49,55,60]

The vast majority of group 4 MBs have a classic histology.

All histologic subtypes can present with this molecular profile, except the desmoplastic one.

These tumors tend to have minimal or no enhancement.[51]

**Molecular profiling: implications in treatment** The identification of different molecular pathways involved in the pathogenesis of MBs provides new therapeutic targets for drug development.[11,46,51,61–63]

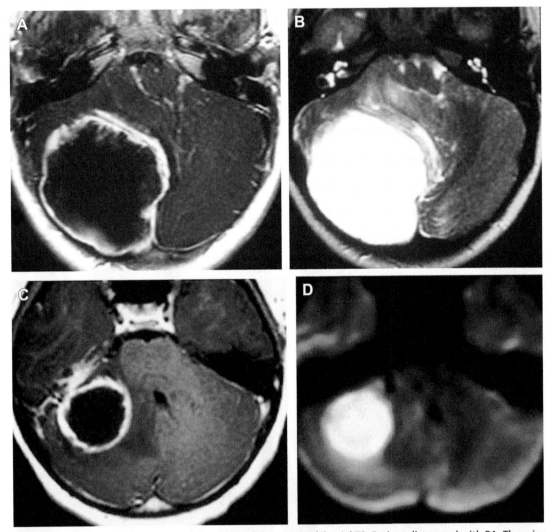

**Fig. 19.** PA: peripheral enhancement. (*A*) Axial T1 with contrast, (*B*) axial T2: Patient diagnosed with PA. There is a large round lesion in the right cerebellar hemisphere presenting with marginal enhancement (*A*) and mild peripheral edema (*B*). (*C, D*) Child diagnosed with right cerebellar abscess presenting with peripheral enhancement (*C*: axial T1 with contrast). There is significant diffusion restriction (*D*: DWI) not typically found in PA.

### Medulloblastomas and associated syndromes

*Basal cell nevus syndrome (Gorlin syndrome)* This is a rare autosomal dominant disorder with high incidence of neoplasms, notably MB. Ten percent of these patients will develop MBs, usually desmoplastic.

Falcine calcification in children with MB may be a marker for basal cell nevus syndrome.[64,65]

*Turcot syndrome* Turcot syndrome is associated with familial colonic polyposis, with high incidence of brain tumors, such as MB and glioma.[66]

*Li-Fraumeni* Germline mutations of the p-53 tumor suppressor gene predisposes to different types of cancer in patients, especially soft tissue sarcomas. Ten percent of these patients develop MB.[67]

*Key points to remember*

- MB is the most common posterior fossa tumor in children
- MB affects mainly boys before 10 years of age
- There is a second peak in adults

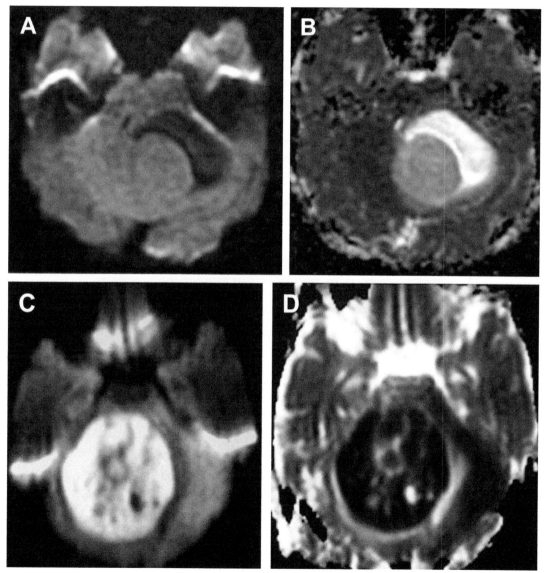

Fig. 20. PA: DWI. (*A, B*) Same patient as Fig. 16A, B. There is no restricted diffusion in the solid component of the PA (*A*: DWI and *B*: ADC map), which helps distinguish PAs from MBs, which typically present with restricted diffusion, due to high cell density (*C*: DWI and *D*: ADC map, same patient as Fig. 16C).

- Lesion is often located in the midline vermis and presents with hyperattenuation on CT, isointense to hypointense on T2, restricted diffusion and high Cho and taurine on MRS
- Perfusion and permeability values are variable
- Look for CSF spread!

- There are imaging features associated with molecular subgroups: SHH involves the cerebellar hemisphere, the WNT pathway involves cerebellar peduncle/CPA cistern, group 3 tumors are ill-defined on imaging, and group 4 tumors have minimal or no enhancement

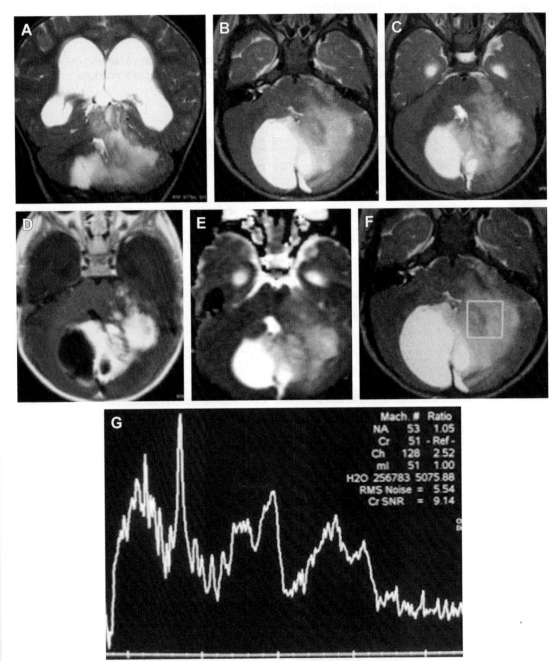

**Fig. 21.** Infiltrative rather than well circumscribed PA. A 23-month-old boy with developmental delay, low stature and low weight for his age. There is a PA infiltrating the left cerebellar hemisphere and vermis, extending anteriorly to the left cerebellopontine angle, compressing the fourth ventricle (*A*: coronal T2, *B*, *C*: axial T2). There is an associated cystic component in the right cerebellar hemisphere. There is striking enhancement in the solid component (*D*: axial T1 with contrast) and no restricted diffusion (*E*: ADC map). MRS (*F*, *G*) demonstrates a large choline peak, along with reduced NAA and Cr, as well as high lipids, very consistent with the diagnosis of PA.

## ATYPICAL TERATOID RHABDOID TUMORS

ATRTs are classified as part of the embryonal tumor group of central nervous system (CNS) tumors.[3]

ATRT is a highly malignant CNS neoplasm that most often occurs in children younger than 2 years.[68,69] ATRTs represent 1.3% of CNS primary brain tumors in the pediatric population, but if one considers only children younger than 3, prevalence rises to 20%.[4,70]

ATRTs are more common in girls than in boys, with 94% in an intra-axial location.[70] A review of 14 histologically confirmed cases of ATRTs demonstrated equal preference for the supratentorial and infratentorial compartments.[71]

These tumors are aggressive lesions with a dismal prognosis, and a 2-year survival of only 17%. Survival improves if the patient is older than 3 years.[4]

Poor prognosis is related to the young age of the affected patients as well as the high propensity for CSF tumor spread.[71] Metastasis to the lungs and abdomen also may be demonstrated.[72,73]

### Imaging Findings

On unenhanced CT, the tumor is usually characterized as hyperdense (**Fig. 14**) and on T2 images, as isointense to hypointense compared with gray matter (**Fig. 15**). These imaging findings are likely secondary to high cell density and high nuclear-to-cytoplasmic ratio and overlap with those described for MBs.

Enhancement is demonstrated in approximately 89% of the cases (see **Fig. 15F**).[71]

Due to high cell density, as well as high nuclear-to-cytoplasmic ratio, restricted diffusion is typically seen (see **Fig. 15G, H**).

MRS shows elevated Cho and reduced NAA as well as a prominent Lip peak. However, there are no reports in the literature that quantify these

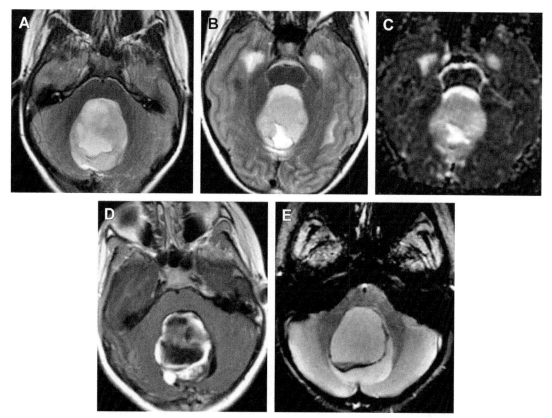

**Fig. 22.** PA: blood. A 10-year-old girl, presenting with headache and dizziness. There is a PA within the cerebellar vermis. The solid portion is hyperintense to the cerebellar cortex on T2 (*A, B*: axial T2) and has no restricted diffusion (*C*: ADC map). There is nonhomogeneous enhancement in the lesion (*D*: axial T1 with contrast) and low signal intensity foci within the solid portion in the gradient echo image (*E*) related to the presence of blood products, as confirmed after surgical resection.

changes or address the presence or size of Tau peaks.[4,36]

### Atypical Teratoid Rhabdoid Tumors Versus Medulloblastoma

The main differential diagnosis for posterior fossa ATRT is MB. If the patient is younger than 3 years, if tumor is located off midline, extending to the CPA, and if blood products are demonstrated in the lesion, one should consider ATRT as the most likely diagnosis.[74]

However, the precise distinction can be made only through immunohistochemistry and genetic analyses. ATRTs frequently demonstrate deletions of chromosome 22q with inactivation of the INI1/hSNF5, thought to be a tumor suppressor gene. Loss of the INI1 gene product is used to diagnose ATRT, although it is not present in all ATRT tumors.[75,76]

# CEREBELLAR PILOCYTIC ASTROCYTOMA

CPA and MB each constitute approximately 35% of all posterior fossa masses in children.[77]

Pilocytic astrocytomas (PAs) are low-grade (grade I) tumors, most often located in the posterior fossa (60%), with 40% involving the cerebellum and 20% involving the brainstem.[4]

CPA has excellent survival after gross total surgical resection.[2,4,78]

Differential diagnosis between PA and MB in the posterior fossa is crucial; the former is a low-grade (WHO grade I) tumor, with excellent prognosis, whereas MB is a grade IV tumor, with poorer prognosis.[36,79]

### Location

Predilection for the cerebellar hemisphere instead of the cerebellar vermis is typically demonstrated.

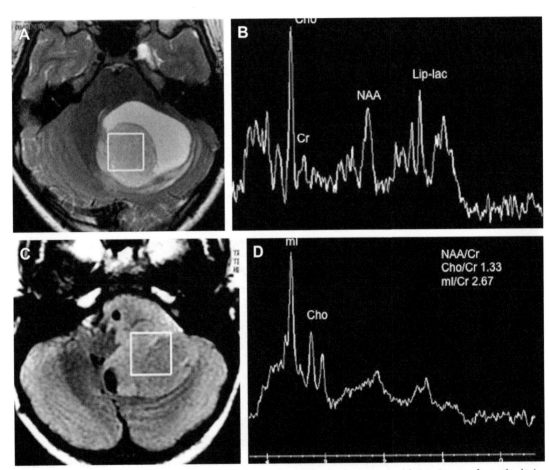

Fig. 23. PA versus ependymoma: MRS. (A, B) Same patient as Fig. 18 diagnosed with PA. Spectra from the lesion (A, B) demonstrates very high Cho peak, reduced NAA and Cr peaks, along with presence of lipids and lactate, typical of PA. (C, D) A 3-year-old boy diagnosed with grade II ependymoma. Spectra from the tumor demonstrates significant elevation of the mI peak as the most striking finding.

The lesion displaces and compresses the fourth ventricle (**Fig. 16**A, B), as opposed to what is typically demonstrated in MB that usually compromises the cerebellar vermis, filling the fourth ventricle (**Fig. 16**C, D).[2,4,79]

## Imaging Findings

CPA often presents with a solid component that is hyperintense to the cerebellar cortex on T2 due to high water content as well as low cell density (see **Fig. 16**A, B).[2,4,79] By contrast, the solid component of MBs is usually isointense or hypointense to normal cerebellar parenchyma on T2 images (see **Fig. 16**C).[2,4] However, higher-grade astrocytomas may manifest lower signal intensity on T2-weighted images, effectively mimicking MBs.[4] On the other hand, some MBs may present with high signal intensity on T2, resembling PA (see **Fig. 16**D).[18]

Cysts associated with PAs are usually larger than those demonstrated in MBs (compare **Fig. 16** A, B vs C).[79]

Some tumors may present with multiple solid and/or cystic components (multinodular/multicystic appearance) (**Fig. 17**).

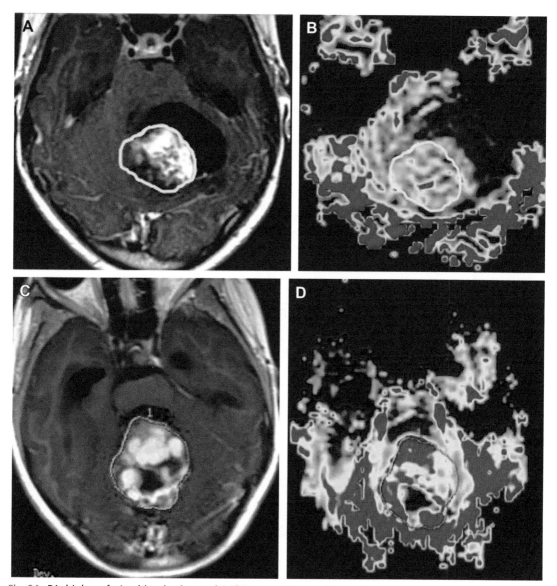

**Fig. 24.** PA: high perfusion blood volumes. (*A, B*) Same patient as **Fig. 18**. The solid enhancing PA (*A*: axial T1 with contrast) demonstrates high blood volume on the DCE perfusion study (*B*: rCBV map). (*C, D*): Same patient as **Fig. 22**. The solid enhancing PA (*C*: axial T1 with contrast) presents with high blood volumes (*D*: rCBV map).

Despite being low-grade (grade I) tumors, striking solid enhancement is characteristic (**Fig. 18**). The amount of gadolinium enhancement matches the T2 abnormality.[79]

Some lesions will present with peripheral enhancement resembling abscesses (**Fig. 19**). Diffusion may help in the differential diagnosis in these cases.[21]

The solid component of PAs has higher ADC values than do other cerebellar tumors, such as MB and ATRT (**Fig. 20**).[21–23]

The typical imaging features described previously may be useful to suggest the diagnosis of a pilocytic tumor and to distinguish this tumor from more aggressive tumors, such as MBs. However, the following are some imaging findings rarely seen that can be considered atypical.[79]

### Infiltrative, rather than well-circumscribed lesion

CPAs are typically well-circumscribed, localized lesions. However, sometimes the tumor may be infiltrative, presenting with ill-defined margins, and hence complete surgical resection is very difficult (**Fig. 21**).

### Presence of blood products

CPAs, despite being grade I (low-grade) tumors may bleed (**Fig. 22**). Knowledge of this "unexpected" finding is essential so as not to change the diagnosis in these cases.

### Restricted diffusion

Diffusion is typically not restricted in PAs (see **Fig. 20**A, B), because these are low cell density lesions.[21–23] Approximately 7% of these tumors may present with restricted diffusion.[21]

### Very high Cho along with presence of lipids and lactate in the magnetic resonance spectroscopy

Brain metabolites may be useful to suggest tumor grade. Among these, Cho is typically related to tumor cell density and, hence, higher Cho/creatine and Cho/NAA ratios are typically demonstrated in higher grade (grade III) than in lower grade (grade II) gliomas. However, tCho is not an effective or accurate biomarker for grade I PAs.[36]

Choline is typically very high in pilocytic tumors, despite the benign clinical course for tumors of this type (**Fig. 23**A, B).[2,4,26,36,80]

Due to the very high Cho peak, the spectral pattern of PAs may overlap with that from MB (see **Fig. 10**).[79] However, the Tau peak, considered very characteristic of MBs, is not typically demonstrated in PAs.[33]

Lipids and lactate are also usually demonstrated in the spectra of PA.[26,79]

The spectral pattern of PAs may be used to distinguish between these tumors and grade II ependymomas (**Fig. 23**C, D).[79]

### High blood volumes in the perfusion study

Despite being low grade (grade I tumors), PAs may present with high blood volumes on dynamic

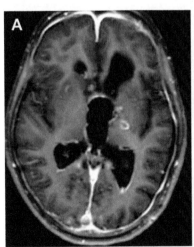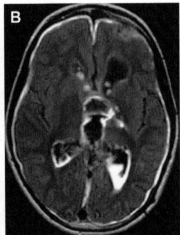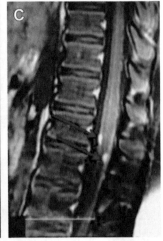

**Fig. 25.** PA: CSF tumor spread. (*A, B*) An 8-year-old girl treated for PA, now presenting with CSF tumor spread with multiple ependymal enhancing nodules in both frontal horns (*A*: axial T1 with contrast) better demonstrated in the axial T2 fluid-attenuated inversion recovery (FLAIR) with contrast (*B*). There is also involvement of the ependyma of the third ventricle and the atrium bilaterally. (*C*) A 6-year-old boy treated for PA presenting with CSF spread. Enhancing nodules are demonstrated adjacent to the conus medullaris (*C*: sagittal T1 with contrast).

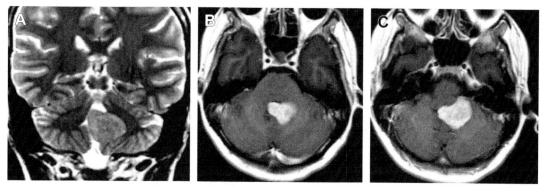

Fig. 26. Ependymoma in the fourth ventricle. Fourth ventricular mass, extending though the foramina of Luschka on the left to the left cerebellopontine angle (CPA). (*A*) Coronal T2, (*B, C*) axial T1 with contrast.

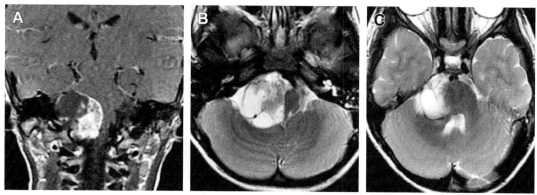

Fig. 27. Ependymoma in the foramina of Luschka. A 4-year-old boy with ataxia and hearing loss. Ependymoma growing in the foramina of Luschka on the right, displacing the medulla and pons. Lesion was mistaken for exophytic BG. (*A*) Coronal T1 with contrast, (*B, C*) axial T2.

susceptibility contrast studies (**Fig. 24**).[79,81–83] This finding is not related to aggressiveness in these lesions.

*Cerebrospinal fluid spread*
Despite the low malignancy grade, PA may spread via CSF dissemination (**Fig. 25**).[4,79]

## EPENDYMOMAS

Ependymomas are characterized by perivascular arrangement of tumor cells.[3] These tumors are most often seen in children younger than 5, with a second peak in adults in the fourth decade.[2,4]

Ependymomas are the fourth most common posterior fossa tumors in children after MB, cerebellar astrocytoma, and BG.[2,4]

There are genetically distinct subgroups that have been identified by genomic studies based on locations in classic grade II and III ependymomas. They are supratentorial ependymomas with C11 or f95-RELA fusion or YAP1 fusion, infratentorial ependymomas

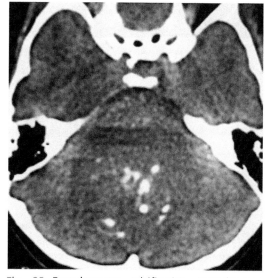

Fig. 28. Ependymoma: calcification. Ependymoma located in the fourth ventricle, presenting with multiple foci of calcification. (*Courtesy of* A. James Barkovich, MD, San Francisco, CA.)

with or without a hypermethylated phenotype (CIMP), and spinal cord ependymomas.[84]

Seventy percent of all ependymomas are in the posterior fossa, with 90% involving the ventricular ependyma (Fig. 26).[2] Ependymomas may also spread through the foramina of Luschka and Magendie (Fig. 27). Punctate calcification is demonstrated in 50% of ependymoma cases on CT (Fig. 28).[4] Calcification is most often seen in ependymomas than in any other posterior fossa tumor in children.

These tumors are heterogeneous on MR imaging (see Fig. 28, see also Fig. 27), reflecting a combination of solid tumor, cyst, calcification, necrosis, edema, or hemorrhage.[4]

The most important imaging finding in identifying an ependymoma is extension of the tumor through the fourth ventricular outflow

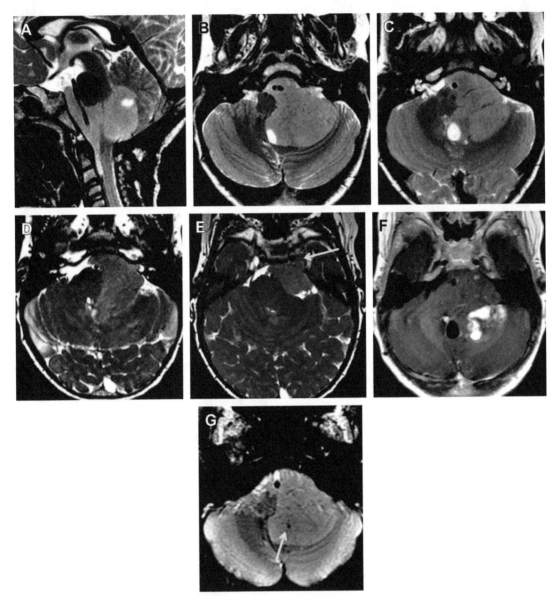

Fig. 29. Ependymoma: MR imaging. MR imaging after surgical resection of an ependymoma in a 3-year old boy demonstrates residual tumor in the fourth ventricle, extending through the foramina of Luschka on the left, encasing the vertebral and basilar arteries, as well as extending inferiorly through the foramina of Magendie and foramen magnum. The lesion is isointense to the cerebellar cortex on T2 (A: sagittal, B, C: axial T2) and presents with a cystic component. High-resolution T2 (D, E) demonstrates encasement of the basilar artery, extension to the left internal auditory canal (IAC) and to left Meckel cave (arrow in E). There is heterogeneous enhancement (F) and a punctate hypointensity likely representing calcification is demonstrated within the lesion (arrow in G).

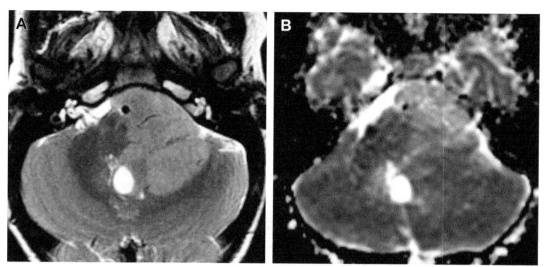

Fig. 30. Ependymoma: DWI. (*A, B*) Same patient as Fig. 29. There is mild restricted diffusion in the lesion (*A*: axial T2, *B*: ADC map).

foramina (see Fig. 26; and Fig. 29)[4]; however, this feature is not entirely pathognomonic, as some MBs may extend through the fourth ventricular exit foramina. In addition, they usually show more bulbous extension and restricted diffusion rather than small amounts of tissue through the foramina that is characteristic of an ependymoma.[4,85] Siderosis[86] may be demonstrated associated with ependymomas.

### Diffusion-Weighted Imaging

Most ependymomas in the posterior fossa are classic (grade II) ependymomas. These tumors usually present with no or mild restricted diffusion (Fig. 30). Jaremko and colleagues[21] demonstrated an overlap between ADC values of the classic type (WHO grade 2, one-half of tumors demonstrating restricted diffusion) and anaplastic type (WHO grade 3, two-thirds of tumors demonstrating restricted diffusion). Given the wide histologic and prognostic spectrum of ependymoma, diffusion characteristics of ependymoma also have a wide range overlapping other tumor types, such as MB.[21,29,87] Because ependymoma shows no distant disease in more than 90% of cases,[85] metastasis favors MB.

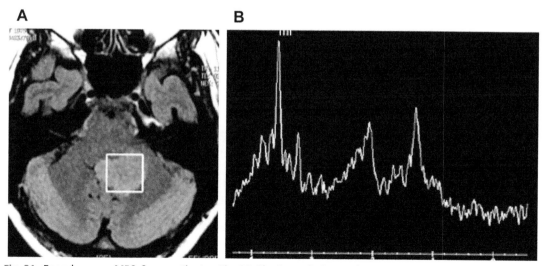

Fig. 31. Ependymoma: MRS. Same patient as Fig. 26. Classic grade II ependymomas typically demonstrate high mI in the spectra (*A*: axial FLAIR, *B*: spectroscopy).

## Magnetic Resonance Spectroscopy

High myo-inositol (mI) levels are typically demonstrated in classic grade II ependymomas.[36,81] In a study by Harris and colleagues,[88] the presence of high mI levels strongly suggested a diagnosis of ependymoma when short TE is used at 1.5 T (Fig. 31 see also Fig. 23C, D). Schneider and colleagues[29] also demonstrated that ependymomas are characterized by an elevation in mI and Glx.

## Perfusion and Permeability Studies

Ependymomas generally demonstrate markedly elevated relative cerebral blood volume (rCBV) (Fig. 32) and, unlike many other glial neoplasms, a poor return to baseline that may be attributable to fenestrated blood vessels and an incomplete blood brain barrier (BBB) (see Fig. 32C).[89–91] This behavior, although very characteristic of ependymomas, is not entirely pathognomonic and also may be demonstrated in other tumors, such as

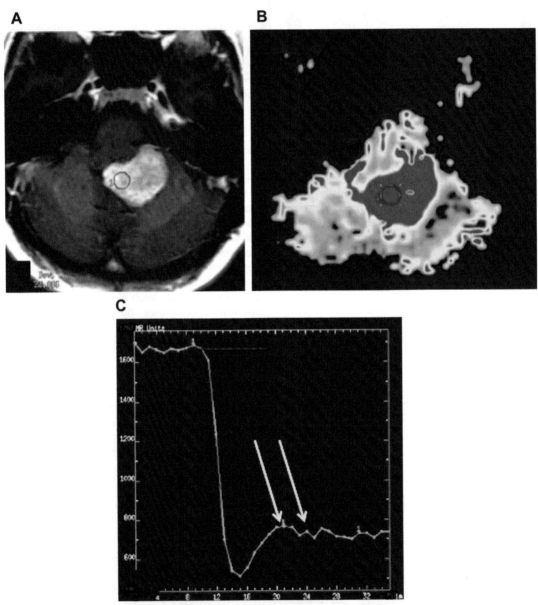

Fig. 32. Ependymoma: perfusion. Same patient as Fig. 26 diagnosed with ependymoma. There is a solid enhancing tumor in the fourth ventricle (A: axial T1 with contrast) presenting with significant elevation of rCBV on perfusion imaging (B: rCBV map) with poor return of the perfusion curve to the baseline (arrows in C: perfusion curve).

embryonal tumors (**Fig. 33**) (Lara A. Brandão, MD, personal communication, 2013).

For the same reason stated previously (fenestrated blood vessels and an incomplete BBB), ependymomas tend to present with very high permeability (**Fig. 34**) (Lara A. Brandão, MD, personal communication, 2013).

## BRAINSTEM GLIOMA AND OTHER BRAINSTEM TUMORS

One narrowly defined group of tumors primarily occurring in children (but sometimes in adults too) is characterized by K27M mutations in the histone H3 gene H3F3A, or less commonly in the related HIST1H3B gene, a diffuse growth pattern, and a midline location (eg, thalamus, brainstem, and spinal cord). This newly defined entity is termed diffuse midline glioma, H3 K27M–mutant and includes tumors previously referred to as diffuse intrinsic pontine glioma.[51] Most of these tumors have poor prognosis but exceptions have been reported.[51]

The identification of this phenotypically and molecularly defined set of tumors provides a

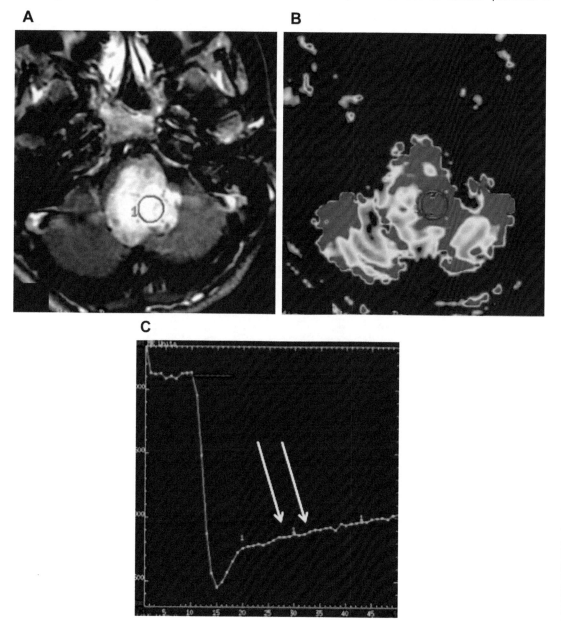

**Fig. 33.** Embryonal tumor: perfusion. Brainstem embryonal tumor presenting with striking enhancement (*A*: axial T1 with contrast) and significant elevation of the rCBV on the perfusion study (*B*: rCBV map) with poor return of the perfusion curve to the baseline (*arrows* in *C*: perfusion curve); similar findings as in ependymomas (see **Fig. 32**).

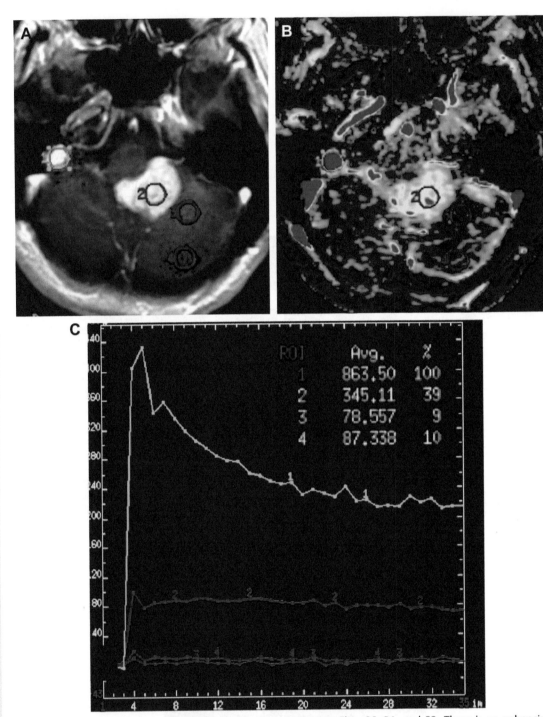

Fig. 34. Ependymoma: permeability (DCE study). Same patient as Figs. 26, 31, and 32. There is an enhancing fourth ventricular ependymoma (A: axial T1 with contrast) with significant elevation of the permeability (B: maximum slope of increase map, C: curves; region of interest [ROI] 1, from the jugular vein; 2, from the tumor; 3, from the cerebellar white matter; 4, from the cerebellar cortex).

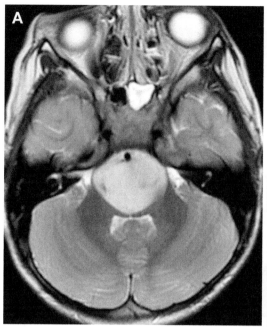
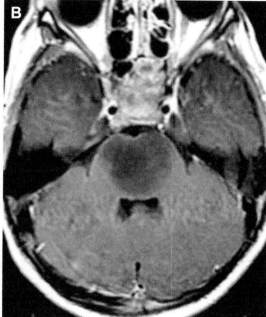

Fig. 35. BG: MR imaging. A 5-year-old girl presenting with headaches and diplopia. There is a midline diffuse glioma with high signal intensity on T2 (*A*: axial) expanding the pons, compressing the fourth ventricle and encasing the basilar artery. There is no enhancement in the lesion (*B*: axial T1 with contrast).

rationale for therapies directed against the effects of these mutations.

Brainstem tumors represent 10% to 20% of all CNS tumors in childhood.[2] Most BGs are diffuse and involve the pons.[4]

Diagnosis is based on the characteristic changes on MR imaging of diffuse T2 hyperintense expansion of the brainstem without biopsy (**Figs. 35** and **36**).[2,4] Enhancement is typically absent (see **Fig. 35**B) or restricted to a small portion of the lesion (**Fig. 36**D).

Five-year survival is related to location, with midbrain lesions having the best outcome (72%–100% of patients alive in 5 years) and pontine lesions having the worst (18% alive in 5 years).[92] Tumor extension also influences survival, with diffuse lesions having the worst survival rates (18%–20%) and focal lesions having the best (56%–199%).[92]

## Diffusion-Weighted Imaging

Areas of restricted diffusion may be demonstrated within a pontine glioma, indicating higher cell density and the best place for biopsy (**Fig. 37**).[79]

ADC measurements in these tumors are closely related to prognosis and survival with lower ADC values associated with poorer survival.[92,93]

## Magnetic Resonance Spectroscopy

Single-voxel MRS (SV-MRS) or multivoxel spectroscopy (chemical shift imaging) can be used to evaluate BGs.[36,94]

Proton MRS and perfusion imaging may be useful in differentiating low-grade (usually focal) pontine tumors, which have lower Cho peaks (as well as Cho/Cr and Cho/NAA ratios) and lower blood volumes, from high-grade tumors in which the Cho/Cr ratio is usually higher (**Fig. 38**).[36]

A citrate peak can be demonstrated at approximately 2.6 ppm and can be used to follow tumor progression (**Fig. 39**).[95–97] Reduced citrate levels may indicate malignant transformation of these tumors, or may be related to chronic administration of steroids, RT, and/or chemotherapy.[96] Although the citrate signal is most prominent and most often observed in diffuse midline gliomas of the pons, it is also noted in other common pediatric brain tumors and in the developing brain of infants younger than 6 months.[97]

Some studies suggest that MRS might be a useful early predictor of disease progression in BGs, preceding clinical and radiological deterioration.[95,98,99] Metabolic changes indicative of malignant transformation include increased levels of tCho, decreased metabolite ratios of NAA/tCho and Cr/tCho, and increased levels of Lips. In addition, a significant reduction in the "apparent" citrate levels also may be associated with malignant transformation.[97]

## Perfusion and Permeability Studies

Available literature suggests that at least a subset of diffuse midline gliomas of the pons

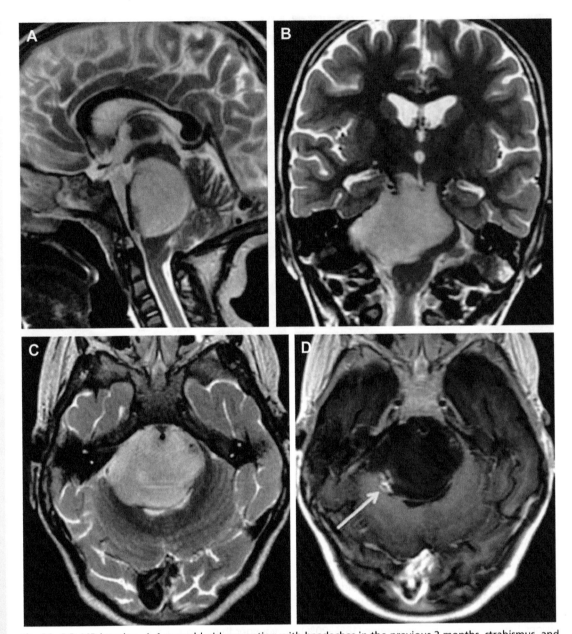

**Fig. 36.** BG: MR imaging. A 4-year-old girl presenting with headaches in the previous 3 months, strabismus, and ataxia. There is a midline diffuse glioma with high signal intensity on T2 (*A*: sagittal, *B*: coronal, *C*: axial T2) expanding the pons, compressing the fourth ventricle and encasing the basilar artery. A small area of enhancement is demonstrated in the lesion (*arrow* in *D*: axial T1 with contrast).

is histologically low grade (WHO grade II) at initial clinical presentation, but rapidly evolves into high-grade neoplasms, with most found to be glioblastoma at postmortem examination.[96,99–105]

Perfusion and permeability are related to tumor grade, with areas of higher blood volumes and higher permeability indicating aggressiveness and the best site for biopsy (**Fig. 40**).[81]

*Treatment considerations*
Radiation therapy is the most used therapy for BGs, with very good response in some patients, especially in those with low cell density tumors (**Fig. 41**).

Enlargement of a pontine glioma during radiation therapy plus chemotherapy and or immunotherapy is not necessarily related to treatment failure and may represent pseudoprogression especially with immunotherapy treatments.[106,107]

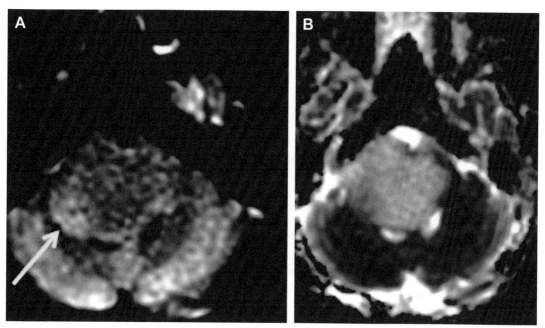

**Fig. 37.** BG: DWI. Same patient as **Fig. 36**. An area of restricted diffusion is demonstrated in the lateral portion of the lesion (*arrow* in A: DWI, *B*: ADC map) indicating high cell density.

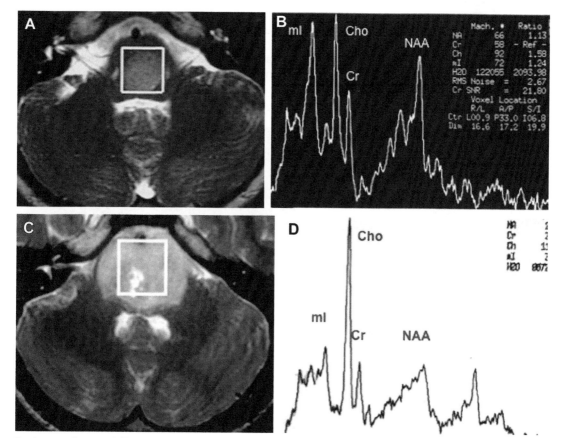

**Fig. 38.** Focal versus diffuse BG: MRS. (*A, B*) Focal BG presenting with more preserved NAA and higher mI than the infiltrative more aggressive pontine glioma (*C, D*). Cho/Cr and Cho/NAA ratios are also higher in the diffuse glioma versus the focal less aggressive one.

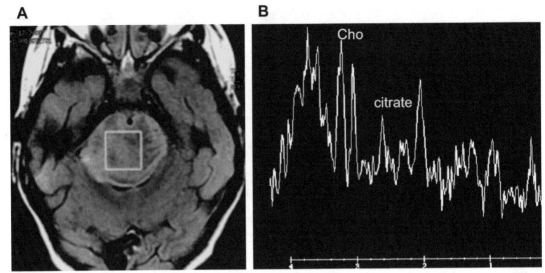

**Fig. 39.** BG: MRS. Same patient as **Figs. 36** and **37**. MRS (*A*: voxel, *B*, curve) shows high Cho along with citrate peak in 2.6 ppm.

### Other brainstem tumors

Tumors in the midbrain and medulla are most often PAs on histology, with a better prognosis than the diffuse midline glioma.[2,4]

Ganglioglioma is another diagnostic consideration for tumors located in the brainstem.

Posterior fossa gangliogliomas (PF GGs) occur less often than supratentorial gangliogliomas (ST GGs).[108]

On imaging, PF GGs are most often infiltrative and expansile solid masses with dorsal predominant "paintbrush" enhancement (**Fig. 42**).

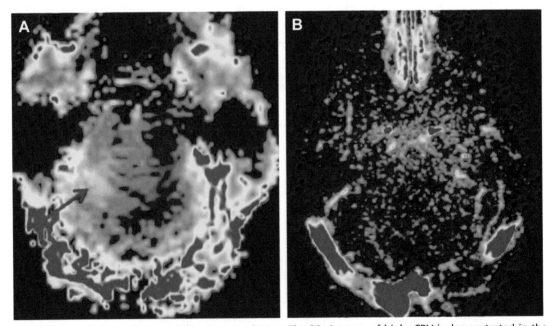

**Fig. 40.** BG: perfusion and permeability. Same patient as **Fig. 36**. An area of high rCBV is demonstrated in the lateral portion of the lesion (*arrow* in *A*: rCBV map). There is no significant elevation of the permeability (*B*: maximum slope of increase map).

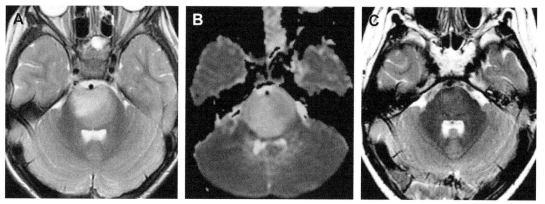

Fig. 41. BG: good response to RT. Same patient as Fig. 35. A 5-year-old boy presenting with headaches and diplopia, diagnosed with diffuse midline glioma of the pons (*A*: axial T2). There is no restricted diffusion in the lesion, indicating low cell density (*B*: ADC map). After RT (*C*: axial T2) the lesion is smaller and less hyperintense, indicating therapeutic response.

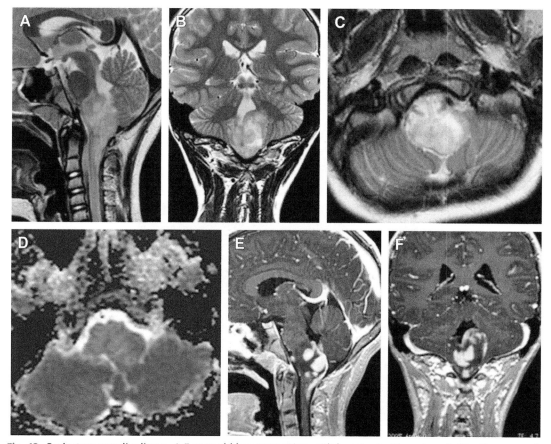

Fig. 42. Brainstem ganglioglioma. A 5-year-old boy presenting with hypotonia. There is an infiltrative expansile ganglioglioma at the cervicomedullary junction, with an exophytic component in the left foramina of Luschka, hyperintense on T2 (*A*: sagittal, *B*: coronal, *C*: axial T2) with no restricted diffusion (*D*: ADC map). There is dorsal linear enhancement, as well as multiple enhancing nodules within the lesion (*E*: sagittal, *F*: coronal T1 with contrast).

PF GGs are not amenable to gross total resection, and have worse progression-free survival and mortality, compared with ST GGs.[107]

These tumors can be grade I or II and have a higher propensity to CSF spread than PA.[109]

If there is evidence of high cell density within the tumor, with restricted diffusion and high Cho in the spectra, one should consider embryonal tumor in the differential diagnosis (**Figs. 43** and **44**).[110]

## EMBRYONAL TUMOR WITH MULTILAYERED ROSETTES C19MC-ALTERED

A new entity, embryonal tumor with multilayered rosettes (ETMR) C19MC-altered, was recently described in children younger than 3 years.[51]

The spectrum of morphologic patterns in this entity includes the following:

- ETANRT (embryonal tumors with abundant neuropil & true rosettes) with variable numbers of rosettes, small blue cells
- Ependymoblastoma (diagnosis removed from WHO 2016)

These are usually large bulk tumors in the supratentorial compartment, but also may be found in the posterior fossa.

They are usually heterogeneous and can have little edema for their size.

A small percentage of pontine gliomas may be diagnosed as ETMR.

Prognosis is dismal despite radiation therapy.

## SUMMARY

Pediatric brain tumors are the most common solid tumor in children and the leading cause of death in

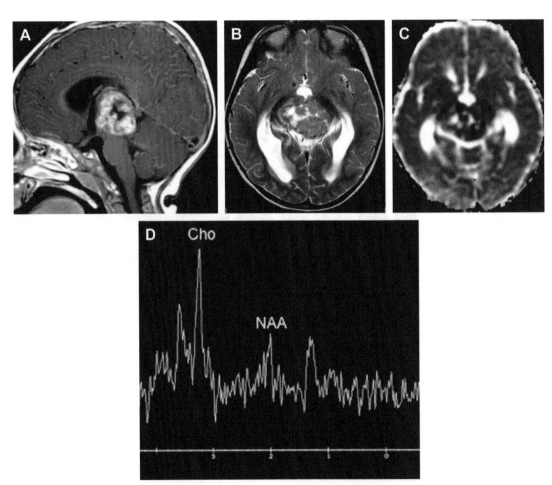

**Fig. 43.** ATRT. There is a heterogeneously enhancing lesion in the midbrain (*A*: sagittal T1 with contrast) mainly hypointense on T2 (*B*: axial) with restricted diffusion (*C*: ADC map) and high Cho on MR spectra (*D*), suggesting high cell density.

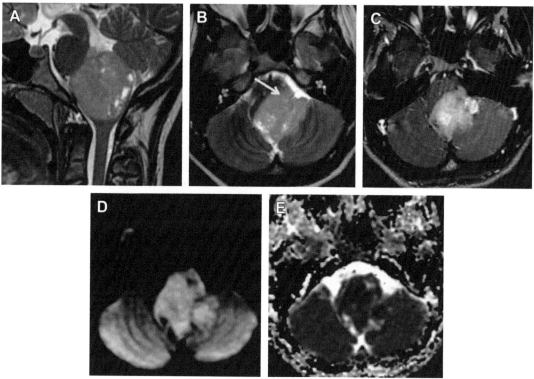

**Fig. 44.** Embryonal tumor. Same patient as **Fig. 33**, diagnosed with embryonal tumor. A 13-year-old girl with headaches, ataxia, and diplopia. There is a solid lesion centered in the medulla, hypointense on T2 (*A*: sagittal, *B*: axial T2) extending to the left cerebellopontine angle (*arrow* in *B*), presenting with significant enhancement (*C*: axial T1 with contrast). Restricted diffusion is demonstrated (*D*: DWI, *E*: ADC map), indicating high cell density.

this patient population. The primary objective of this article was to offer a detailed overview of the most common brain tumors affecting the posterior fossa in children. The respective imaging features on CT, cMR imaging, and advanced MR imaging studies, may help suggest the most likely diagnosis leading to early and appropriate treatment.

## REFERENCES

1. Ostrom QT, Gittleman H, Fulop J, et al. CBTRUS statistical report. Neuro Oncol 2015;17:iv1–62.
2. Poussaint TY. Pediatric brain tumors. In: Newton HB, Jolesz FA, editors. Handbook of neuro-oncology neuroimaging. New York: Elsevier; 2008. p. 469–84.
3. Louis DN, Ohgaki H, Wiestler OD, et al, editors. WHO classification of tumours of the central nervous system. Lyon (France): IARC; 2007.
4. Barkovich AJ, Raybaud C. Intracranial, orbital and neck masses of childhood. In: Pediatric neuroimaging. 5th edition. Philadelphia: Lippincott Williams & Wilkins and Wolters Kluwer; 2012. p. 637–711.
5. Najel BJ, Palmer SL, Reddick WE, et al. Abnormal hippocampal development in children with medulloblastoma treated with risk-adapted irradiation. AJNR Am J Neuroradiol 2004;25:1575–82.
6. Khong P, Kwong DL, Chan GC, et al. Diffusion-tensor imaging for the detection and quantification of treatment-induced white matter injury in children with medulloblastoma: a pilot study. AJNR Am J Neuroradiol 2003;24:734–40.
7. Kovantikaya A, Panigrahy A, Krieger MD, et al. Untreated pediatric primitive neuroectodermal tumor in vivo: quantification of taurine with MR spectroscopy. Radiology 2005;236:1020–5.
8. Annette C, akinwandea D, Paynerb TD, et al. Medulloblastoma mimicking Lhermitte-Duclos disease on MRI and CT. Clin Neurol Neurosurg 2009;111:536–53.
9. Koeller KK, Rushing EF. Medulloblastoma: a comprehensive review with radiologic-pathologic correlation. Radiographics 2003;23:1613–37.
10. Wilne S, Collier J, Kennedy C, et al. Progression from first symptom to diagnosis in childhood brain tumors. Eur J Pediatr 2012;171(1):87–93.
11. Lamont JM, McManamy CS, Pearson AD, et al. Combined histopathological and molecular

cytogenetic stratification of medulloblastoma patients. Clin Cancer Res 2004;10:5482–93.

12. Bourgouin PM, Tampieri D, Grahovac SZ, et al. CT and MR imaging findings in adults with cerebellar medulloblastoma: comparison with findings in children. AJR Am J Roentgenol 1992;159:609–12.

13. Koci TM, Chiang F, Mehringer CM, et al. Adult cerebellar medulloblastoma: imaging features with emphasis on MR findings. AJNR Am J Neuroradiol 1993;14:929–39.

14. Meyers SP, Kemp SS, Tarr RW. MR imaging features of medulloblastomas. AJR Am J Roentgenol 1992;158:859–65.

15. Rollins N, Mendelshon D, Mulne A, et al. Recurrent medulloblastoma: frequency of tumor enhancement on Gd-DTPA MR imaging. AJNR Am J Neuroradiol 1990;11:583–7.

16. Zerbini C, Gelber RD, Weinberg D, et al. Prognostic factors in medulloblastoma, including DNA ploidy. J Clin Oncol 1993;11:616–22.

17. Kuhl J. Modern treatment strategies in medulloblastoma. Childs Nerv Syst 1998;14:2–5.

18. Aliye O, Bricker MD, Manzoor Ahmed MD, Medulloblastoma: spectrum of imaging appearances with focus on atypical findings. The Cleveland Clinic foundation- Presented at the ASNR 50th Annual Meeting and The Foundation of the ASNR Symposium 2012. New York, April 21–26, 2012.

19. Naitoh Y, Kinouchi H, Mikawa S, et al. Medulloblastoma with extensive nodularity: single photon emission CT study with iodine-123 metaiodobenzylguanidine. AJNR Am J Neuroradiol 2002;23(9): 1564–7.

20. Pizer BL, Clifford SC. The potential impact of tumour biology on improved clinical practice for medulloblastoma: progress towards biologically driven clinical trials. Br J Neurosurg 2009;23(4): 364–75.

21. Jaremko JL, JAns LBO, Coleman LT, et al. Value and limitations of diffusion-weighted imaging in grading and diagnosis of pediatric posterior fossa tumors. AJNR Am J Neuroradiol 2010;31:1613–6.

22. Rumboldt Z, Camacho DL, Lake D, et al. Apparent diffusion coefficients for differentiation of cerebellar tumors in children. AJNR Am J Neuroradiol 2006; 27:1362–9.

23. Yamasaki F, Kurisu K, Satoh K, et al. Apparent diffusion coefficient of human brain tumors at MR imaging. Radiology 2005;235:985–91.

24. Panigrahy A, Krieger I, Gonzalez G, et al. Quantitative short echo time 1H-MR spectroscopy of un-treated pediatric brain tumors: preoperative diagnosis and characterization. AJNR Am J Neuroradiol 2006;27:560–72.

25. Wang Z, Sutton LN, Cnaan A, et al. Proton MR spectroscopy of pediatric cerebellar tumors. AJNR Am J Neuroradiol 1995;16:1821–33.

26. Brandão L, Domingues R. Intracranial neoplasms. In: McAllister L, Lazar T, Cook RE, editors. MR Spectroscopy of the brain. Philadelphia: Lippincott Williams & Wilkins; 2003. p. 130–67.

27. Majo ós C, Alonso J, Aguilera C, et al. Adult primitive neuroectodermal tumor: proton MR spectroscopic findings with possible application for differential diagnosis. Radiology 2002;225: 556–66.

28. Tong Z, Yamaki T, Harada K, et al. In vivo quantification of the metabolites in normal brain and brain tumors by proton MR spectroscopy using water as an internal standard. Magn Reson Imaging 2004; 22:1017–24.

29. Schneider JF, Gouny C, Viola A, et al. Multiparametric differentiation of posterior fossa tumors in children using diffusion-weighted imaging and short echo-time 1H-MR spectroscopy. J Magn Reson Imaging 2007;26:1390–8.

30. Panigrahy A, Nelson M, Blüml S. Magnetic resonance spectroscopy in pediatric neuroradiology: clinical and research applications. Pediatr Radiol 2010;40:3–30.

31. Majós C, Aguilera C, Cos M, et al. In vivo proton magnetic resonance spectroscopy of intraventricular tumors of the brain. Eur Radiol 2009;19: 2049–59.

32. Jouanneau E, Tovar RA, Desuzinges C. Very late frontal relapse of medulloblastoma mimicking a meningioma in an adult. Usefulness of 1H magnetic resonance spectroscopy and diffusion-perfusion magnetic resonance imaging for preoperative diagnosis: case report. Neurosurgery 2006;58:E789–90.

33. Moreno-Torres A, Martinez-Perez I, Baquero M, et al. Taurine detection by proton magnetic resonance spectroscopy in medulloblastoma: contribution to noninvasive differential diagnosis with cerebellar astrocytoma. Neurosurgery 2004;55: 824–9.

34. Wilke M, Eidenschink A, Muller-Weihrich S, et al. MR diffusion imaging and 1H spectroscopy in a child with medulloblastoma: a case report. Acta Radiol 2001;42:39–42.

35. Peeling J, Sutherland G. High-resolution 1H NMR spectroscopy studies of extracts of human cerebral neoplasms. Magn Reson Med 1992;24:123–6.

36. Brandão L, Poussaint T. Pediatric brain tumors. In: MR spectroscopy of the brain. Neuroimaging Clin N Am 2013;23:499–523.

37. Peet AC, Daviesa NP, Lee R, et al. Magnetic resonance spectroscopy suggests key differences in the metastatic behaviour of medulloblastoma. Eur J Cancer 2007;43:1037–44.

38. Lindskog M, Kogner P, Ponthan F, et al. Non invasive estimation of tumour viability in a xenograft model of human neuroblastoma with proton

magnetic resonance spectroscopy (1H MRS). Br J Caner 2003;88:478–85.

39. Peet AC, Wilson M, Levine B, et al. 1H NMR spectroscopy identifies differences in choline metabolism related to the MYCN oncogene in neuroblastoma. Proc Intl Soc Mag Reson Med 2005;13:2489.

40. De Souza RM, Jones BRT, Kathreena MK. Pediatric medulloblastoma–update on molecular classification driving targeted therapies. Front Oncol 2014;4:176.

41. Giangaspero F, Perilongo G, Fondelli MP, et al. Medulloblastoma with extensive nodularity: a variant with favorable prognosis. J Neurosurg 1999;91:971–7.

42. Kool M, Korshunov A, Remke M, et al. Molecular subgroups of medulloblastoma: an international meta-analysis of transcriptome, genetic aberrations, and clinical data of WNT, SHH, Group 3, and Group 4 medulloblastomas. Acta Neuropathol 2012;123:473–84.

43. Haberler C, Slavc I, Czech T, et al. Histopathological prognostic factors in medulloblastoma: high expression of survivin is related to unfavourable outcome. Eur J Cancer 2006;42(17):2996–3003.

44. Giangaspero F, Wellek S, Masuoka J, et al. Stratification of medulloblastoma on the basis of histopathological grading. Acta Neuropathol 2006;112(1):5–12.

45. Northcott PA, Korshunov A, Witt H, et al. Medulloblastoma comprises four distinct molecular variants. J Clin Oncol 2011;29:1408–14.

46. Robinson G, Parker M, Kranenburg TA, et al. Novel mutations target distinct subgroups of medulloblastoma. Nature 2012;488(7409):43–8.

47. Ellison DW, Kocak M, Dalton J, et al. Definition of disease-risk stratification groups in childhood medulloblastoma using combined clinical, pathologic, and molecular variables. J Clin Oncol 2011;29:1400–7.

48. Pugh TJ, Weeraratne SD, Archer TC, et al. Medulloblastoma exome sequencing uncovers subtype-specific somatic mutations. Nature 2012;488(7409):106–10.

49. MAGIC – Medulloblastoma Advanced. Genomics International Consortium Stratifying and Targeting Pediatric Medulloblastoma through Genomics. Available at: http://www.bcgsc.ca/project/magic. Accessed May 21, 2016.

50. Cho YJ, Tsherniak A, Tamayo P, et al. Integrative genomic analysis of medulloblastoma identifies a molecular sub-group that drives poor clinical outcome. J Clin Oncol 2011;29:1424–30.

51. Louis DN, Perry A, Reifenberger G, et al. The 2016 World Health Organization Classification of Tumors of the Central Nervous System: a summary. Acta Neuropathol 2016;131:803–20.

52. Taylor MD, Northcott PA, Korshunov A, et al. Molecular subgroups of medulloblastoma: the current consensus. Acta Neuropathol 2012;123:465–72.

53. Samakari A, White JC, Packer RJ. Medulloblastoma: toward biologically based management. Semin Pediatr Neurol 2015;22(1):6–13.

54. Samakari A, White J, Packer R. SHH inhibitors for the treatment of medulloblastoma. Expert Rev Neurother 2015;31:1–8.

55. Perrealut S, Ramaswamy V, Achrol AS, et al. MRI surrogates for molecular subgroups of medulloblastoma. AJNR Am J Neuroradiol 2014;35(7):1263–9.

56. Baryawno N, Sveinbjörnsson B, Eksborg S, et al. Small-molecule inhibitors of phosphatidylinositol 3-kinase/Akt signaling inhibit Wnt/beta-catenin pathway cross-talk and suppress medulloblastoma growth. Cancer Res 2010;70(1):266–76.

57. Chiang C, Litingtung Y, Lee E, et al. Cyclopia and defective axial patterning in mice lacking Sonic hedgehog gene function. Nature 1996;383:407–13.

58. Von Hoff DD, LoRusso PM, Rudin CM, et al. Inhibition of the hedgehog pathway in advanced basal-cell carcinoma. N Engl J Med 2009;361(12):1164–72.

59. Kool M, Koster J, Bunt J, et al. Integrated genomics identifies five medulloblastoma subtypes with distinct genetic profiles, pathway signatures and clinicopathological features. PLoS One 2008;3(8):e3088.

60. Ellison DW, Dalton J, Kocak M, et al. Medulloblastoma: clinicopathological correlates of SHH, WNT, and non-SHH/WNT molecular subgroups. Acta Neuropathol 2011;121(3):381–96.

61. Hyman JM, Firestone AJ, Heine VM, et al. Small-molecule inhibitors reveal multiple strategiesfor Hedgehog pathway blockade. Proc Natl Acad Sci U S A 2009;106(33):14132–7.

62. Packer RJ, Macdonald T, Vezina G, et al. Medulloblastoma and primitive neuroectodermal tumors. Handb Clin Neurol 2012;105:529–48.

63. Clifford SC, Lusher ME, Lindsey JC, et al. Wnt/Wingless pathway activation and chromosome 6 loss characterize a distinct molecular sub-group of medulloblastomas associated with a favorable prognosis. Cell Cycle 2006;5(22):2666–70.

64. Gorlin RJ, Goltz RW. Multiple nevoid basal-cell epithelioma, jaw cysts and bifid rib. A syndrome. N Engl J Med 1960;262:908–12.

65. Stavrou T, Dubovsky EC, Reaman GH, et al. Intracranial calcifications in childhood medulloblastoma: relation to nevoid basal cell carcinoma syndrome. AJNR Am J Neuroradiol 2000;21:790–4.

66. Hamilton SR, Liu B, Parsons RE, et al. The molecular basis of Turcot's syndrome. N Engl J Med 1995;332:839–47.

67. Michael T, Todd M, James R, et al. Molecular insight into medulloblastoma and central nervous system primitive neuroectodermal tumor biology from hereditary syndromes: a review [Topic Review]. Neurosurgery 2000;47(4):888–901.

68. Rorke LB, Packer RJ, Biegel JA. Central nervous system atypical teratoid/rhabdoid tumors of infancy and childhood: definition of an entity. J Neurosurg 1996;85:56–65.

69. Burger PC, Yu IT, Tihan T, et al. Atypical teratoid/rhabdoid tumors of the central nervous system: a highly malignant tumor of infancy and childhood frequently mistaken for medulloblastoma: a Pediatric Oncology Group study. Am J Surg Pathol 1998; 22:1083–92.

70. Meyers SP, Khademian ZP, Biegel JA, et al. Primary intracranial atypical teratoid/rhabdoid tumors of infancy and childhood: MRI features and patient outcomes. AJNR Am J Neuroradiol 2006;27:962–71.

71. Mazumder AA, Adams A, Paine SML, et al. Atypical teratoid/rhabdoid tumor. Review of 14 pathologic confirmed cases. Presented at the ASNR 51th Annual Meeting and The Foundation of the ASNR Symposium 2013. San Diego, May 18–23, 2013.

72. Lee YK, Choi CG, Lee JH. Atypical teratoid/rhabdoid tumor of the cerebellum: report of two infantile cases. AJNR Am J Neuroradiol 2004;25:481–3.

73. Moeller KK, Coventry S, Jernigan S, et al. Atypical teratoid/rhabdoid tumor of the spine. AJNR Am J Neuroradiol 2007;28:593–5.

74. Jin B, Feng Y. MRI features of atypical teratoid/rhabdoid tumor in children. Pediatr Radiol 2013; 43:1001–8.

75. Biegel JA, Zhou JY, Rorke LB, et al. Germ-line and acquired mutations of INI1 in atypical teratoid and rhabdoid tumors. Cancer Res 1999;59(1):74–9.

76. Versteege I, Sévenet N, Lange J, et al. Truncating mutations of hSNF5/INI1nin aggressive paediatric cancer. Nature 1998;394(6689):203–6.

77. Poretti A, Meoded A, Huisman TA. Neuroimaging of pediatric posterior fossa tumors including review of the literature. J Magn Reson Imaging 2012;35(1): 32–47.

78. Pencalet P, Maixner W, Sainte-Rose C, et al. Benign cerebellar astrocytomas in children. J Neurosurg 1999;90:265–73.

79. Brandao LA, Rossi A. A pictorial review of typical and atypical/bizarre imaging findings, as well as post-treatment changes in pilocytic astrocytomas in children. Presented as eEdE 18 at ASNR 53rd Annual Meeting and The Foundation of the ASNR Symposium 2015. Chicago, IL, April 25–30, 2015.

80. Porto L, Kieslich M, Franz K, et al. Spectroscopy of untreated pilocytic astrocytomas: do children and adults share some metabolic features in addition to their morphologic similarities? Childs Nerv Syst 2010;26:801–6.

81. Brandão LA, Shiroishi M, Law M. Brain tumors: a multimodality approach with diffusion-weighted imaging, diffusion tensor imaging, magnetic resonance spectroscopy, dynamic susceptibility contrast and dynamic contrast-enhanced magnetic resonance imaging. In: Mukherji AK, Steinbach L, editors. Modern imaging evaluation of the brain, body and spine. Philadelphia (PA): Elsevier; 2013. p. 199–240. MRI Clin NA.

82. Ball WS, Holland SK. Perfusion imaging in the pediatric patient. Magn Reson Imaging Clin N Am 2001; 9(1):207–30.

83. Provenzale JM, Mukundan S, Barboriak DP. Diffusion-weighted and perfusion MR imaging for brain tumor characterization and assessment of therapeutic response. Radiology 2006;239(3): 632–49.

84. Wu J, Armstrong TS, Gilbert MR. Biology and management of ependymomas. Neuro Oncol 2016; 18(7):902–13.

85. Blaser SI, Harwood-Nash DC. Neuroradiology of pediatric posterior fossa medulloblastoma. J Neurooncol 1996;29:23–34.

86. Salem A, Krainik A, Helias A, et al. MRI findings in a case of a superficial siderosis associated with an ependymoma. J Neuroradiol 2002;29(2):136–8.

87. Bouffet E, Perilongo G, Canete A, et al. Intracranial ependymomas in children: a critical review of prognostic factors and a plea for cooperation. Med Pediatr Oncol 1998;30:319–29 [discussion: 329–31].

88. Harris L, Davies N, MacPherson L, et al. The use of short-echo time 1H MRS for childhood with cerebellar tumors prior to histopathological diagnosis. Pediatr Radiol 2007;37:1101–9.

89. Yuh EL, Barkovich AJ, Gupta N. Imaging of ependymomas: MRI and CT. Childs Nerv Syst 2009; 25:1203–13.

90. Uematsu Y, Hirano A, Llena JF. Electron microscopic observations of blood vessels in ependymoma. No Shinkei Geka 1988;16:1235–42 [in Japanese].

91. Chen CJ, Tseng YC, Hsu HL, et al. Imaging predictors' intracranial ependymomas. J Comput Assist Tomogr 2004;28:407–13.

92. Lober RM, Cho YJ, Tang Y. Diffusion-weighted MRI derived apparent diffusion coefficient identifies prognostically distinct subgroups of pediatric diffuse intrinsic pontine glioma. J Neurooncol 2014;117(1):175–82.

93. Poussaint TY, Vajapeyam S, Ricci KI, et al. Apparent diffusion coefficient histogram metrics correlate with survival in diffuse intrinsic pontine glioma: a report from the Pediatric Brain Tumor Consortium. Neuro Oncol 2015;18(5):725–34.

94. Panigrahy A, Nelson MD Jr, Finlay JL, et al. Metabolism of diffuse intrinsic brainstem gliomas in children. Neuro Oncol 2008;10:32–44.

95. Lobel U, Sedlacik J, Reddick WE, et al. Quantitative diffusion-weighted and dynamic susceptibility-weighted contrast-enhanced perfusion MR imaging analysis of T2 hypointense lesion components in pediatric diffuse intrinsic pontine glioma. AJNR Am J Neuroradiol 2011;32:315–22.

96. Chen HJ, Panigrahy A, Dhall G, et al. Apparent diffusion and fractional anisotropy of diffuse intrinsic brain stem gliomas. AJNR Am J Neuroradiol 2010;31:1879–85.

97. Seymour ZA, Panigrahy A, Finlay JL, et al. Citrate in pediatric CNS tumors? AJNR Am J Neuroradiol 2008;29:1006–11.

98. Laprie A, Pirzkall A, Haas-Kogan DA, et al. Longitudinal multivoxel MR spectroscopy study of pediatric diffuse brainstem. Int J Radiat Oncol Biol Phys 2005;62:20–31.

99. Thakur SB, Karimi S, Dunkel IJ, et al. Longitudinal MR spectroscopic imaging of pediatric diffuse pontine tumors to assess tumor aggression and progression. AJNR Am J Neuroradiol 2006;27:806–9.

100. Pan E, Prados M, Gupta N, et al, editors. Pediatric CNS tumors, vol. 3. Berlin: Springer-Verlag; 2004. p. 49–61.

101. Farmer JP, Montes JL, Freeman CR, et al. Brainstem gliomas. A 10-year institutional review. Pediatr Neurosurg 2001;34:206–14.

102. Freeman CR, Farmer JP. Pediatric brain stem gliomas: a review. Int J Radiat Oncol Biol Phys 1998;40:265–71.

103. Mandell LR, Kadota R, Freeman C, et al. There is no role for hyperfractionated radiotherapy in the management of children with newly diagnosed diffuse intrinsic brainstem tumors: results of a pediatric oncology group phase III trial comparing conventional vs. hyperfractionated radiotherapy. Int J Radiat Oncol Biol Phys 1999;43:959–64.

104. Nelson MD, Soni D, Baram TZ. Necrosis in pontine gliomas: radiation induced or natural history? Radiology 1994;191:279–82.

105. Yoshimura J, Onda K, Tanaka R, et al. Clinicopathological study of diffuse type brainstem gliomas: analysis of 40 autopsy cases. Neurol Med Chir 2003;43:375–82.

106. Ceschin R, Kurland BF, Abberbock SR, et al. Parametric response mapping of apparent diffusion coefficient as an imaging biomarker to distinguish pseudoprogression from true tumor progression in peptide-based vaccine therapy for pediatric diffuse intrinsic pontine glioma. AJNR Am J Neuroradiol 2015;36:2170–6.

107. Chassot A, Canale S, Varlet P, et al. Radiotherapy with concurrent adjuvant temozolamide in children with newly diagnosed diffuse intrinsic pontine glioma. J Neurooncol 2012;106(2):399–407.

108. Lindsay AJ, Rush SZ, Fenton LZ. Pediatric posterior fossa ganglioglioma: unique MRI features and correlation with BRAF V600E mutation status. J Neurooncol 2014;118(2):395–404.

109. Jay V, Squire J, Blaser S, et al. Intracranial and spinal metastases from a ganglioglioma with unusual cytogenetic abnormalities in a patient with complex partial seizures. Childs Nerv Syst 1997;13(10):550–5.

110. Buczkowicz P, Bartels U, Bouffet E, et al. Histopathological spectrum of paediatric diffuse intrinsic pontine glioma: diagnostic and therapeutic implications. Acta Neuropathol 2014;128:573–81.

# Supratentorial Tumors in Pediatric Patients

Carlos Zamora, MD, PhD[a,b], Thierry A.G.M. Huisman, MD[c], Izlem Izbudak, MD[a,*]

## KEYWORDS

- Astrocytoma • Brain tumors • Desmoplastic infantile tumors • Ependymoma • Glioma
- Neuroepithelial tumors • Supratentorial • Embryonal tumors

## KEY POINTS

- Anaplastic transformation of diffuse astrocytomas is a much less common event in children compared with adults.
- Both subependymal nodules and subependymal giant cell tumors can show contrast enhancement.
- Contrast enhancement and calcifications in pediatric oligodendrogliomas are less common than in adults.
- Almost all gangliogliomas are low grade and present as cystic and solid mass lesions, most frequently arising in the temporal lobes.
- Up to one-third of dysembryoplastic neuroepithelial tumors may show contrast enhancement that may be nodular or ring-like.

## INTRODUCTION

Brain and central nervous system (CNS) tumors continue to represent a significant source of morbidity and mortality in the pediatric population. They are the most common solid tumors in children between 0 to 14 years of age, and their incidence is highest during the first year of life. These tumors account for the most cancer-related deaths in the 0 to 14 age group according to the Central Brain Tumor Registry of the United States (CBTRUS).[1] Overall, most brain tumors in children are gliomas, with roughly half of them consisting of pilocytic astrocytomas or other low-grade neoplasms, followed by embryonal tumors. Approximately 21% of all gliomas have a high-grade histology[1] and are associated with an aggressive clinical behavior and a dismal prognosis.[2] When brain stem tumors are excluded, high-grade gliomas are most commonly supratentorial, occurring in the cerebral hemispheres, followed by central gray matter structures.[2]

Fifteen percent of all CNS neoplasms are embryonal tumors,[1] a heterogeneous group of lesions that arise from undifferentiated small round cells, tend to occur in small children, and are associated with a poor prognosis and

Conflict of Interest: The authors have no commercial or financial interest to disclose.
[a] Section of Pediatric Neuroradiology, Division of Neuroradiology, The Russell H. Morgan Department of Radiology and Radiological Science, The Johns Hopkins School of Medicine, 600 North Wolfe Street, Baltimore, MD 21287-0842, USA; [b] Division of Neuroradiology, Department of Radiology, University of North Carolina School of Medicine, 3326 Old Infirmary Road, Chapel Hill, NC 27514, USA; [c] Division of Pediatric Radiology, Section of Pediatric Neuroradiology, The Russell H. Morgan Department of Radiology and Radiological Science, The Johns Hopkins School of Medicine, 600 North Wolfe Street, Phipps B-126-B, Baltimore, MD 21287-0842, USA
* Corresponding author.
*E-mail address:* iizbuda@jhmi.edu

a tendency to disseminate throughout the neuraxis.[3] With the exception of medulloblastomas, embryonal tumors are predominantly supratentorial. Finally, although neuronal and mixed neuronal-glial tumors are not as common, accounting for less than 5% of all neoplasms,[1] they may nonetheless lead to significant morbidity in many patients due to intractable seizures. Many of these lesions share similar clinical and imaging presentations making their prospective diagnosis challenging. This article reviews the neuroimaging characteristics of these entities with particular attention to relevant features that may aid in narrowing the differential diagnosis, including demographics and clinical presentation.

## GLIAL CELL TUMORS
### Low-Grade Gliomas

World Health Organization (WHO) grade 1 and 2 gliomas roughly account for 60% of all gliomas in children.[1] They are considered benign and usually follow a relatively indolent course with an overall 10-year survival exceeding 80%.[4] However, these tumors may be associated with significant morbidity and even mortality with increasingly recognized leptomeningeal spread in pilocytic astrocytomas and malignant transformation in diffuse astrocytomas, although the latter is less commonly seen than in adults.[4,5]

### Pilocytic astrocytoma

Pilocytic astrocytomas account for one-third of all gliomas in children from 0 to 14 years of age and constitute the most common primary brain tumor in this population.[1] Their incidence is relatively evenly distributed across this age group after the first year of life.[1] They are histologically benign (WHO grade I) and demonstrate slow growth over time. Pilocytic astrocytomas have an excellent prognosis, with survival rates as high as 95% at 10 years.[6] They most commonly occur in the cerebellar hemispheres (about two-thirds of lesions in pediatric patients), followed by optic chiasm and nerves and hypothalamus, but they can rarely develop in the cerebral hemispheres (particularly in older children and adults, accounting for half of all tumors in the latter group).[6,7] Most pilocytic astrocytomas are sporadic, but there is a higher incidence in neurofibromatosis type 1, where they occur in up to 20% of patients.[8] Notably, approximately one-third of patients with an optic pathway glioma (the majority of which are pilocytic) have neurofibromatosis type 1.[9] Most pilocytic astrocytomas harbor a

BRAF-KIAA1549 fusion gene mutation, which may be associated with improved clinical outcomes.[10,11]

Nearly all pilocytic astrocytomas are well circumscribed on imaging, and approximately two-thirds of those in the cerebellum present with the characteristic appearance of a cystic mass with an avidly enhancing mural nodule.[7,12] The cyst wall rarely enhances. In the cerebral hemispheres, the frequency of this appearance is unknown but appears to be less common than in the posterior fossa. A prior study has shown that approximately 36% of all cerebral astrocytomas present with cystic changes (Fig. 1).[13] Pilocytic astrocytomas may also appear as solid enhancing masses (Fig. 2). On occasion they may demonstrate an infiltrating pattern in the surrounding tissue and even leptomeningeal spread, which renders their distinction from high-grade tumors challenging (Fig. 3).[7] An additional characteristic feature is the lack of significant vasogenic edema in the surrounding parenchyma. When edema does occur, it tends to be limited in relation to the size of the tumor.[12]

Pilocytic astrocytomas are exceptional tumors in that they commonly show avid enhancement despite their benign and relatively indolent biology. They can also show an aggressive profile on magnetic resonance spectroscopy (MRS) that may be mistaken for a high-grade tumor, with increased choline, decreased N-acetylaspartate, and a lipid-lactate peak.[14] However, recent data suggest that pilocytic astrocytomas have higher lipid–lactate/creatine ratios compared with high-grade tumors.[15] The enhancing components of pilocytic astrocytomas tend to have low perfusion with decreased relative cerebral blood volumes (rCBV),[16] although nodules with increased perfusion may at times be encountered. They also show significantly higher apparent diffusion coefficient (ADC) values compared with high-grade tumors by virtue of their low cellularity.[15] Malignant transformation of pilocytic astrocytomas has been described but is an unusually rare event. Some studies suggest that this may be much more common in adults.[17,18]

### Diffuse astrocytomas

Diffuse astrocytomas are low-grade tumors (WHO grade II) that are several times less common in children than pilocytic astrocytomas.[4] They can occur anywhere in the CNS, but one-third arise in the frontal or parietal lobes, which represent the most common location.[4] On MR imaging, they have relatively ill-defined margins but are homogeneously hypointense on T1- and hyperintense on T2-weighted sequences, without

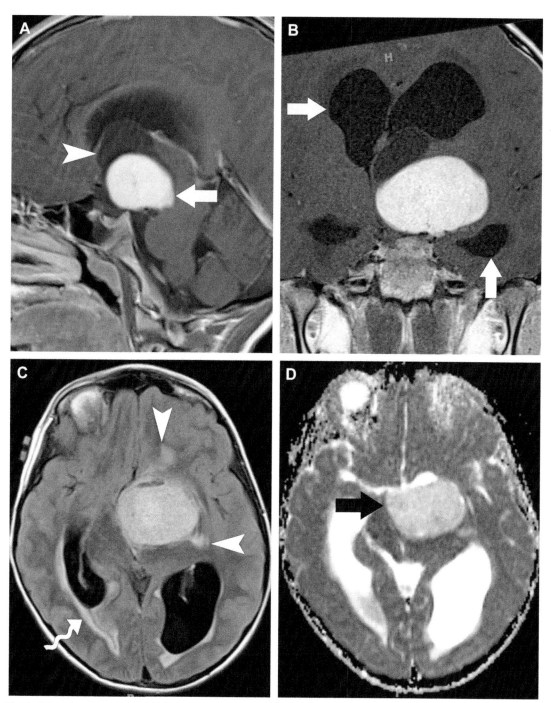

Fig. 1. Pilocytic astrocytoma. (*A*) Postcontrast T1 image demonstrates a partially cystic (*arrowhead*) mass with an avidly enhancing solid component (*arrow*) centered in the hypothalamic region and basal ganglia. (*B*) Coronal T1 image shows marked mass effect on the ventricular system with obstructive hydrocephalus (*arrows*). (*C*) Axial FLAIR (fluid attenuated inversion recovery) shows the mass to have minimal surrounding edema (*arrowheads*). Note periventricular signal due to transependymal flow/interstitial edema (*wavy arrow*). (*D*) Corresponding ADC (apparent diffusion coefficient) map shows no evidence of restricted diffusion (*arrow*).

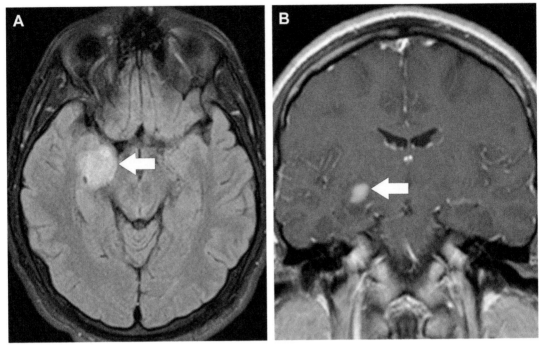

Fig. 2. Predominantly solid pilocytic astrocytoma. (*A*) Axial FLAIR shows a mildly expansile infiltrative lesion centered in the right uncus (*arrow*). (*B*) Corresponding coronal postcontrast T1 image shows a small focus of enhancement (*arrow*) within the lesion.

contrast enhancement or restricted diffusion (Fig. 4).[19] Interestingly, while in adults most diffuse low-grade astrocytomas eventually undergo anaplastic transformation, progression to a higher-grade tumor is a rare event in children and accounts for only about 10% of cases.[5,20] Diffuse astrocytomas do not show significantly increased rCBV and may show elevated myoinositol on MRS.[15,21]

### High-Grade Gliomas

High-grade gliomas are significantly less common in children than in adults, yet they constitute 11% of all CNS neoplasms in the pediatric population, with an estimated incidence of 0.59 per 100,000 person–years.[1] Supratentorial high-grade gliomas comprise one-third of all pediatric high-grade gliomas and occur most commonly in adolescents.[22] They may be related to prior radiation exposure or occur in the setting of rare syndromes such as Li Fraumeni.[23] Most-high grade gliomas in children are purely astrocytic and classified as either anaplastic astrocytomas (WHO grade III) or glioblastomas (WHO grade IV), with other mixed or nonastrocytic types being rare in this population.[22] Notably, evidence shows that pediatric high-grade gliomas are

genetically and molecularly distinct from their adult counterparts.[24]

### Anaplastic astrocytoma

Anaplastic astrocytomas represent close to 2% of all CNS tumors in children.[25] They are rapidly growing and infiltrative lesions with poorly circumscribed margins and are most commonly found in the cerebral hemispheres (particularly frontal and temporal lobes), although they can occur in the deep midline structures, brain stem, or cerebellum.[19,20] They do not show significant contrast enhancement, hemorrhage, or necrosis, features that are associated with glioblastomas (Fig. 5).[19] ADC values of anaplastic astrocytomas are lower than those of pilocytic or diffuse astrocytomas, and they also show increased rCBV compared with lower-grade histologies (Fig. 6).[15] On MRS, anaplastic astrocytomas show increased choline and decreased N-acetylaspartate, with decreased myoinositol compared with the spectra of lower-grade gliomas.[15,21]

### Glioblastoma

Glioblastomas are rare in children, in whom they constitute about 3% of primary brain tumors.[26] Survival is poor but better than that of adult

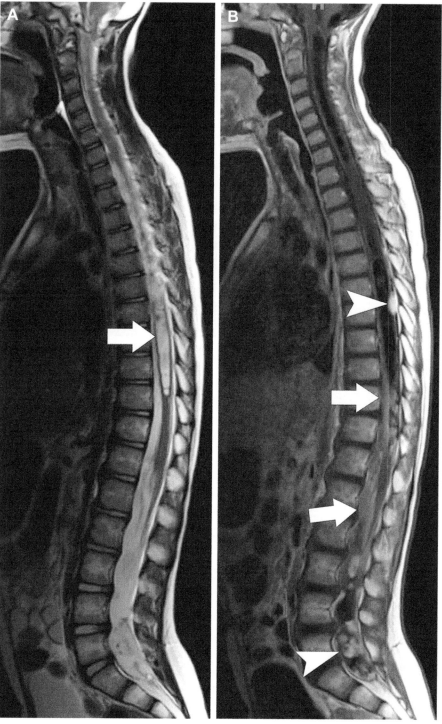

**Fig. 3.** Spinal leptomeningeal metastases from pilocytic astrocytoma. (*A*) Sagittal T2 image of the entire spine demonstrates areas of heterogeneity within the spinal canal and presence of a thoracic syrinx (*arrow*). (*B*) Sagittal postcontrast T1 image shows thick leptomeningeal enhancement surrounding the cord (*arrows*) and numerous enhancing nodules (*arrowheads*).

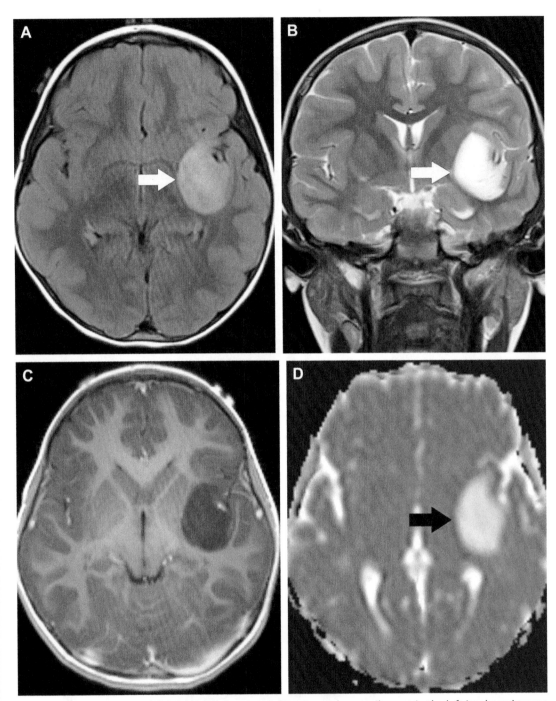

**Fig. 4.** Diffuse astrocytoma. (*A*) Axial FLAIR shows an infiltrative and expansile mass in the left insula and tempo-ral lobe (*arrow*). (*B*) Coronal T2 image shows the lesion to be very bright (*arrow*). (*C*) Axial postcontrast T1 image demonstrates that the mass is markedly hypointense and does not enhance. (*D*) The mass has high signal on the ADC map in keeping with its low grade.

glioblastomas.[27] Most glioblastomas occur in the frontotemporal region but can also affect other lobes or the deep gray structures. The imaging hallmark of glioblastoma is that of heterogeneous enhancement with necrosis and marked peritu-moral edema (**Fig. 7**).[4] The solid components show restricted diffusion with low ADC values as well as increased MR imaging perfusion and

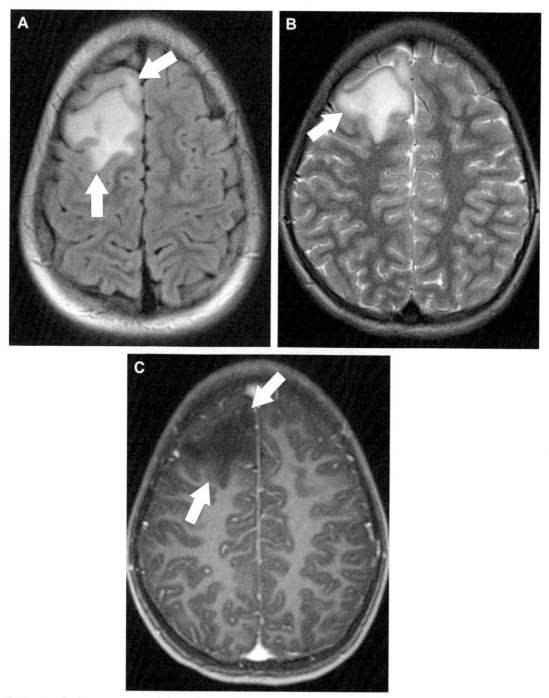

Fig. 5. Anaplastic astrocytoma. (A) Axial FLAIR shows an infiltrative mass in the right frontal lobe (arrows). (B) Axial T2 image at a slightly lower level shows mild heterogeneity within the lateral aspect of the lesion (arrow). (C) Corresponding postcontrast T1 image shows no evidence of enhancement (arrows).

permeability parameters (such as rCBV and $K^{trans}$), which may be helpful in differentiating them from low-grade gliomas or for evaluation of tumor recurrence versus treatment response.[28]

On MRS, in addition to decreased myoinositol, decreased N-acetylaspartate, and elevated choline, glioblastomas typically have elevated lactate due to anaerobic metabolism and

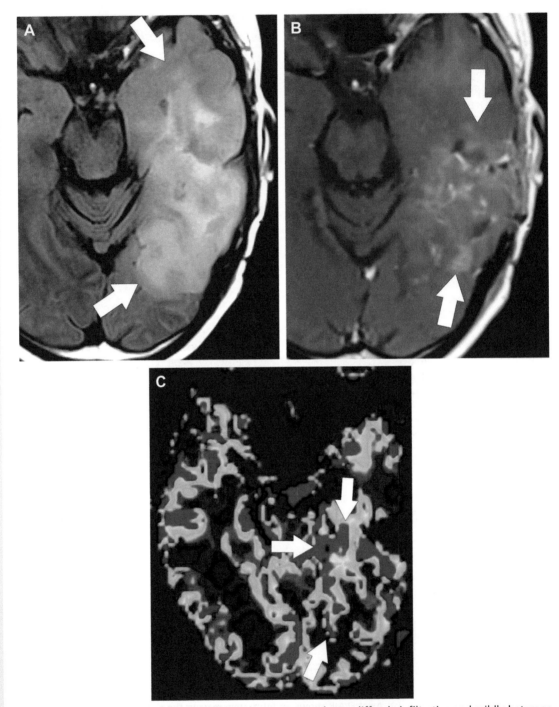

**Fig. 6.** Anaplastic astrocytoma. (*A*) Axial FLAIR demonstrates a large, diffusely infiltrative and mildly heterogeneous mass involving the entire left temporal lobe (*arrows*). (*B*) Axial postcontrast T1 image shows small foci of heterogeneous enhancement within the lesion (*arrows*). (*C*) MR rCBV map shows areas of increased perfusion (*arrows*).

elevated lipids due to the presence of necrosis.[15] Note that most of these studies have been performed in adults due to the rarity of these tumors in children.

## Subependymal giant cell tumor

Subependymal giant cell tumors (SGCTs) are slow-growing neoplasms characterized as WHO grade I. They show mixed glioneuronal lineage

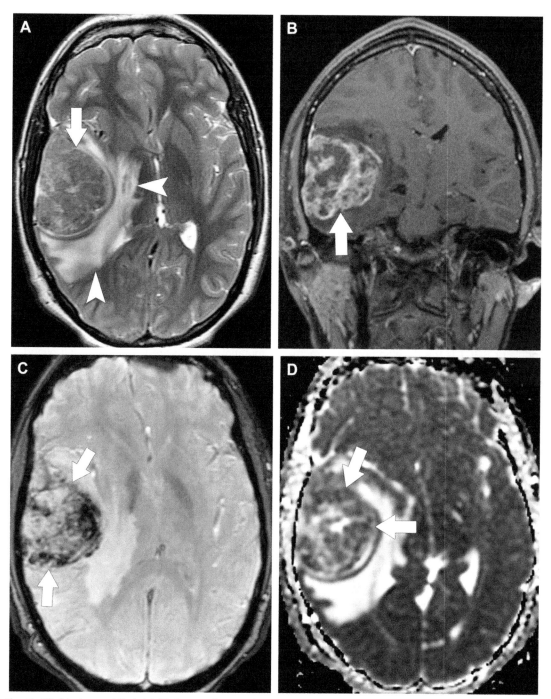

Fig. 7. Glioblastoma. (*A*) Axial T2 image shows a heterogeneous mass that is predominantly hypointense to cortex and relatively well-circumscribed (*arrow*). Note moderate peritumoral edema (*arrowheads*). (*B*) Coronal postcontrast T1 image heterogeneous but avid enhancement throughout the mass (*arrow*). (*C*) Axial susceptibility-weighted image shows areas of increased susceptibility within the tumor due to hemorrhage (*arrows*). (*D*) ADC map shows low signal within the lesion in keeping with restricted diffusion (*arrows*).

and are not pure astrocytomas. SGCTs are most commonly seen in children and adolescents with tuberous sclerosis complex (TSC), in whom they constitute the most common CNS neoplasm (5%–20% of patients).[29] It is unusual to develop an SGCT after age 21 years if not already present, although tumors that have been diagnosed in childhood can become symptomatic later.[30]

Several cases of solitary SGCTs have been described in patients without other manifestations of TSC.[31,32] However, genetic testing in some isolated SGCTs has demonstrated mutations in the TSC-1 and TSC-2 genes, suggesting that at least some of these tumors may represent a forme fruste of TSC in patients without other clinical manifestations of the disease.[33] They are supratentorial and virtually always located in a lateral ventricle near the foramen of Monro,[34] although they may rarely occur in other locations. SGCTs appear to arise from neoplastic transformation of existing subependymal nodules,[35] but the reason why some nodules grow and others do not is not clear. Enhancement is variable but usually avid and heterogeneous (Fig. 8). However, in and of itself, contrast enhancement is not sufficient for diagnosis, as many subependymal nodules have also been shown to enhance.[36] Both subependymal nodules and SGCTs can calcify and hemorrhage.[37] From a clinical standpoint, the most important factor in the evaluation of a subependymal nodule or SGCT is the development of intracranial hypertension with new papilledema or obstructive hydrocephalus, or growth over serial imaging.[38]

### Pleomorphic xanthoastrocytoma

Pleomorphic xanthoastrocytomas (PXAs) are rare tumors that account for less than 1% of all astrocytic neoplasms.[39] They have a wide range of age at presentation, from early infancy to the ninth decade of life, with a median of 20 years at the time of diagnosis.[40] Most are classified as WHO grade II and have a relatively favorable prognosis, with 5- and 10-year survival rates of 75% and 67%, respectively.[40] However, between 10% and 23% display a more aggressive behavior with histologically malignant features, and prognosis seems to be worse in males and with increasing age.[40–42] Anaplastic pleomorphic xanthoastrocytoma, WHO grade III, has been added to the 2016 CNS WHO as a distinct entity. Patients with such tumors have shorter survival times when compared to those with WHO grade II PXAs.[43] Seventy percent to 80% of patients present with seizures.[44]

The imaging features of PXAs are variable.[45] PXAs occur most commonly in the temporal (39%), followed by the frontal (19%) and parietal (14%) lobes.[40] They are overwhelmingly supratentorial, with only 2 cerebellar tumors out of 213 PXAs in the largest single series published to date.[40] These tumors favor a peripheral location and may scallop the inner table of the calvarium,

reflecting their slow growth.[45] Most are heterogeneous, and the solid components show avid enhancement and may characteristically abut the meninges (Fig. 9).[45,46]

### Oligodendroglial tumors

The peak incidence of oligodendroglial tumors is between the fifth and sixths decades of life. They are rare in children, in whom they represent 2% to 4% of brain tumors, with the majority being low grade (WHO grade II).[47–49] In contrast to their adult counterparts, in whom 1p19q codeletions are common and associated with increased chemosensitivity and improved prognosis, such alteration is rare in pediatric oligodendrogliomas.[50] Other molecular features that have been associated with increased overall and progression-free survival in adult oligodendrogliomas, namely Isocitrate dehydrogenase 1 (IDH1) mutations and methylguanine-methyltransferase (MGMT) promoter methylation, appear to have a distinct presentation in the pediatric population. IDH1 mutations, which are frequent in adult oligodendrogliomas, are notoriously rare in children, while MGMT promoter methylation appears to be as common.[50] Oligodendroglial tumors occur most commonly in the frontal lobe, followed by the temporal and parietal lobes.[47,49] Other locations such as the brain stem, cerebellopontine angle, optic nerve, and spinal cord are rare.[51] The imaging characteristics of oligodendrogliomas are nonspecific, but they tend to be relatively well circumscribed and typically expand the cortex with variable degrees of white matter involvement.[49,51] Enhancement is less common than in adult oligodendrogliomas and is heterogeneous when present.[19,49] Susceptibility-weighted imaging (SWI) may be helpful to detect calcification, but this feature also appears to be less common in children (Fig. 10).[19,52] As opposed to astroglial tumors, where increased perfusion correlates with tumor grade, high rCBV is often found in low-grade oligodendrogliomas.[53] Regardless, perfusion parameters may still have a role in assessing treatment response or disease progression or possibly in predicting malignant transformation.[53,54]

### Ependymoma

Ependymomas constitute 10% of all primary CNS neoplasms in children.[1] Most occur in the posterior fossa, and 40% are supratentorial, half of which are situated within the brain parenchyma.[55] A rare subset of supratentorial ependymomas may selectively involve the cortex and is more commonly associated with seizures.[56] They are

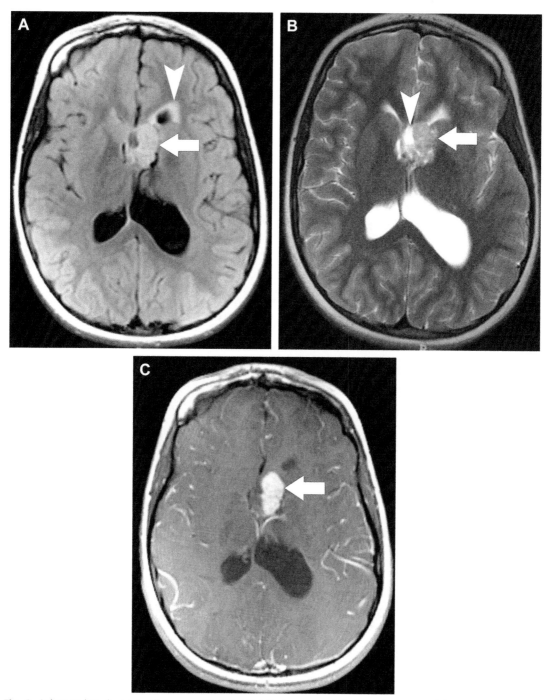

**Fig. 8.** Subependymal giant cell tumor. (*A*) Axial FLAIR shows a mildly hyperintense and heterogeneous mass projecting into the left foramen of Monro (*arrow*). Note obstructive hydrocephalus with transependymal flow/interstitial edema (*arrowhead*). (*B*) Axial T2 shows the mass to be slightly hyperintense relative to cortex (*arrow*). Note small cystic changes (*arrowhead*). (*C*) Postcontrast T1 image shows avid enhancement (*arrow*).

found most commonly in the frontal lobes, followed by the parietal lobes.[57] It is believed that parenchymal ependymomas may arise from embryonic ependymal rests trapped during development of the cerebral hemispheres.[34] Due to their parenchymal location, extraventricular ependymomas tend to be larger at presentation than intraventricular ones, which more commonly

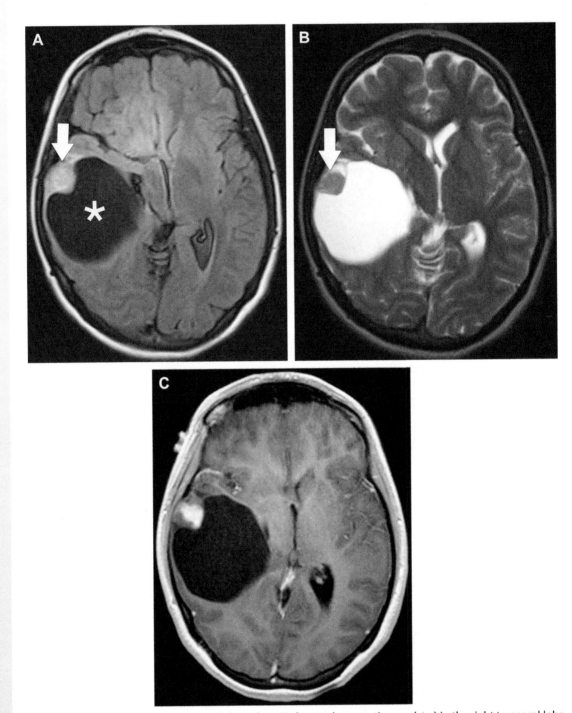

**Fig. 9.** Pleomorphic xanthoastrocytoma. (*A*) Axial FLAIR shows a large cystic mass (*star*) in the right temporal lobe with a peripheral solid component abutting the meningeal surface (*arrow*). (*B*) Axial T2 image shows the nodule to be only slightly hyperintense relative to the cerebral cortex (*arrow*). (*C*) Axial postcontrast T1 image shows avid enhancement of the nodule.

result in obstructive hydrocephalus.[58] On imaging, ependymomas are usually well circumscribed but heterogeneous tumors that show variable degrees of inhomogeneous contrast enhancement.[55] They have a higher incidence of cysts compared with infratentorial ependymomas; about 50% show areas of calcification, and hemorrhage may occur (**Fig. 11**).[59,60] Although their imaging appearance

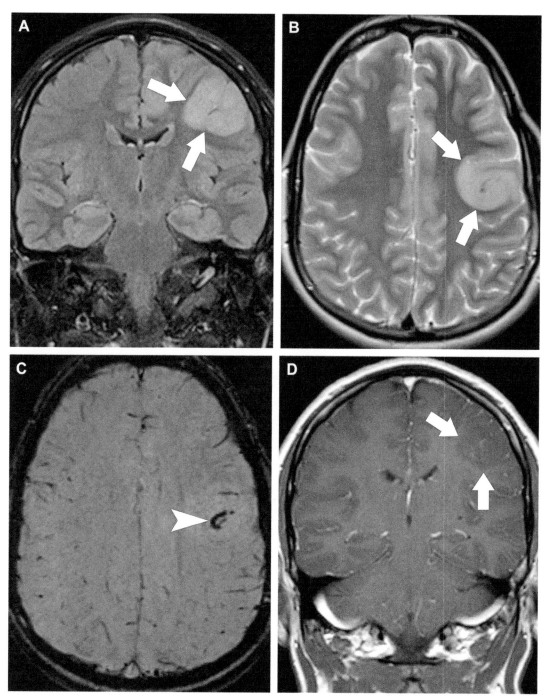

**Fig. 10.** Oligodendroglioma. (*A*) Coronal FLAIR and (*B*) axial T2 images show a mildly hyperintense cortically based and expansile mass in the left frontal lobe (*arrows*). (*C*) Susceptibility-weighted image minimum-intensity projection (minIP) shows curvilinear artifact within the mass (*arrowhead*) due to a gyriform calcification. (*D*) Coronal postcontrast T1 shows that the tumor does not enhance (*arrows*).

is similar to that of ependymoblastomas and other embryonal tumors, there is suggestion that ependymomas have a higher incidence of cysts that are more often peripherally located and that their enhancement is more commonly inhomogeneous.[60] Similar to their infratentorial counterpart, the solid components of supratentorial ependymomas show low ADC signal due to restricted

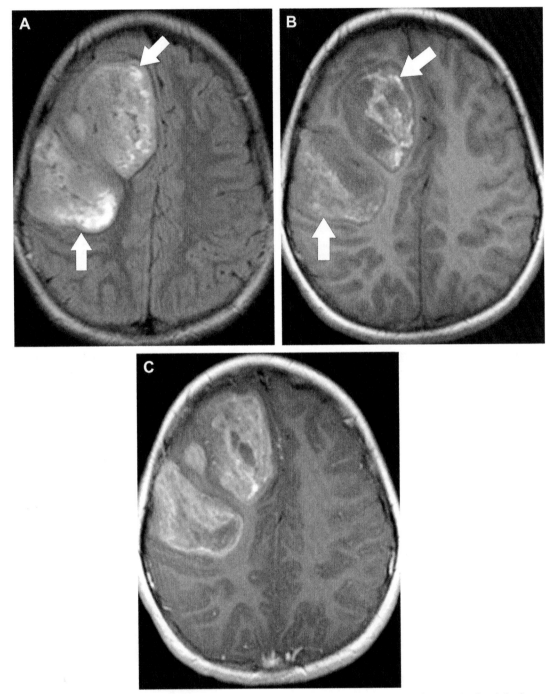

**Fig. 11.** Ependymoma. (*A*) Axial FLAIR shows a relatively well-circumscribed intra-axial tumor in the right frontal and parietal lobes (*arrows*). (*B*) Axial noncontrast T1 image shows large areas of intrinsic hyperintensity related to hemorrhage (*arrows*). (*C*) Axial postcontrast T1 demonstrates superimposed enhancement of the lesion.

diffusion.[60] However, ADC values of ependymomas are usually higher than those of embryonal tumors.[61–63] Perfusion is rarely performed but has been shown to be high with a slow return to baseline.[57,59] MRS characteristics are nonspecific, with increased choline and reduced N-acetylaspartate, but may be useful for follow-up and determination of tumor recurrence.[57,59]

## Angiocentric glioma

Angiocentric gliomas are now recognized as a distinct subset of glial tumors with uncertain histogenesis but with some degree of astrocytic and ependymal differentiation.[64] Two independent case series were first described in 2005, and these lesions were listed as a new entity in the WHO classification of tumors of the CNS in

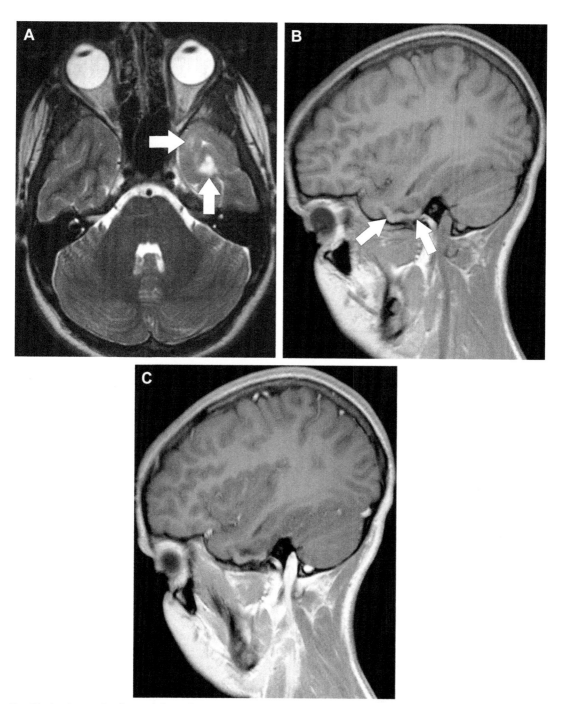

**Fig. 12.** Angiocentric glioma. (*A*) Axial T2 image shows a heterogeneous mass in the left temporal lobe (*arrows*). (*B*) Sagittal noncontrast T1 image shows a component of the lesion to be cortically based and to demonstrate intrinsic hyperintensity (*arrows*). (*C*) Corresponding postcontrast T1 image shows no evidence of superimposed enhancement.

2007.[65,66] Angiocentric gliomas are by far tumors of children and less commonly young adults, although a few cases in older patients have also been described.[67] They are relatively indolent and slow growing (WHO grade I), and most come to attention due to longstanding or intractable seizures.[68] Except for 1 tumor that occurred in the midbrain and was characterized pathologically as angiocentric glioma-like, all other reported cases in the literature have been located in the supratentorial brain, most commonly involving the frontal and temporal followed by parietal and occipital lobes.[67,69] Angiocentric gliomas are superficial nonenhancing cortical lesions, although a few cases showing subtle to mild enhancement have been reported.[67] Some of them may be intrinsically hyperintense on T1-weighted sequences and have a stalk-like extension to the adjacent ventricle on T2-weighted sequences, features thought to be characteristic but inconsistently present (**Fig. 12**).[64,68] A recent study using MRS has found a myoinositol and/or glycine peak in an angiocentric glioma, but for the most part their spectral characteristics overlap with those of other low-grade neoplasms.[70] Information on MR imaging diffusion features is scarce in the literature due to the paucity of published cases. However, no significant restricted diffusion should be expected due to the low-grade histology of this lesion, as shown in 1 reported case where DWI (diffusion weighted imaging) showed facilitated diffusion.[71]

## NEURONAL AND MIXED NEURONAL–GLIAL TUMORS

Neuronal and mixed neuronal–glial cell tumors are rare, representing nearly 1% of all primary brain tumors in children, with a median age of 9 years at presentation.[1] In the pediatric population, their incidence is highest in the 10 to 14 years age group, among whom they constitute 6.5% of brain tumors.[1] The more relevant neuronal–glial tumors will be discussed, while recognizing that various other entities may be included under the same classification.

### Ganglioglioma

Gangliogliomas are composed of neoplastic neuronal elements and astrocytes. Most are relatively indolent and have a natural history that is comparable to that of pilocytic astrocytomas, with an overall survival of 98% at 7.5 years.[72] Almost all of these tumors are

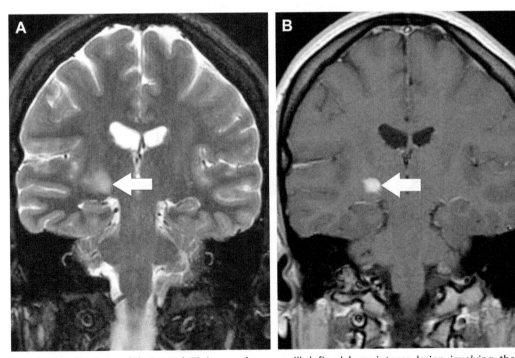

**Fig. 13.** Ganglioglioma. (*A*) Coronal T2 image shows an ill-defined hyperintense lesion involving the right insula and temporal stem (*arrow*). (*B*) Coronal postcontrast T1 shows a focus of avid enhancement within the lesion (*arrow*).

**Table 1**
Pediatric supratentorial brain tumors and their neuroimaging key features

| Tumor | Key Features |
|---|---|
| **Glial cell tumors** | |
| Pilocytic astrocytoma | Most common primary tumor in children<br>Excellent prognosis<br>Cystic with enhancing mural nodule or solid mass<br>Lack of significant vasogenic edema |
| Diffuse astrocytoma | Much less common in children than in adults<br>Relatively ill defined without contrast enhancement<br>Dedifferentiation rarely seen in children |
| Anaplastic astrocytoma | Poorly circumscribed margins<br>No hemorrhage or necrosis<br>Usually no contrast enhancement |
| Glioblastoma | Rare in children<br>Heterogeneous enhancement<br>Necrosis and marked peritumoral edema |
| Subependymal giant cell tumor | Associated with the tuberous sclerosis complex<br>Avid enhancement<br>Virtually always in a lateral ventricle near foramen of Monro |
| Pleomorphic xanthoastrocytoma | Almost always supratentorial<br>Solid components show avid enhancement<br>Peripheral location abutting meningeal surface |
| Oligodendroglial tumors | Relatively well circumscribed, expanded cortex<br>Enhancement and calcification less common than in adults<br>High rCBV often found in low-grade tumors |
| Ependymoma | Half of supratentorial tumors are parenchymal<br>Higher incidence of cysts than infratentorial ones<br>Calcifications, hemorrhage andinhomogeneous enhancement<br>ADC values usually higher than embryonal tumors |
| Angiocentric glioma | Superficial cortical lesions<br>T1 hyperintensity is a characteristic but infrequent feature<br>Usually no contrast enhancement |
| **Neuronal and mixed neuronal glial tumors** | |
| Ganglioglioma | Most common in temporal lobes<br>Mixed cystic and solid masses with avidly enhancing nodule<br>Calcifications are common |
| Desmoplastic infantile tumors | Very rare, typically 18 months of age or younger<br>Predominantly cystic with solid nodules located near cortex<br>Solid components may show low ADC values even if benign |
| Dysembryoplastic neuroepithelial tumors | Cortically based, favor temporal lobes<br>30% associated with cortical dysplasia<br>May have a characteristic bubbly appearance<br>Can rarely have nodular or ring-like enhancement |
| **Embryonal tumors** | |
| Embryonal tumors not otherwise specified | Usually children <5 y of age<br>Large at presentation with little surrounding edema<br>Intense and heterogeneous contrast enhancement<br>Low ADC values |

*(continued on next page)*

| Table 1 *(continued)* | |
|---|---|
| **Tumor** | **Key Features** |
| Atypical teratoid rhabdoid tumor | 10% of CNS tumors in children <12 mo of age <br> Rare aggressive neoplasms <br> Large and predominantly solid with minimal edema <br> Common calcifications, hemorrhage, and cysts <br> Moderate to marked enhancement and low ADC values |

low grade: 1 large series with 184 patients classified 93% of gangliogliomas as WHO grade I, 6% as grade II (atypical), and 1% as grade III (anaplastic), with frank glioblastoma documented in a patient who presented with recurrent disease after treatment.[72] They occur most commonly in the temporal lobes, particularly mesial regions (79%), followed by the frontal lobes,[72] and they may be incidentally found after temporal lobectomies in patients with intractable epilepsy (Fig. 13, Table 1). Interestingly, tumors previously diagnosed as other low-grade histologies have been reclassified as gangliogliomas after the 2000 WHO classification system was introduced, and newer and more specific immunohistochemical profiles became available (expression of CD34 and lack of MAP2 expression).[72] Eighty-five percent of these lesions are associated with long-standing seizures.[72]

The conventional imaging characteristics of gangliogliomas are nonspecific. Most of them will present as mixed cystic and solid masses with avidly enhancing tumoral components, and calcifications are a common feature (Figs. 14 and 15).[73] As with other lesions, ADC values tend to decrease with higher tumor grades, which may aid in their preoperative evaluation.[74]

## Desmoplastic Infantile Tumors

Desmoplastic infantile tumors (DITs) are classified as WHO grade I and include desmoplastic infantile astrocytomas and desmoplastic infantile gangliogliomas, with the latter featuring a neuronal component.[65,75] They are rare and occur most frequently in children 18 months old or younger.[75] Despite their benign classification and usually favorable prognosis, several cases with aggressive pathologic

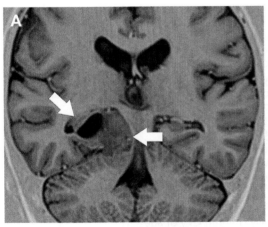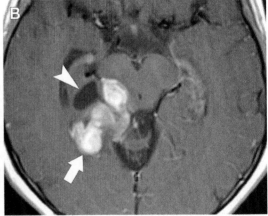

**Fig. 14.** Ganglioglioma. (*A*) Coronal T1 inversion recovery sequence shows a partially solid and partially cystic mass centered in the mesial right temporal lobe (*arrows*) that results in compression of the brain stem. (*B*) Corresponding axial postcontrast T1 image shows avid enhancement of the solid components of the tumor (*arrow*) with a nonenhancing cystic component (*arrowhead*).

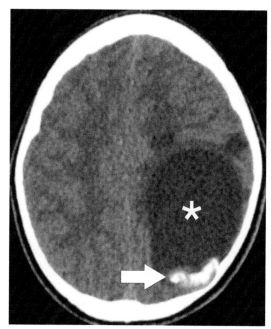

Fig. 15. Ganglioglioma. Axial noncontrast CT image demonstrates a large cystic mass (*star*) with coarse peripheral calcifications posteriorly (*arrow*).

features and/or a malignant clinical course have been described.[76–78] DITs are typically large at presentation and are frequently multilobar, most commonly involving the frontal and parietal lobes.[75,79] Occasionally they may be located in the suprasellar region.[80] DITs are heterogeneous and tend to be peripherally located, characteristically involving the cortex, leptomeninges, and dura, which may show variable degrees of thickening and enhancement.[81,82] Most DITs are predominantly cystic with solid nodules that tend to be located near the cortex and which represent tumor with intermixed desmoplasia, although some may be entirely solid.[80,83,84] The solid components are hyperdense on computed tomography (CT), iso-to hypointense on T2-weighted MR imaging, and show avid contrast enhancement (**Fig. 16**).[82,83] Hemorrhage is rare, and peritumoral edema is variable and in many cases mild or absent.[75,80] Despite their benign histology, the solid components of DITs may show restricted diffusion.[82]

## Dysembryoplastic Neuroepithelial Tumor

Dysembryoplastic neuroepithelial tumors (DNETs) are benign glioneuronal neoplasms (WHO grade I) most commonly seen in children and adolescents who present with intractable seizures.[85] They have a peak incidence during the second decade of life and are more common in males.[86] The great majority of DNETs are cortically based lesions and, while they can occur anywhere in the supratentorial brain, they preferentially arise in the temporal lobes.[85] Less common locations include the brain stem, cerebellum, and striatum.[86] DNETs are virtually always solitary, but rare cases of multifocal lesions have been reported.[87,88] Approximately 30% are associated with adjacent cortical dysplasia.[86] On CT, these lesions are hypodense[89] but may be difficult to visualize unless large. They have minimal if any associated mass effect or edema.[85,89] On MR imaging, they are well-circumscribed, iso-to hypointense on T1-, and hyperintense on T2-weighted sequences and may show a triangular configuration (**Fig. 17**).[85] Forty percent of them are cystic, sometimes with a typical bubbly appearance, and the rest are nodular or diffuse (**Fig. 18**).[86] Calcifications are seen in 40% of cases.[90] Although most DNETs do not enhance, contrast enhancement has been described in up to one-third of cases and may be nodular or ring-like.[90,91] These tumors do not show restricted diffusion, and therefore ADC values are high.[92] Spontaneous intralesional hemorrhage may occur but is exceedingly rare.[93] DNETs are benign tumors, but presumed malignant transformation has been reported in a few cases.[94] Notably, contrast enhancement can develop over time in some tumors without necessarily indicating malignant transformation.[90,95] MR imaging perfusion shows low rCBV and rCBF values relative to brain.[92] MRS demonstrates a normal spectrum, but elevated myoinositol has also been reported.[92]

## EMBRYONAL TUMORS
### Embryonal Tumors Not Otherwise Specified

One of the major changes in the 2016 CNS WHO classification has been the removal of primitive neuroectodermal tumors (PNETs), which accounted for 15% of all embryonal neoplasms and which are now included within the category of embryonal tumors not otherwise specified (NOS).[43] Embryonal tumors themselves represent 15% of all CNS neoplasms in children.[1] They are usually seen in children less than 5 years of age but can also occur in adults, who appear to have a worse prognosis.[96] Embryonal tumors NOS comprise a heterogeneous group of aggressive malignancies (WHO grade IV) that are biologically distinct from medulloblastomas and histologically include

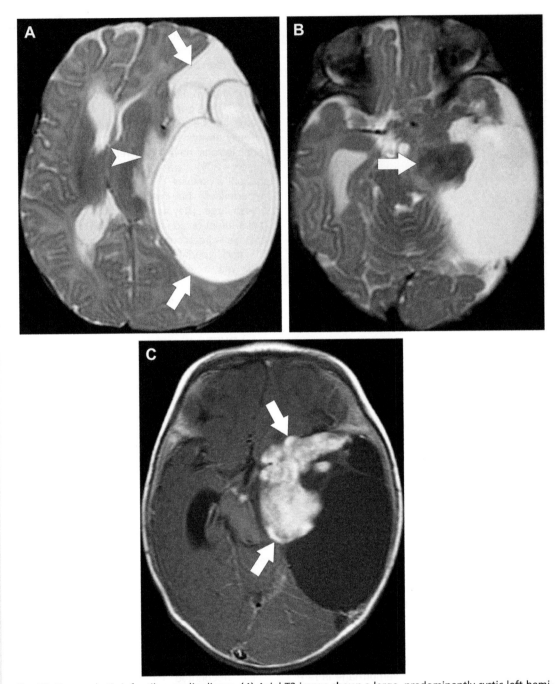

**Fig. 16.** Desmoplastic infantile ganglioglioma. (*A*) Axial T2 image shows a large, predominantly cystic left hemispheric mass (*arrows*) resulting in shift of midline structures and hydrocephalus. Note the minimal amount of edema (*arrowhead*) for the size of the tumor. (*B*) Axial T2 image at a lower level shows a hypointense solid component (*arrow*). (*C*) Axial postcontrast T1 image shows avid enhancement of the solid components of the lesion (*arrows*).

neuroblastomas, ganglioneuroblastomas, ependymoblastomas, and medulloepitheliomas.[3] They are typically large at presentation and can arise in the cerebral hemispheres (most commonly), pineal gland, brain stem, or spinal cord.[96] On imaging, they are frequently large, well demarcated, and heterogeneous due to frequent cystic changes and calcifications

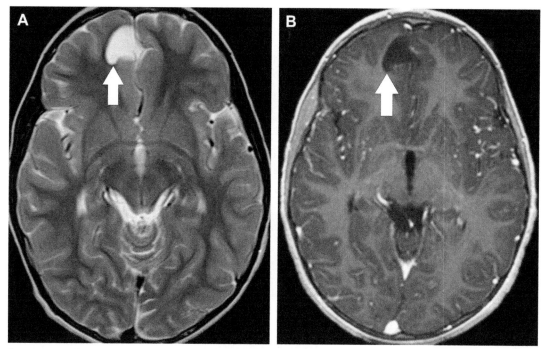

Fig. 17. Dysembryoplastic neuroepithelial tumor. (*A*) Axial T2 image shows a well-circumscribed hyperintense mass with a somewhat triangular morphology (*arrow*). (*B*) Axial postcontrast T1 image shows the lesion to be hypointense and without evidence of enhancement (*arrow*).

(**Fig. 19**).[19,97,98] Hemorrhage may be present but is relatively rare, and there is typically little surrounding edema (**Fig. 20**).[98,99] As is the case with other high-grade malignancies, embryonal tumors also show restricted diffusion with low ADC values and are hyperdense on CT due to high cellularity.[98,100] Contrast enhancement is generally intense and heterogeneous, and these tumors have a propensity for leptomeningeal spread.[19,60] One study using dynamic susceptibility contrast MR imaging perfusion has described increased relative cerebral blood flow and perfusion parameters, features that are also seen in other high-grade lesions.[99] While the MRS pattern of these tumors is nonspecific and generally follows that of other high grade malignancies, the presence of a taurine peak, deemed to be highly characteristic of medulloblastomas, has also been described in at least 1 supratentorial embryonal tumor previously classified as a PNET.[101,102]

## Atypical Teratoid Rhabdoid Tumor

These are rare but aggressive tumors with a poor prognosis that are most frequently seen in children no more than 3 years of age.[103,104] They constitute less than 2% of all CNS tumors in the pediatric population but account for 10% of those seen in children under 1 year of age.[104] They are formed by a combination of rhabdoid cells, peripheral neuroepithelial elements, and mesenchymal elements but lack the divergent cellular features of teratomas.[105] Their hallmark genetic feature is alteration of the SMARCB1 tumor suppressor gene.[106] By histopathology they may be confused with other embryonal tumors, including medulloblastomas, a distinction that has clinical relevance, because atypical teratoid rhabdoid tumors (ATRTs) have a much worse prognosis.[103,105] According to 1 meta-analysis, roughly one-half of reported ATRTs are supratentorial, one-third infratentorial, and 7% occur in the spine.[103] Rare cases of primarily extra-axial ATRTs have also been reported.[107,108] The appearance of these tumors on imaging is nonspecific. They tend to be large and predominantly solid but heterogeneous due to the presence of hemorrhage, cysts (sometimes peripherally located), and calcifications, which are common.[109–111] Most ATRTs show inhomogeneous areas of moderate to marked contrast

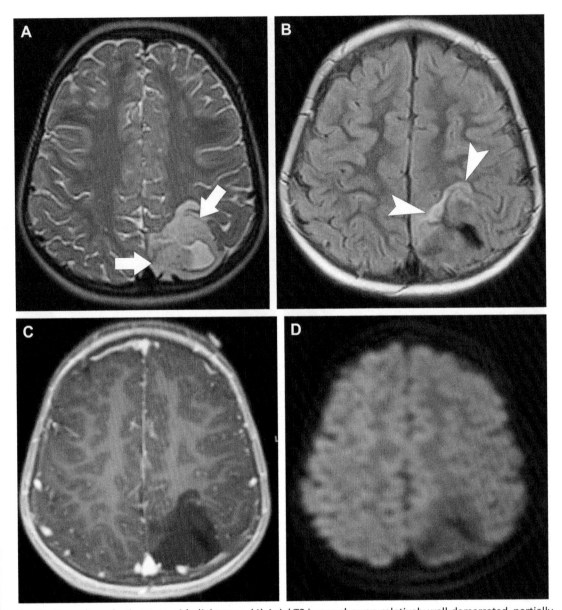

**Fig. 18.** Dysembryoplastic neuroepithelial tumor. (*A*) Axial T2 image shows a relatively well-demarcated, partially cystic and partially solid mass in the left parietal lobe (*arrows*). (*B*) Corresponding axial FLAIR image demonstrates minimal surrounding edema (*arrowheads*). (*C*) Axial postcontrast T1 and (*D*) diffusion tensor images demonstrate no evidence of enhancement or restricted diffusion, respectively.

enhancement and have an increased tendency for leptomeningeal spread.[108,109] As opposed to glial and neuroepithelial tumors, transgression of the dura with bone invasion may be a more common phenomenon in ATRTs.[111,112] As is the case with medulloblastomas and due to their high cellularity, the solid components of ATRTs show low ADC values in keeping with restricted diffusion.[109,113,114] Tumors are also predominantly hypointense on T2-weighted sequences and

hyperdense on CT, presumably on the same basis.[108,115] Even when large, peritumoral edema in ATRTs may be mild or absent (**Fig. 21**).[109] Although the imaging characteristics of medulloblastomas and ATRTs are similar, the latter may more commonly involve the cerebellopontine angle and show intratumoral hemorrhage.[113] Their MRS features are nonspecific with decreased N-acetyl aspartate, elevated choline, and lipid peaks in some patients.[109]

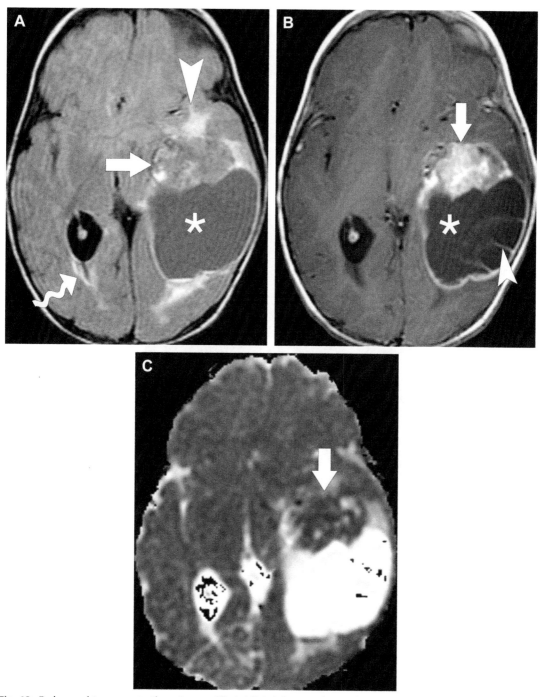

**Fig. 19.** Embryonal tumor not otherwise specified. (*A*) Axial FLAIR shows a lesion that is partially cystic (*star*) and partially solid (*arrow*) centered in the left temporoparietal region. Note that the signal of the cyst is higher than that of cerebrospinal fluid. There is little peritumoral edema (*arrowhead*) for the size of the lesion, as well as obstructive hydrocephalus with transependymal flow/interstitial edema (*wavy arrow*). (*B*) Axial postcontrast T1 image demonstrates avid enhancement of the solid component of the tumor (*arrow*) and enhancing septations (*arrowhead*) within the cyst (*star*). (*C*) ADC map shows low signal from the solid component due to restricted diffusion (*arrow*).

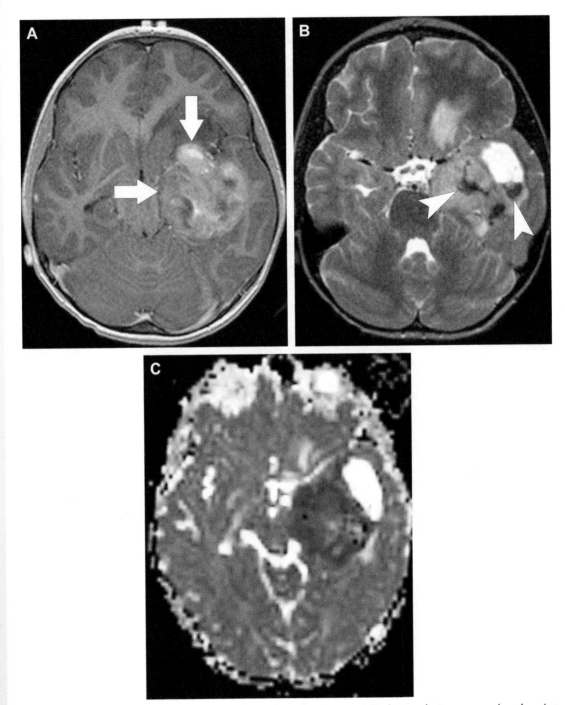

Fig. 20. Embryonal tumor not otherwise specified. (*A*) Axial postcontrast T1 shows a heterogeneously enhancing mass in the left temporal lobe (*arrows*). (*B*) Axial T2 image shows multiple foci of hypointensity within the mass due to hemorrhage (*arrowheads*). (*C*) ADC map shows low signal caused by restricted diffusion.

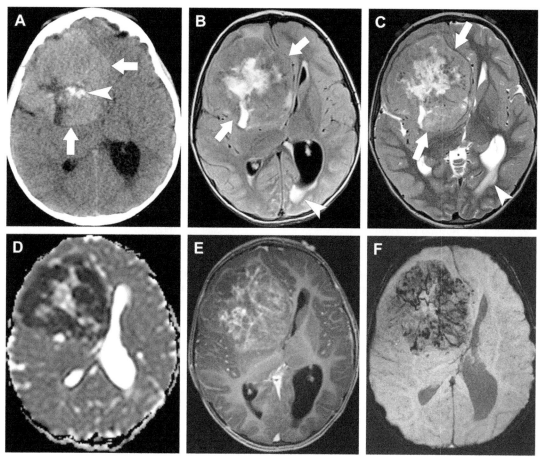

**Fig. 21.** Atypical teratoid rhabdoid tumor. (*A*) Axial noncontrast CT shows a predominantly hyperdense mass (*arrows*) with small foci of calcification (*arrowhead*). (*B*) Axial FLAIR and (*C*) axial T2 images show that the mass (*arrows*) is relatively well circumscribed with large areas of necrosis. There is little peritumoral edema. Note shift of midline structures and obstructive hydrocephalus with transependymal flow/interstitial edema (*arrowhead*). (*D*) Corresponding ADC map shows profound hypointensity in keeping with restricted diffusion. (*E*) Postcontrast T1 image shows heterogeneous enhancement throughout the tumor. (*F*) Susceptibility-weighted image demonstrates numerous prominent vessels within the tumor due to hypervascularity and scattered puddles of hypointensity related to hemorrhage.

## SUMMARY

The breadth of tumors that can arise in the supratentorial brain in children is extensive. With the exception of those that result in seizures and the highly malignant histologies, supratentorial tumors may come to medical attention later as they are less commonly associated with ventricular obstruction. Although there is overlap in the imaging appearance of some of these entities, many have relatively characteristic features that in combination with the patient's demographics and clinical presentation may aid in narrowing the differential diagnosis.

## REFERENCES

1. Ostrom QT, de Blank PM, Kruchko C, et al. Alex's lemonade stand foundation infant and childhood primary brain and central nervous system tumors diagnosed in the United States in 2007-2011. Neuro Oncol 2015;16(Suppl 10):x1–36.

2. Fangusaro J. Pediatric high grade glioma: a review and update on tumor clinical characteristics and biology. Front Oncol 2012;2:105.

3. McGovern SL, Grosshans D, Mahajan A. Embryonal brain tumors. Cancer J 2014;20(6): 397–402.

4. Pfister S, Witt O. Pediatric gliomas. Recent Results Cancer Res 2009;171:67–81.

5. Nakamura M, Shimada K, Ishida E, et al. Molecular pathogenesis of pediatric astrocytic tumors. Neuro Oncol 2007;9(2):113–23.

6. Burkhard C, Di Patre PL, Schuler D, et al. A population-based study of the incidence and survival rates in patients with pilocytic astrocytoma. J Neurosurg 2003;98(6):1170–4.

7. Chourmouzi D, Papadopoulou E, Konstantinidis M, et al. Manifestations of pilocytic astrocytoma: a pictorial review. Insights Imaging 2014;5(3): 387–402.

8. Fried I, Tabori U, Tihan T, et al. Optic pathway gliomas: a review. CNS Oncol 2013;2(2):143–59.

9. Dutton JJ. Gliomas of the anterior visual pathway. Surv Ophthalmol 1994;38(5):427–52.

10. Collins VP, Jones DT, Giannini C. Pilocytic astrocytoma: pathology, molecular mechanisms and markers. Acta Neuropathol 2015;129(6):775–88.

11. Hawkins C, Walker E, Mohamed N, et al. BRAF-KIAA1549 fusion predicts better clinical outcome in pediatric low-grade astrocytoma. Clin Cancer Res 2011;17(14):4790–8.

12. Koeller KK, Rushing EJ. From the archives of the AFIP: pilocytic astrocytoma: radiologic-pathologic correlation. Radiographics 2004;24(6):1693–708.

13. Hirsch JF, Sainte Rose C, Pierre-Kahn A, et al. Benign astrocytic and oligodendrocytic tumors of the cerebral hemispheres in children. J Neurosurg 1989;70(4):568–72.

14. Hwang JH, Egnaczyk GF, Ballard E, et al. Proton MR spectroscopic characteristics of pediatric pilocytic astrocytomas. AJNR Am J Neuroradiol 1998; 19(3):535–40.

15. de Fatima Vasco Aragao M, Law M, Batista de Almeida D, et al. Comparison of perfusion, diffusion, and MR spectroscopy between low-grade enhancing pilocytic astrocytomas and high-grade astrocytomas. AJNR Am J Neuroradiol 2014; 35(8):1495–502.

16. Grand SD, Kremer S, Tropres IM, et al. Perfusion-sensitive MRI of pilocytic astrocytomas: initial results. Neuroradiology 2007;49(7):545–50.

17. Ellis JA, Waziri A, Balmaceda C, et al. Rapid recurrence and malignant transformation of pilocytic astrocytoma in adult patients. J Neurooncol 2009; 95(3):377–82.

18. Stuer C, Vilz B, Majores M, et al. Frequent recurrence and progression in pilocytic astrocytoma in adults. Cancer 2007;110(12):2799–808.

19. Borja MJ, Plaza MJ, Altman N, et al. Conventional and advanced MRI features of pediatric intracranial tumors: supratentorial tumors. AJR Am J Roentgenol 2013;200(5):W483–503.

20. Pfister S, Hartmann C, Korshunov A. Histology and molecular pathology of pediatric brain tumors. J Child Neurol 2009;24(11):1375–86.

21. Castillo M, Smith JK, Kwock L. Correlation of myo-inositol levels and grading of cerebral astrocytomas. AJNR Am J Neuroradiol 2000; 21(9):1645–9.

22. Broniscer A, Gajjar A. Supratentorial high-grade astrocytoma and diffuse brainstem glioma: two challenges for the pediatric oncologist. Oncologist 2004;9(2):197–206.

23. Cage TA, Mueller S, Haas-Kogan D, et al. High-grade gliomas in children. Neurosurg Clin N Am 2012;23(3):515–23.

24. Paugh BS, Qu C, Jones C, et al. Integrated molecular genetic profiling of pediatric high-grade gliomas reveals key differences with the adult disease. J Clin Oncol 2010;28(18):3061–8.

25. Kaatsch P, Rickert CH, Kuhl J, et al. Population-based epidemiologic data on brain tumors in German children. Cancer 2001;92(12):3155–64.

26. Perkins SM, Rubin JB, Leonard JR, et al. Glioblastoma in children: a single-institution experience. Int J Radiat Oncol Biol Phys 2011;80(4):1117–21.

27. Song KS, Phi JH, Cho BK, et al. Long-term outcomes in children with glioblastoma. J Neurosurg Pediatr 2010;6(2):145–9.

28. Shin KE, Ahn KJ, Choi HS, et al. DCE and DSC MR perfusion imaging in the differentiation of recurrent tumour from treatment-related changes in patients with glioma. Clin Radiol 2014;69(6):e264–72.

29. Hallett L, Foster T, Liu Z, et al. Burden of disease and unmet needs in tuberous sclerosis complex with neurological manifestations: systematic review. Curr Med Res Opin 2011;27(8):1571–83.

30. Goh S, Butler W, Thiele EA. Subependymal giant cell tumors in tuberous sclerosis complex. Neurology 2004;63(8):1457–61.

31. Beaumont TL, Godzik J, Dahiya S, et al. Subependymal giant cell astrocytoma in the absence of tuberous sclerosis complex: case report. J Neurosurg Pediatr 2015;16(2):134–7.

32. Kashiwagi N, Yoshihara W, Shimada N, et al. Solitary subependymal giant cell astrocytoma: case report. Eur J Radiol 2000;33(1):55–8.

33. Ichikawa T, Wakisaka A, Daido S, et al. A case of solitary subependymal giant cell astrocytoma: two somatic hits of TSC2 in the tumor, without evidence of somatic mosaicism. J Mol Diagn 2005;7(4): 544–9.

34. Koeller KK, Sandberg GD, Armed Forces Institute of Pathology. From the archives of the AFIP. Cerebral intraventricular neoplasms: radiologic-pathologic correlation. Radiographics 2002;22(6): 1473–505.

35. Shepherd CW, Scheithauer BW, Gomez MR, et al. Subependymal giant cell astrocytoma: a clinical, pathological, and flow cytometric study. Neurosurgery 1991;28(6):864–8.

36. O'Callaghan FJ, Martyn CN, Renowden S, et al. Subependymal nodules, giant cell astrocytomas and the tuberous sclerosis complex: a population-based study. Arch Dis Child 2008; 93(9):751–4.

37. Mizuguchi M, Takashima S. Neuropathology of tuberous sclerosis. Brain Dev 2001;23(7):508–15.

38. Rovira A, Ruiz-Falco ML, Garcia-Esparza E, et al. Recommendations for the radiological diagnosis

and follow-up of neuropathological abnormalities associated with tuberous sclerosis complex. J Neurooncol 2014;118(2):205–23.

39. Rao AA, Laack NN, Giannini C, et al. Pleomorphic xanthoastrocytoma in children and adolescents. Pediatr Blood Cancer 2010;55(2):290–4.

40. Perkins SM, Mitra N, Fei W, et al. Patterns of care and outcomes of patients with pleomorphic xanthoastrocytoma: a SEER analysis. J Neurooncol 2012;110(1):99–104.

41. Kahramancetin N, Tihan T. Aggressive behavior and anaplasia in pleomorphic xanthoastrocytoma: a plea for a revision of the current WHO classification. CNS Oncol 2013;2(6):523–30.

42. Marton E, Feletti A, Orvieto E, et al. Malignant progression in pleomorphic xanthoastrocytoma: personal experience and review of the literature. J Neurol Sci 2007;252(2):144–53.

43. Louis DN, Perry A, Reifenberger G, et al. The 2016 World Health Organization classification of tumors of the central nervous system: a summary. Acta Neuropathol 2016;131(6):803–20.

44. Wallace DJ, Byrne RW, Ruban D, et al. Temporal lobe pleomorphic xanthoastrocytoma and chronic epilepsy: long-term surgical outcomes. Clin Neurol Neurosurg 2011;113(10):918–22.

45. Moore W, Mathis D, Gargan L, et al. Pleomorphic xanthoastrocytoma of childhood: MR imaging and diffusion MR imaging features. AJNR Am J Neuroradiol 2014;35(11):2192–6.

46. Yu S, He L, Zhuang X, et al. Pleomorphic xanthoastrocytoma: MR imaging findings in 19 patients. Acta Radiol 2011;52(2):223–8.

47. Wesseling P, van den Bent M, Perry A. Oligodendroglioma: pathology, molecular mechanisms and markers. Acta Neuropathol 2015;129(6):809–27.

48. Sievert AJ, Fisher MJ. Pediatric low-grade gliomas. J Child Neurol 2009;24(11):1397–408.

49. Rodriguez FJ, Tihan T, Lin D, et al. Clinicopathologic features of pediatric oligodendrogliomas: a series of 50 patients. Am J Surg Pathol 2014; 38(8):1058–70.

50. Suri V, Jha P, Agarwal S, et al. Molecular profile of oligodendrogliomas in young patients. Neuro Oncol 2011;13(10):1099–106.

51. Wagner MW, Poretti A, Huisman TA, et al. Conventional and advanced (DTI/SWI) neuroimaging findings in pediatric oligodendroglioma. Childs Nerv Syst 2015;31(6):885–91.

52. Zulfiqar M, Dumrongpisutikul N, Intrapiromkul J, et al. Detection of intratumoral calcification in oligodendrogliomas by susceptibility-weighted MR imaging. AJNR Am J Neuroradiol 2012;33(5):858–64.

53. Khalid L, Carone M, Dumrongpisutikul N, et al. Imaging characteristics of oligodendrogliomas that predict grade. AJNR Am J Neuroradiol 2012; 33(5):852–7.

54. Danchaivijitr N, Waldman AD, Tozer DJ, et al. Low-grade gliomas: do changes in rCBV measurements at longitudinal perfusion-weighted MR imaging predict malignant transformation? Radiology 2008;247(1):170–8.

55. Reni M, Gatta G, Mazza E, et al. Ependymoma. Crit Rev Oncol Hematol 2007;63(1):81–9.

56. Liu Z, Li J, Liu Z, et al. Supratentorial cortical ependymoma: case series and review of the literature. Neuropathology 2014;34(3):243–52.

57. Mangalore S, Aryan S, Prasad C, et al. Imaging characteristics of supratentorial ependymomas: Study on a large single institutional cohort with histopathological correlation. Asian J Neurosurg 2015; 10(4):276–81.

58. Mermuys K, Jeuris W, Vanhoenacker PK, et al. Best cases from the AFIP: supratentorial ependymoma. Radiographics 2005;25(2):486–90.

59. Yuh EL, Barkovich AJ, Gupta N. Imaging of ependymomas: MRI and CT. Childs Nerv Syst 2009; 25(10):1203–13.

60. Nowak J, Seidel C, Pietsch T, et al. Systematic comparison of MRI findings in pediatric ependymoblastoma with ependymoma and CNS primitive neuroectodermal tumor not otherwise specified. Neuro Oncol 2015;17(8):1157–65.

61. Bull JG, Saunders DE, Clark CA. Discrimination of paediatric brain tumours using apparent diffusion coefficient histograms. Eur Radiol 2012;22(2): 447–57.

62. Gauvain KM, McKinstry RC, Mukherjee P, et al. Evaluating pediatric brain tumor cellularity with diffusion-tensor imaging. AJR Am J Roentgenol 2001;177(2):449–54.

63. Koral K, Alford R, Choudhury N, et al. Applicability of apparent diffusion coefficient ratios in preoperative diagnosis of common pediatric cerebellar tumors across two institutions. Neuroradiology 2014;56(9):781–8.

64. Preusser M, Hoischen A, Novak K, et al. Angiocentric glioma: report of clinico-pathologic and genetic findings in 8 cases. Am J Surg Pathol 2007;31(11): 1709–18.

65. Louis DN, Ohgaki H, Wiestler OD, et al. The 2007 WHO classification of tumours of the central nervous system. Acta Neuropathol 2007;114(2): 97–109.

66. Brat DJ, Scheithauer BW, Fuller GN, et al. Newly codified glial neoplasms of the 2007 WHO classification of tumours of the central nervous system: angiocentric glioma, pilomyxoid astrocytoma and pituicytoma. Brain Pathol 2007;17(3): 319–24.

67. Ni HC, Chen SY, Chen L, et al. Angiocentric glioma: a report of nine new cases, including four with atypical histological features. Neuropathol Appl Neurobiol 2015;41(3):333–46.

68. Shakur SF, McGirt MJ, Johnson MW, et al. Angiocentric glioma: a case series. J Neurosurg Pediatr 2009;3(3):197–202.

69. Covington DB, Rosenblum MK, Brathwaite CD, et al. Angiocentric glioma-like tumor of the midbrain. Pediatr Neurosurg 2009;45(6):429–33.

70. Whitehead MT, Vezina G. MR spectroscopic profile of an angiocentric glioma. Anticancer Res 2015; 35(11):6267–70.

71. Koral K, Koral KM, Sklar F. Angiocentric glioma in a 4-year-old boy: imaging characteristics and review of the literature. Clin Imaging 2012;36(1):61–4.

72. Luyken C, Blumcke I, Fimmers R, et al. Supratentorial gangliogliomas: histopathologic grading and tumor recurrence in 184 patients with a median follow-up of 8 years. Cancer 2004;101(1):146–55.

73. Adachi Y, Yagishita A. Gangliogliomas: characteristic imaging findings and role in the temporal lobe epilepsy. Neuroradiology 2008;50(10): 829–34.

74. Kralik SF, Taha A, Kamer AP, et al. Diffusion imaging for tumor grading of supratentorial brain tumors in the first year of life. AJNR Am J Neuroradiol 2014;35(4):815–23.

75. Hummel TR, Miles L, Mangano FT, et al. Clinical heterogeneity of desmoplastic infantile ganglioglioma: a case series and literature review. J Pediatr Hematol Oncol 2012;34(6):e232–6.

76. Darwish B, Arbuckle S, Kellie S, et al. Desmoplastic infantile ganglioglioma/astrocytoma with cerebrospinal metastasis. J Clin Neurosci 2007;14(5): 498–501.

77. De Munnynck K, Van Gool S, Van Calenbergh F, et al. Desmoplastic infantile ganglioglioma: a potentially malignant tumor? Am J Surg Pathol 2002;26(11):1515–22.

78. Hoving EW, Kros JM, Groninger E, et al. Desmoplastic infantile ganglioglioma with a malignant course. J Neurosurg Pediatr 2008;1(1):95–8.

79. Trehan G, Bruge H, Vinchon M, et al. MR imaging in the diagnosis of desmoplastic infantile tumor: retrospective study of six cases. AJNR Am J Neuroradiol 2004;25(6):1028–33.

80. Jurkiewicz E, Grajkowska W, Nowak K, et al. MR imaging, apparent diffusion coefficient and histopathological features of desmoplastic infantile tumors-own experience and review of the literature. Childs Nerv Syst 2015;31(2):251–9.

81. Tamburrini G, Colosimo C Jr, Giangaspero F, et al. Desmoplastic infantile ganglioglioma. Childs Nerv Syst 2003;19(5–6):292–7.

82. Bader A, Heran M, Dunham C, et al. Radiological features of infantile glioblastoma and desmoplastic infantile tumors: British Columbia's Children's Hospital experience. J Neurosurg Pediatr 2015;16(2): 119–25.

83. Tenreiro-Picon OR, Kamath SV, Knorr JR, et al. Desmoplastic infantile ganglioglioma: CT and MRI features. Pediatr Radiol 1995;25(7):540–3.

84. Martin DS, Levy B, Awwad EE, et al. Desmoplastic infantile ganglioglioma: CT and MR features. AJNR Am J Neuroradiol 1991;12(6):1195–7.

85. Zhang JG, Hu WZ, Zhao RJ, et al. Dysembryoplastic neuroepithelial tumor: a clinical, neuroradiological, and pathological study of 15 cases. J Child Neurol 2014;29(11):1441–7.

86. O'Brien DF, Farrell M, Delanty N, et al. The Children's Cancer and Leukaemia Group guidelines for the diagnosis and management of dysembryoplastic neuroepithelial tumours. Br J Neurosurg 2007;21(6):539–49.

87. Krossnes BK, Wester K, Moen G, et al. Multifocal dysembryoplastic neuroepithelial tumour in a male with the XYY syndrome. Neuropathol Appl Neurobiol 2005;31(5):556–60.

88. Whittle IR, Dow GR, Lammie GA, et al. Dsyembryoplastic neuroepithelial tumour with discrete bilateral multifocality: further evidence for a germinal origin. Br J Neurosurg 1999;13(5):508–11.

89. Stanescu Cosson R, Varlet P, Beuvon F, et al. Dysembryoplastic neuroepithelial tumors: CT, MR findings and imaging follow-up: a study of 53 cases. J Neuroradiol 2001;28(4):230–40.

90. Mano Y, Kumabe T, Shibahara I, et al. Dynamic changes in magnetic resonance imaging appearance of dysembryoplastic neuroepithelial tumor with or without malignant transformation. J Neurosurg Pediatr 2013;11(5):518–25.

91. Tailor JK, Kim AH, Folkerth RD, et al. The development of ring-shaped contrast enhancement in a case of cerebellar dysembryoplastic neuroepithelial tumor: case report. Neurosurgery 2008;63(3): E609–10 [discussion: E610].

92. Fellah S, Callot V, Viout P, et al. Epileptogenic brain lesions in children: the added-value of combined diffusion imaging and proton MR spectroscopy to the presurgical differential diagnosis. Childs Nerv Syst 2012;28(2):273–82.

93. Thom M, Gomez-Anson B, Revesz T, et al. Spontaneous intralesional haemorrhage in dysembryoplastic neuroepithelial tumours: a series of five cases. J Neurol Neurosurg Psychiatry 1999;67(1):97–101.

94. Ray WZ, Blackburn SL, Casavilca-Zambrano S, et al. Clinicopathologic features of recurrent dysembryoplastic neuroepithelial tumor and rare malignant transformation: a report of 5 cases and review of the literature. J Neurooncol 2009;94(2): 283–92.

95. Jensen RL, Caamano E, Jensen EM, et al. Development of contrast enhancement after long-term observation of a dysembryoplastic neuroepithelial tumor. J Neurooncol 2006;78(1):59–62.

96. Lester RA, Brown LC, Eckel LJ, et al. Clinical outcomes of children and adults with central nervous system primitive neuroectodermal tumor. J Neurooncol 2014;120(2):371–9.

97. Poussaint TY. Magnetic resonance imaging of pediatric brain tumors: state of the art. Top Magn Reson Imaging 2001;12(6):411–33.

98. Dai AI, Backstrom JW, Burger PC, et al. Supratentorial primitive neuroectodermal tumors of infancy: clinical and radiologic findings. Pediatr Neurol 2003;29(5):430–4.

99. Law M, Kazmi K, Wetzel S, et al. Dynamic susceptibility contrast-enhanced perfusion and conventional MR imaging findings for adult patients with cerebral primitive neuroectodermal tumors. AJNR Am J Neuroradiol 2004;25(6):997–1005.

100. Yamasaki F, Kurisu K, Satoh K, et al. Apparent diffusion coefficient of human brain tumors at MR imaging. Radiology 2005;235(3):985–91.

101. Chawla A, Emmanuel JV, Seow WT, et al. Paediatric PNET: pre-surgical MRI features. Clin Radiol 2007; 62(1):43–52.

102. Kovanlikaya A, Panigrahy A, Krieger MD, et al. Untreated pediatric primitive neuroectodermal tumor in vivo: quantitation of taurine with MR spectroscopy. Radiology 2005;236(3):1020–5.

103. Athale UH, Duckworth J, Odame I, et al. Childhood atypical teratoid rhabdoid tumor of the central nervous system: a meta-analysis of observational studies. J Pediatr Hematol Oncol 2009;31(9): 651–63.

104. Ostrom QT, Chen Y, M de Blank P, et al. The descriptive epidemiology of atypical teratoid/ rhabdoid tumors in the United States, 2001-2010. Neuro Oncol 2014;16(10):1392–9.

105. Ho DM, Hsu CY, Wong TT, et al. Atypical teratoid/ rhabdoid tumor of the central nervous system: a comparative study with primitive neuroectodermal tumor/medulloblastoma. Acta Neuropathol 2000; 99(5):482–8.

106. Torchia J, Picard D, Lafay-Cousin L, et al. Molecular subgroups of atypical teratoid rhabdoid tumours in children: an integrated genomic and clinicopathological analysis. Lancet Oncol 2015; 16(5):569–82.

107. Bing F, Nugues F, Grand S, et al. Primary intracranial extra-axial and supratentorial atypical rhabdoid tumor. Pediatr Neurol 2009;41(6):453–6.

108. Parmar H, Hawkins C, Bouffet E, et al. Imaging findings in primary intracranial atypical teratoid/ rhabdoid tumors. Pediatr Radiol 2006;36(2): 126–32.

109. Jin B, Feng XY. MRI features of atypical teratoid/ rhabdoid tumors in children. Pediatr Radiol 2013; 43(8):1001–8.

110. Zhao RJ, Wu KY, Zhang JG, et al. Primary intracranial atypical teratoid/rhabdoid tumors: a clinicopathologic and neuroradiologic study. J Child Neurol 2015;30(8):1017–23.

111. Arslanoglu A, Aygun N, Tekhtani D, et al. Imaging findings of CNS atypical teratoid/rhabdoid tumors. AJNR Am J Neuroradiol 2004;25(3):476–80.

112. Warmuth-Metz M, Bison B, Gerber NU, et al. Bone involvement in atypical teratoid/rhabdoid tumors of the CNS. AJNR Am J Neuroradiol 2013;34(10): 2039–42.

113. Koral K, Gargan L, Bowers DC, et al. Imaging characteristics of atypical teratoid-rhabdoid tumor in children compared with medulloblastoma. AJR Am J Roentgenol 2008;190(3):809–14.

114. Rumboldt Z, Camacho DL, Lake D, et al. Apparent diffusion coefficients for differentiation of cerebellar tumors in children. AJNR Am J Neuroradiol 2006; 27(6):1362–9.

115. Warmuth-Metz M, Bison B, Dannemann-Stern E, et al. CT and MR imaging in atypical teratoid/rhabdoid tumors of the central nervous system. Neuroradiology 2008;50(5):447–52.

# Brain Tumors in the Neonate

Karuna V. Shekdar, MD*, Erin Simon Schwartz, MD

## KEYWORDS

- Brain tumor • Neonate • Fetus • Computed tomography • Magnetic resonance imaging

## KEY POINTS

- Neonatal brain tumors are rare and account for fewer than 2% of all pediatric brain tumors.
- Most brain tumors that present within the neonatal period (first 4 weeks after delivery) develop prenatally and may be diagnosed in utero with obstetric ultrasound imaging or fetal MR imaging.
- Teratoma, a subtype of germ cell tumors, is the most common brain tumor in neonates. On imaging, teratomas typically are well-defined, large, heterogeneous masses with contrast-enhancing solid portions, nonenhancing cystic portions, fatty tissue, and mineralization.
- Choroid plexus tumors are the second most common brain tumors found in neonates, commonly found in the lateral ventricle and often presenting with hydrocephalus. On MR imaging, they demonstrate a typical frondlike appearance, and avid contrast enhancement.
- Atypical teratoid/rhabdoid tumor (ATRT) is a primitive neoplasm that is a World Health Organization grade IV and is markedly aggressive with a universally dismal prognosis. The imaging appearance of ATRT is very similar to that of other embryonal tumors; however, ATRT often demonstrates a dramatically rapid growth pattern not seen with other tumors.

## INTRODUCTION

The neonatal period is defined as the period of first 4 weeks after delivery. Brain tumors that present within the neonatal period are discussed in this article. Most of these develop prenatally and may be diagnosed in utero with obstetric ultrasound imaging or fetal MR imaging. Neonatal brain tumors are rare and represent 0.5% to 1.9% of all pediatric brain tumors.[1–3] Several of the previously published series on neonatal brain tumors relied on data collected before the wide availability of neuroimaging with computed tomography (CT) or MR.[3–5] The availability of high-resolution imaging during the fetal and neonatal periods makes the early diagnosis of these tumors possible, often at a subclinical stage. Advanced neuroimaging techniques have improved our understanding of the histologic and anatomic distribution and behavior of these tumors. With this improved understanding of neonatal brain tumors. it is likely that the previously published prevalence may not be a true reflection of the incidence of neonatal brain tumors.

Wakai and colleagues[5] presented their categorization of congenital brain tumors to include brain tumor cases in infants presenting up to the first 2 months of life. Clearly tumors presenting at birth are congenital brain tumors. Thereafter, the confidence regarding the congenital or neonatal origin of brain tumors decreases with the increase in time between birth and presentation. More slowly growing brain tumors that develop during the neonatal period may not become apparent until the child is a year or older. Hence, several neonatal brain tumors that grow slowly may not be included

Conflict of Interest/Author Disclaimer: None.
The Children's Hospital of Philadelphia, Perelman School of Medicine at University of Pennsylvania, # 2115 Wood building, 34 and Civic Center Boulevard, Philadelphia, PA 19146, USA
* Corresponding author.
*E-mail address:* shekdar@email.chop.edu

Neuroimag Clin N Am 27 (2017) 69–83
http://dx.doi.org/10.1016/j.nic.2016.09.001

neuroimaging.theclinics.com

in this category. In this article, we review imaging features of the brain tumors when they present in the neonatal age group.

The most recent update (2016) in the World Health Organization (WHO) classification of central nervous system (CNS) tumors has significantly changed the classification of a number of tumor families. This 2016 update has, for the first time, included molecular parameters into the diagnostic scheme.[6] The most common neonatal brain tumor is teratoma, a subtype of germ cell tumors,[3,5,7] followed by choroid plexus tumors.[6] Another large group of neonatal brain tumors, the embryonal tumors, include embryonal tumors with multilayered rosettes (formerly known as primitive neuroectodermal tumor [PNET]), medulloblastomas, and atypical teratoid/rhabdoid tumors (ATRTs). ATRTs are a unique group of embryonal tumors that tend to occur in young children and neonates. The astrocytic tumors and tumors of neuronal and mixed neuronal-glial neuronal tumors, such as desmoplastic infantile astrocytomas (DIA) and gangliogliomas (DIG), are also typically found in the neonates. Meningeal tumors and hematopoietic tumors also can rarely present in the neonatal period. The more commonly occurring brain tumors in the neonate are presented in **Box 1**.

## CLINICAL PRESENTATION

Clinical presentation of neonatal brain tumors varies depending on the type, size, and location of the tumor. Most common presenting signs are increasing head circumference, vomiting, and lethargy.[5,8] A bulging fontanelle and setting-sun sign may also frequently be noted. Other presenting signs may include seizures, focal motor deficits, hemiparesis, cranial nerve palsy, and nystagmus.[5] Cases diagnosed prenatally may have delivery complications including prolonged labor, fetal distress, and failure of labor progression, typically related to large head size.[5,9]

## IMAGING

Head ultrasound and unenhanced brain CT are the most common initial imaging modalities when neonatal brain tumors are suspected.[10] In utero detection of congenital brain tumors is most often incidental, with screening or routine obstetric ultrasound, and better characterized with the increasing use of fetal MR imaging.[11] The neonatal brain can be assessed with head ultrasound via the sonographic window created by the open fontanelles.[10] Although detection of a mass is possible with ultrasound, cross-sectional imaging is required for further evaluation.[10] CT imaging is quick and usually can be performed with swaddling of the neonate, without requiring sedation. Calcification and acute hemorrhage are easily detected with CT; however, CT scanning exposes the neonate to ionizing radiation. MR imaging with its multiplanar imaging capability, high signal-to-noise ratio, and superior ability to characterize tumors and their impact on surrounding structures, does not involve ionizing radiation. However, MR imaging may require sedation or, in some cases, general anesthesia. Advanced imaging sequences, such as perfusion, diffusion tensor imaging, and susceptibility weighted imaging can be extremely helpful in better characterizing the tumor types and their relationship(s) to eloquent brain regions. Volumetric acquisitions facilitate intraoperative imaging guidance, and can be performed with CT and MR imaging.

Regardless of the tumor type, the dominant imaging appearance of neonatal brain tumors is that of a large, heterogeneous-appearing mass, usually with hydrocephalus and macrocephaly.

## GERM CELL TUMORS

Teratomas, a subtype of germ cell tumors are the most common brain tumor in neonates, accounting for approximately 33% to 50% of cases.[6,9] Intracranial is the third most common location, after sacrococcygeal and cervico-facial.[9] Teratomas arise from multipotent cells and, as a result, usually produce tissues that represent an admixture of 2 or more of the embryologic layers of ectoderm, mesoderm, and endoderm. A supratentorial location is seen in approximately in two-thirds of cases, most commonly associated with the

---

**Box 1**
**Congenital and neonatal brain tumors**

- Germ cell tumors: teratoma (mature and immature)

- Choroid plexus tumors (papilloma and carcinoma)

- Embryonal tumors

  ○ Embryonal tumors with multilayered rosettes (formerly primitive neuroectodermal tumor)

  ○ Atypical teratoid/rhabdoid tumor

  ○ Medulloblastoma

- Astrocytic tumors

- Neuronal and mixed neuronal-glial tumors:

  ○ Desmoplastic infantile tumors (astrocytomas and gangliogliomas)

structures about the third ventricle; the pineal gland region is the leading site of origin, followed by the suprasellar region.[7,9] Congenital teratomas also may involve the cerebral hemispheres more extensively.[7]

Mature (benign) teratomas are composed exclusively of well-differentiated, "adult-type" tissue elements. Mitotic activity is low or absent. The more common ectodermal components encountered in such tumors include skin, teeth, neural elements, and choroid plexus.[12,13] Mesodermal representatives include cartilage, bone, fat, smooth and striated muscle, and choroid plexus (noting its dural embryologic origin).[12] Cysts lined by respiratory or enteric epithelium account for endodermal elements and have been reported to contain thyroid, pancreatic, or hepatic tissue.[12]

Immature (malignant) teratomas contain incompletely differentiated components, resembling fetal tissue.[7,14] Presence of any incompletely differentiated areas mandate classification of the lesion as immature, even a small component in an otherwise well-differentiated tumor.[15–17] Some immature teratomas contain malignant cells of conventional somatic type. The most common of these are rhabdomyosarcoma and undifferentiated sarcoma.[15–17] Production of alpha-fetoprotein by the glandular epithelium in an immature teratoma may result in elevated levels of this biomarker in the serum and cerebrospinal fluid (CSF). Increased serum carcinoembryonic antigen (CEA) also may be commonly found in patients with teratoma.[16]

On imaging, mature teratomas typically are well-defined, T1 and T2 heterogeneous masses with contrast-enhancing solid portions, nonenhancing cystic portions, fatty tissue, and mineralization. On CT they commonly appear as mixed density masses with any fatty components appearing hypodense; CT also has a high sensitivity for mineralization. This association of fat, mineralization, and heterogeneous solid and cystic tissue is highly suggestive of a teratoma.[7,10] On MR images, mineralization may be more challenging to detect than on CT. However, with the use of T2 gradient echo and susceptibility weighted imaging, it is possible to reliably identify mineralization in teratomas on MR imaging. MR fat-suppression techniques and CT may be useful in differentiating fat from hemorrhage. Contrast enhancement is usually heterogeneous and is limited to the solid areas and along the walls of the cystic spaces[7] (Fig. 1). Immature teratomas may show less well-defined margins and larger solid to cystic portion ratios. They are typically large and usually lacking in calcification and fat (Fig. 2). Immature teratomas are often larger than mature teratomas at presentation and infiltrate surrounding structures.[7,10] Peritumoral edema is often observed around immature teratomas; this is usually absent with mature teratomas.[7] CSF dissemination is common with immature teratomas.[7] Imaging characteristics may suggest the type of teratoma; however, classification requires histologic examination.[7] Intracranial teratomas are increasingly being diagnosed antenatally (Figs. 3–5).

The histologic subtype is the most important factor in predicting outcome. Mature teratomas are potentially curable by gross total resection. Prognosis with immature teratomas is generally poor, often due to extensive local invasion and/or CSF dissemination. However, the advent of improved adjuvant chemotherapy may improve the prognosis for the immature teratoma.

## CHOROID PLEXUS TUMORS

Choroid plexus tumors are intraventricular, papillary neoplasms derived from the choroid plexus epithelium. Choroid plexus papillomas (CPP) are graded by WHO as grade I, atypical CPP as grade II, and the choroid plexus carcinoma (CPC) as grade III.[6,18]

Overall, the choroid plexus tumors comprise 0.3% to 0.6% of all brain tumors; however, they account for 2% to 4% of all brain tumors in children.[7] Most choroid plexus tumors are CPPs and they are frequently congenital, as CPP has been reported to account for up to 42% of all neonatal brain tumors.[7] In neonates, CPP is most commonly found in the lateral ventricle. Hydrocephalus is a common feature of CPP, and may be caused by mechanical obstruction of CSF pathways, due to adhesions resulting from hemorrhage, overproduction of CSF by the papilloma, or a combination thereof. CT imaging of choroid plexus tumors typically shows a large, isodense to hyperdense mass with well-delineated, lobulated margins and may be associated with foci of mineralization, and avid contrast enhancement. On MRI, they are generally T1 isointense and T2 hyperintense with well-delineated margins, a typical frondlike appearance, and avid contrast enhancement (Figs. 6 and 7).[1] Differentiation between the subtypes of choroid plexus tumors on neuroimaging often is not possible and is usually determined on histopathological study (Fig. 8). It should be noted that, although histologically benign, CPP may seed the CSF due to its intraventricular location. The CPC is commonly associated with leptomeningeal spread of disease. Ventriculoperitoneal shunt-related metastatic spread in the abdomen and extracranial metastases in the lung have rarely been described with CPC.

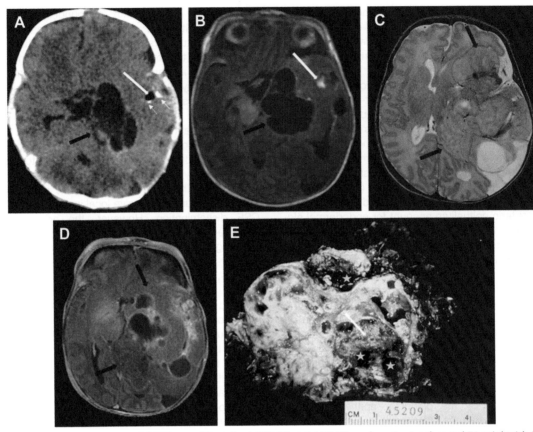

**Fig. 1.** Mature teratoma. Axial CT image (*A*) and axial T1 (*B*), axial T2 (*C*), and contrast-enhanced T1 axial with fat suppression (*D*) MR imaging demonstrates a large, heterogeneous, solid and cystic mass nearly completely filling the left hemi-calvarium (*black arrows*) containing fat components (*thick white arrows*) and mineralization (*small white arrows*). Gross pathologic specimen (*E*) of a teratoma with solid and cystic components containing hemorrhagic (*white star*) and fatty components (*white arrow*). (*Courtesy of* Dr Mariarita Santi, MD, Philadelphia, PA.)

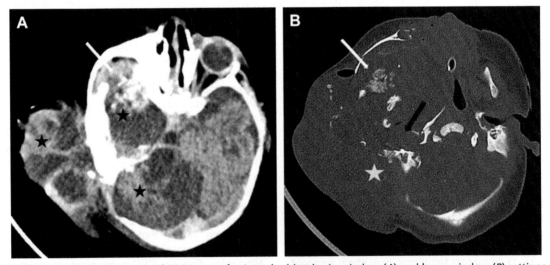

**Fig. 2.** Immature teratoma. Axial CT images of a 1-week-old at brain window (*A*) and bone window (*B*) settings demonstrating a large teratoma (*black star*) involving the right supratentorial and infratentorial compartments of the brain with large exophytic component extending laterally and inferiorly into the cervical region. Extension into the right orbit (*white arrow*), infratemporal fossa, and skull base (*black arrow*) is also evident. Note destruction of the right petrous temporal bone (*white star*) and involvement of the right external auditory canal.

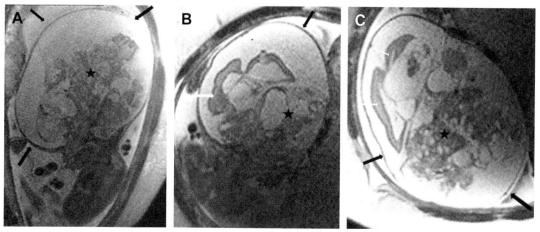

Fig. 3. Teratoma. Three-plane ([A] sagittal, [B] coronal, [C] axial) half-Fourier acquisition single-shot turbo spin-echo (HASTE) images from MR imaging of the brain of a 24-week fetus showing marked macrocephaly (*black arrows*) due to large, complex solid and cystic mass consistent with an intracranial teratoma occupying most of the cranial cavity (*black star*). Only thin bands of residual brain parenchyma can be seen at the periphery (*white arrows*).

CPP has an excellent prognosis when successfully treated surgically, with a 5-year survival rate of up to 100%. Atypical histology with increased mitotic features, brain invasion, and dissemination or frank CPC portend a poorer prognosis.

## EMBRYONAL TUMORS

Embryonal tumors comprise a heterogeneous group of tumors composed of undifferentiated or poorly differentiated neuro-epithelial cells that display divergent differentiation along neuronal, astrocytic, and ependymal lines. Among this group of embryonal tumors, the ATRTs and the medulloblastoma are most commonly encountered in the neonatal population. The new WHO classification of brain tumors has removed the term PNET from the diagnostic lexicon. Many of these tumors display amplification on the C19 MC region on chromosome 19. The presence of C19 MC amplification results in a diagnosis of embryonal tumor with multilayered rosettes (ETMR) C19MC-altered. In the absence of C19 MC amplification, a tumor with histologic features conforming to

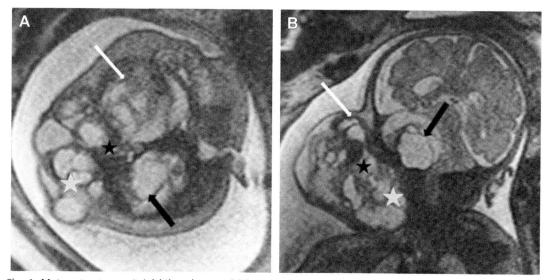

Fig. 4. Mature teratoma. Axial (*A*) and coronal (*B*) HASTE images of fetal MR imaging study show a large solid and cystic teratoma (*black star*) involving right infratemporal fossa (*white arrow*), posterior fossa (*black arrow*) with exophytic extension extending laterally and inferiorly along the right neck (*white star*).

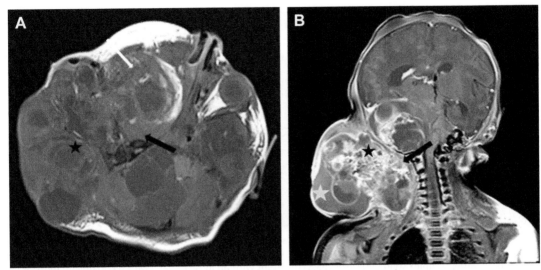

Fig. 5. Mature teratoma. Axial T1 (*A*) and coronal postcontrast T1 (*B*) images from postnatal MR imaging (same patient as Fig. 4) demonstrating a large teratoma (*black star*) involving the right supratentorial and infratentorial compartments of the brain with large exophytic component extending laterally and inferiorly into the neck (*white star*). Extension into the right infratemporal fossa (*white arrow*) and skull base (*black arrow*) is also evident.

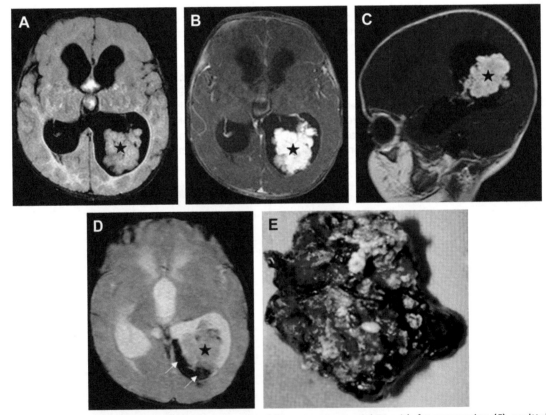

Fig. 6. CPP. Axial fluid-attenuated inversion recovery (*A*), postcontrast axial T1 with fat suppression (*B*), sagittal postcontrast T1 (*C*), and axial T2 gradient echo (*D*) MR images show a lobulated, homogeneously enhancing, mass in the atrium and occipital horn of the left lateral ventricle, in continuity with the choroid plexus (*black star*) containing calcifications/hemorrhage (*white arrows*), compatible with a choroid plexus papilloma. Secondary obstructive hydrocephalus is evident. Gross pathologic specimen (*E*) reveals the typical lobulated frond pattern. (*Courtesy* of Dr Mariarita Santi, CHOP.)

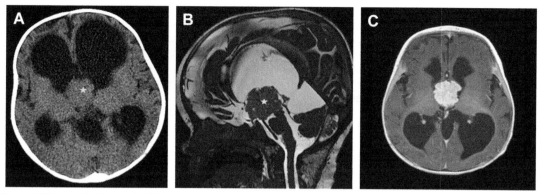

Fig. 7. CPP. Mass (*white star*) within the third ventricle as seen on axial noncontrast CT (*A*) and MR sagittal T2 (*B*) and axial postcontrast T1 (*C*).

ETMR should be diagnosed as ETMR not otherwise specified (NOS).

A new 2016 WHO update on the terminology of CNS tumors has been released recently and has been adhered to in this review article.[6]

### Atypical Teratoid/Rhabdoid Tumor

The ATRT is a primitive neoplasm that may arise in intra-axial or extra-axial spaces of the CNS as well as several other organs in the body. All are WHO grade IV tumors, being[19,20] markedly aggressive with a universally dismal prognosis. Macroscopically, ATRTs are solid tumors with a variable-sized foci of cystic-necrotic change. On histopathology the presence of rhabdoid cells is the hallmark of these tumors. Other cell types may be found in association with rhabdoid cells, such as the primitive neuroectodermal cells, malignant mesenchymal cells, and malignant epithelium.[19,20] Mutation or loss of the INI1/hSNF5

gene locus at chromosome 22 q11.2 is the genetic hallmark of the ATRT.[7,21,22]

Published large series of pediatric ATRT have shown a supratentorial preponderance.[7] When supratentorial, they are usually located in the cerebral hemispheres, and less frequently intraventricular, suprasellar, or pineal. Infratentorial ATRTs can be located in the cerebellum, cerebellopontine angle, or brainstem; primary spinal ATRT is less common. CSF dissemination is frequent at presentation.

Neuroimaging of ATRT frequently demonstrates a large, heterogeneous mass with solid, cystic, and necrotic components, mineralization, and intralesional hemorrhage. The imaging appearance of ATRT is similar to that of other embryonal tumors; however, ATRT often demonstrates a dramatically rapid growth pattern not seen with other tumors.[7,23] On unenhanced CT, solid portions demonstrate isodense to hyperdense attenuation relative to gray matter due to the presence of

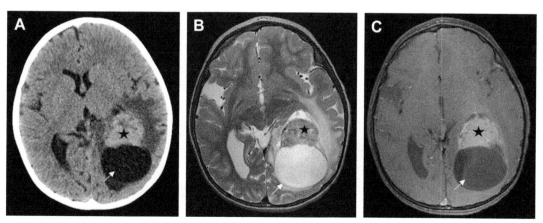

Fig. 8. CPC. Axial noncontrast CT (*A*) and axial T2 (*B*) and axial postcontrast T1 with fat suppression (*C*) MR imaging reveals a homogeneously enhancing lobulated mass (*black star*) within the atrium and occipital horn of the left lateral ventricle along with a large cystic component (*white arrow*).

tightly packed cells with high nuclear-to-cytoplasmic ratio. Contrast enhancement is variable and heterogeneous. Mineralization is often present. On MRI, ATRTs are isointense to hypointense on unenhanced T1-weighted images relative to gray matter, and generally isointense to hypointense on T2-weighted images, in keeping with the high nuclear-to-cytoplasmic ratio, and low free water content within the rhabdoid cells. Cystic-necrotic portions are well demonstrated on MRI. Contrast enhancement is heterogeneous, similar to that seen on CT, and can be mild and/or only involve portions of the solid mass. Solid portions nearly always demonstrate diffusion restriction[24] (Fig. 9). Contrast-enhanced MRI of the entire cranio-spinal axis is mandated in ATRT evaluation to assess for leptomeningeal spread of disease, which is usually present in approximately 33% of cases at presentation[7] (Fig. 10). Multiple sites of synchronous ATRTs suggest an underlying germ-line mutation.[7]

## Medulloblastoma

In children, medulloblastomas are predominantly cerebellar, commonly arising from the vermis; however,[7] in neonates medulloblastomas are more often supratentorial.[25] Other sites in neonates include the pineal region, the suprasellar region, and spinal cord. Regardless of location, the imaging features of CNS medulloblastomas are similar. They are isodense to hyperdense on CT due to the tightly packed, small, round blue cells. They may appear as entirely solid masses or may contain cystic or necrotic areas. Mineralization and/or hemorrhage may be present (Fig. 11). On MRI, medulloblastomas are

hypointense to gray matter on T1-weighted images, and isointense to hypointense on T2-weighted images with any cystic or necrotic areas appearing T2 hyperintense. Contrast enhancement is usually present within the solid portions. Diffusion restriction is a hallmark of medulloblastomas[7] (see Fig. 11; Fig. 12). CSF dissemination is common; hence, MRI of the entire cranio-spinal axis is warranted.[7] A more detailed description of medulloblastomas can be found in other articles of this issue.

## Embryonal Tumor with Multilayered Rosettes

Formerly known as PNET, ETMRs are typically seen in children younger than 4 years and may be either supratentorial or located in the posterior fossa.

These are very aggressive lesions with dismal prognosis.

## ASTROCYTIC TUMORS

Neuroepithelial tumors constitute a large group of neonatal brain tumors. Most of these are glial in origin, most commonly astrocytomas.[5] As with many of the neonatal tumors, a supratentorial location is common, including the suprasellar/hypothalamic region. Astrocytomas also may involve the cerebral hemispheres, optic nerves, thalami, mesencephalon, and the pons. Neonatal astrocytomas involving the cerebral hemisphere are often very large at presentation and commonly involve more than one lobe.[2,26] The imaging appearance of astrocytoma is typically that of a solid or mixed solid and cystic mass, generally hypodense on unenhanced CT with

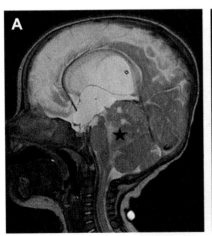
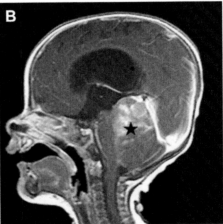
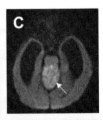
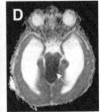

Fig. 9. ATRT. Heterogeneous predominantly solid mass (*black star*) with patchy enhancement and diffusion restriction (*white arrow*) as seen on sagittal T2 (*A*), sagittal postcontrast T1 (*B*), and axial diffusion (*C*) and apparent diffusion coefficient (ADC) map (*D*) in a 4-week-old girl.

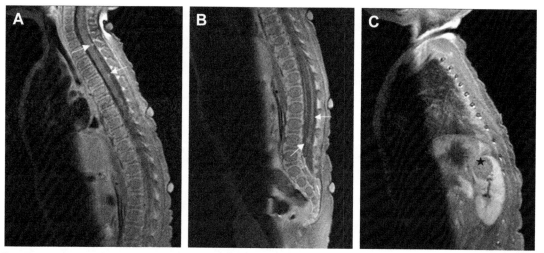

**Fig. 10.** ATRT. Sagittal post-contrast T1 images (*A, B*) through the spine demonstrate multiple enhancing nodules on the surface of the spinal cord and along the cauda equina nerve roots (*white arrows* in *A* and *B*). Note upper pole right renal mass (*black star*) in the para sagittal post-contrast T1 image (*C*) of the spine in the same patient.

variable contrast enhancement. MR imaging of astrocytoma usually demonstrates T1 hypointensity, T2 hyperintensity, and variable contrast enhancement (**Fig. 13**).[1,8,27]

Special mention must be made of astrocytomas, which may be seen in the setting of tuberous sclerosis complex (TSC), along with other stigmata of TSC, which include cortical tubers and

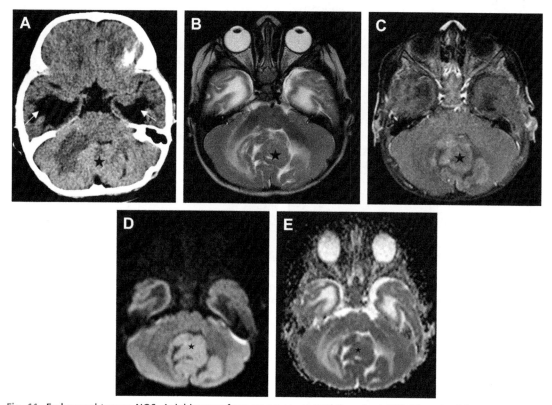

**Fig. 11.** Embryonal tumor, NOS. Axial images from noncontrast CT (*A*) and axial T2 (*B*) and axial postcontrast T1 (*C*) MR imaging demonstrate a hyperdense lobulated mass (*black star*) in the cerebellar vermis with intermediate to mildly hyperintense signal on T2 and patchy enhancement following contrast. Note the obstructive hydrocephalus and transependymal CSF flow (*white arrows*). Axial diffusion-weighted image (*D*) and ADC map (*E*) through the mass reveal diffusion restriction of the solid portion of the mass.

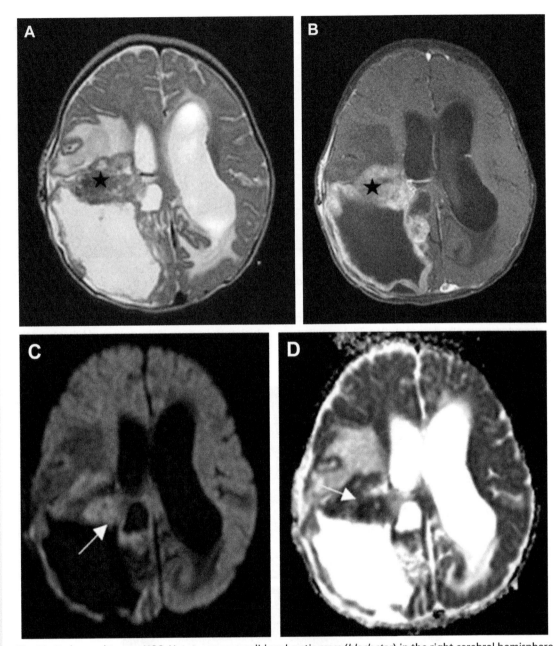

**Fig. 12.** Embryonal tumor, NOS. Heterogeneous solid and cystic mass (*black star*) in the right cerebral hemisphere demonstrating restricted diffusion in the solid component (*white arrow*) and contrast enhancement within solid components of the mass as seen on axial T2 (*A*), axial postcontrast T1 with fat suppression (*B*), axial diffusion (*C*), and ADC map (*D*).

subependymal nodules, and the subependymal giant cell astrocytoma (SEGA), also known as mixed giant cell tumors, typically located at the foramina of Monro (**Fig. 14**). The SEGA can block the flow of CSF, resulting in ventricular trapping and hydrocephalus. It is possible to now identify the SEGAs on antenatal MR imaging, although prenatal and neonatal obstructive hydrocephalus

in TSC is rare. Use of mammalian target of Rapamycin pathway inhibitors, such as Everolimus, has revolutionized the care of patients with TSC; successful treatment of neonatal SEGA and non-CNS tumors has been reported.[28]

Hamartomas are a group of benign tumors that represent heterotopic accumulations of normal brain tissue. Common locations include

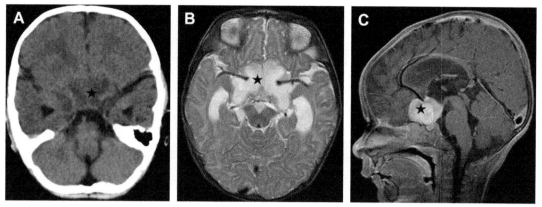

**Fig. 13.** Pilocytic astrocytoma. Axial image from noncontrast CT (*A*) and axial T2 (*B*) and sagittal postcontrast T1 (*C*) MR imaging reveals a lobulated, midline, butterfly-shaped mass (*black star*) with nearly homogeneous contrast enhancement centered at the hypothalamic chiasmatic region.

intraventricular and hypothalamic (**Fig. 15**). Hamartomas may be detected on antenatal or neonatal brain imaging. Hypothalamic hamartoma is the primary feature of Pallister-Hall syndrome, with other major manifestations including polydactyly, dysplastic nails, bifid epiglottis, imperforate anus, renal anomalies, pituitary dysplasia, and hypopituitarism (**Fig. 16**).[29]

## NEURONAL AND MIXED NEURONAL-GLIAL TUMORS

DIAs and DIGs are the most common among the "neuronal and mixed neuronal-glial tumor" group that are found in the neonatal population. DIAs and DIGs are large intracranial cystic tumors of infancy that involve the superficial cerebral cortex and leptomeninges, often also being attached to

the dura via a desmoplastic reaction.[30] DIAs and DIGs are classified as WHO grade I. The DIG is almost exclusively found in infants younger than 6 months and, in most cases, is a congenital tumor. The histopathology of the DIG differs from the DIA by the presence of a neural component with glial differentiation; however, both have similar clinical and neuroimaging features, and favorable prognoses. These tumors typically are supratentorial and involve more than one lobe, most commonly the frontal and parietal, followed by the temporal and, least frequently, the occipital lobe. On CT, DIAs and DIGs are seen as large, cystic, hypodense masses with solid isodense or slightly hyperdense superficial solid components extending to the overlying meninges and demonstrate contrast enhancement of the solid portion.[26,30,31] MR imaging demonstrates

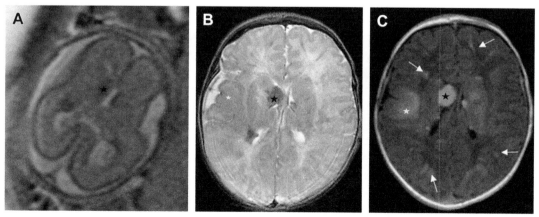

**Fig. 14.** Tuberous sclerosis complex. Axial T2 HASTE images from fetal MR imaging (*A*) and axial T2 (*B*) and postcontrast axial T1 (*C*) from postnatal MR imaging reveal a T2 hypointense mass with contrast enhancement at the right foramen of Monro (*black star*) along with multiple enhancing subependymal nodules as well as radial migration lines (*white arrows*) and cortical tubers (*white star*).

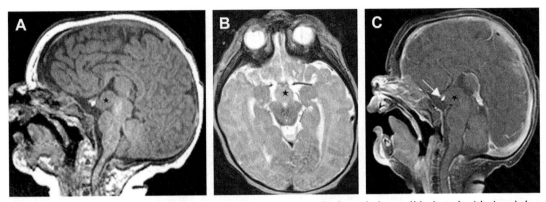

Fig. 15. Hypothalamic hamartoma. Nonenhancing round mass in the hypothalamus (*black star*) with signal characteristics similar to the brain parenchyma as seen on sagittal T1 (*A*), axial T2 (*B*), and sagittal postcontrast T1 (*C*) MR imaging in this 7-day-old. Note the ectopic location of the neurohypophysis (*white arrow*) at the superior infundibular/anterior hypothalamic location, and the hypoplastic pituitary gland.

hypointensity of the cystic components and isointensity of solid components on T1-weighted imaging. On T2-weighted imaging the cystic components are hyperintense and the solid portion is heterogeneously hyperintense.[30,31] Edema is usually absent or disproportionately less compared with the size of the mass[27,30] (**Figs. 17** and **18**).

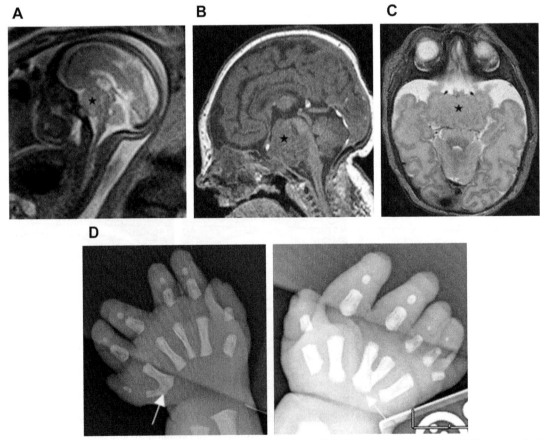

Fig. 16. Pallister-Hall syndrome. Large hypothalamic hamartoma (*black star*) as seen on fetal MR imaging study sagittal T2 HASTE (*A*) and on postnatal MR imaging (sagittal T1 [*B*], axial T2 [*C*]). Radiographs of the hands (*D*) reveal bilateral metacarpal syndactyly.

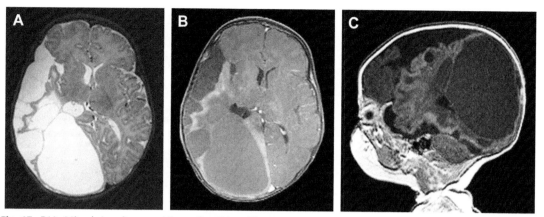

**Fig. 17.** DIA. Mixed signal mass with small solid and large cystic locules almost occupying the entire right supratentorial brain on MR imaging in this 6-week-old on axial T2 (*A*), postcontrast axial T1 with fat suppression (*B*), and sagittal T1 (*C*). Mass was seen to be largely nonenhancing with minimal enhancement along the margin of the cystic locules.

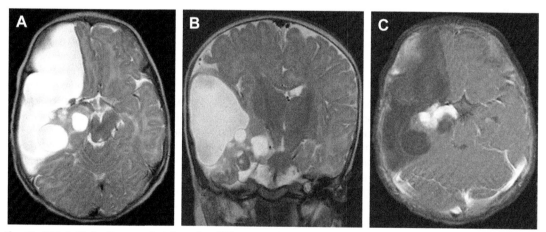

**Fig. 18.** DIG. Initially diagnosed at 4 weeks of life as seen here on follow-up MR imaging on axial (*A*) and coronal T2 (*B*), and axial postcontrast T1 with fat suppression (*C*) with contrast-enhancing solid and large nonenhancing cystic components.

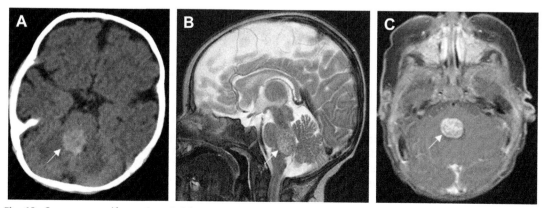

**Fig. 19.** Cavernous malformation. Axial noncontrast CT (*A*) and sagittal T2 (*B*) and axial postcontrast T1 with fat suppression (*C*). MR imaging reveals a hyperdense mass (*white arrow*) on CT within the dorsal pons with a slightly heterogeneous appearance on T2-weighted imaging and homogeneous contrast enhancement.

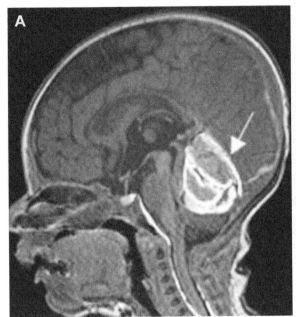
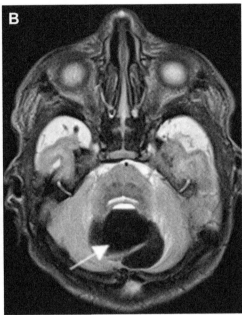

**Fig. 20.** Hematoma. When large, a hematoma can mimic a brain tumor, as seen in this MR image (sagittal T1 [*A*], axial T2 [*B*]) performed on a 6-day-old with a large posterior fossa hemorrhage. No underlying mass or vascular malformation was present.

## BRAIN TUMOR MIMICS

Several entities can mimic the appearance of a neonatal brain tumor on imaging. Moderate to large-size cavernous malformations, hemangiomas, and hemangioendotheliomas can sometimes be mistaken for a neoplasm (**Fig. 19**). Parenchymal hemorrhage can be a perplexing imaging feature because hemorrhage can mask an underlying brain tumor or vascular malformation (**Fig. 20**). Among the neonatal brain tumors, parenchymal hemorrhage has been commonly seen as a presenting feature of the medulloblastoma subtype of embryonal tumors. Follow-up imaging, and in some cases vascular imaging, may be necessary to make the distinction between an underlying tumor and a vascular malformation.

## SUMMARY

Neuroimaging features play an important role in the early detection and characterization of antenatal and neonatal brain tumors. Imaging studies can assess the morphology of the tumor, hydrocephalus, local invasion, and distant spread. A reasonable differential diagnosis of the most likely tumor types can be derived from imaging characteristics. The practicing radiologist should be familiar with the characteristic imaging features of the more common neonatal brain tumors.

## REFERENCES

1. Mazewski CM, Hudgins RJ, Reisner A, et al. Neonatal brain tumors: a review. Semin Perinatol 1999;23(4):286–98.
2. Radkowski MA, Naidich TP, Tomita T, et al. Neonatal brain tumors: CT and MR findings. J Comput Assist Tomogr 1988;12(1):10–20.
3. Buetow PC, Smirniotopoulos JG, Done S. Congenital brain tumors: a review of 45 cases. AJR Am J Roentgenol 1990;155(3):587–93.
4. Arnstein LH, Boldrey E, Naffziger HC. A case report and survey of brain tumors during the neonatal period. J Neurosurg 1951;8(3):315–9.
5. Wakai S, Arai T, Nagai M. Congenital brain tumors. Surg Neurol 1984;21(6):597–609.
6. Louis DN, Perry A, Reifenberger G, et al. The 2016 World Health Organization classification of tumors of the central nervous system: a summary. Acta Neuropathol 2016;131(6):803–20.
7. Tortori-Donati P, Rossi A, Biancheri R, et al. Pediatric neuroradiology. In: Tortori-Donati P, editor. Pediatric Neuroradiology-Brain. Berlin: Springer Verlag; 2005. p. 329–429.
8. Buetow PC, Smirniotopoulos JG, Done S. Congenital brain tumors: a review of 45 cases. AJNR Am J Neuroradiol 1990;11(4):793–9.
9. Chien YH, Tsao PN, Lee WT, et al. Congenital intracranial teratoma. Pediatr Neurol 2000;22(1):72–4.
10. Parmar HA, Pruthi S, Ibrahim M, et al. Imaging of congenital brain tumors. Semin Ultrasound CT MR 2011;32(6):578–89.

11. Milani HJ, Araujo Júnior E, Cavalheiro S, et al. Fetal brain tumors: prenatal diagnosis by ultrasound and magnetic resonance imaging. World J Radiol 2015; 7(1):17–21.

12. Geethanath RM, Abdel-Salam F. Congenital intracranial teratoma. BMJ Case Rep 2010;2010.

13. O'Grady J, Kobayter L, Kaliaperumal C, et al. 'Teeth in the brain' - a case of giant intracranial mature cystic teratoma. BMJ Case Rep 2012;2012.

14. Kentab OY. Congenital intracranial immature teratoma: a case report and review of the literature. Ann Saudi Med 1996;16(2):193–6.

15. Takeuchi J, Handa H, Oda Y, et al. Alpha-fetoprotein in intracranial malignant teratoma. Surg Neurol 1979;12(5):400–4.

16. Diengdoh JV, Buxton PH, Foy PM. Intracranial malignant teratoma. Neuropathol Appl Neurobiol 1985; 11(3):245–50.

17. Uken P, Sato Y, Smith W. MR findings of malignant intracranial teratoma in a neonate. Pediatr Radiol 1986;16(6):504–5.

18. Severino M, Schwartz ES, Thurnher MM, et al. Congenital tumors of the central nervous system. Neuroradiology 2010;52(6):531–48.

19. Ho DM, Hsu CY, Wong TT, et al. Atypical teratoid/ rhabdoid tumor of the central nervous system: a comparative study with primitive neuroectodermal tumor/medulloblastoma. Acta Neuropathol 2000; 99(5):482–8.

20. Rorke LB, Packer R, Biegel J. Central nervous system atypical teratoid/rhabdoid tumors of infancy and childhood. J Neurooncol 1995;24(1):21–8.

21. Judkins AR, Burger PC, Hamilton RL, et al. INI1 protein expression distinguishes atypical teratoid/rhabdoid tumor from choroid plexus carcinoma. J Neuropathol Exp Neurol 2005;64(5):391–7.

22. Biegel JA, Tan L, Zhang F, et al. Alterations of the hSNF5/INI1 gene in central nervous system atypical teratoid/rhabdoid tumors and renal and extrarenal rhabdoid tumors. Clin Cancer Res 2002;8(11): 3461–7.

23. Rai S. Primitive neuroectodermal tumor (MB) versus atypical teratoid/rhabdoid tumors, an imaging dilemma! J Pediatr Neurosci 2009;4(1):48–9.

24. Cheng YC, Lirng JF, Chang FC, et al. Neuroradiological findings in atypical teratoid/rhabdoid tumor of the central nervous system. Acta Radiol 2005; 46(1):89–96.

25. Becker LE, Hinton D. Primitive neuroectodermal tumors of the central nervous system. Hum Pathol 1983;14(6):538–50.

26. Subaramanian MV, Raja Reddy D, Prabhakar V, et al. Congenital astrocytoma. Indian Pediatr 1971;8(6): 200–2.

27. Koeller KK, Henry JM. From the archives of the AFIP: superficial gliomas: radiologic-pathologic correlation. Armed Forces Institute of Pathology. Radiographics 2001;21(6):1533–56.

28. Goyer I, Dahdah N, Major P, et al. Use of mTOR inhibitor everolimus in three neonates for treatment of tumors associated with tuberous sclerosis complex. Pediatr Neurol 2015;52(4):450–3.

29. Kuo JS, Casey SO, Thompson L, et al. Pallister-Hall syndrome: clinical and MR features. AJNR Am J Neuroradiol 1999;20(10):1839–41.

30. Rypens F, Esteban MJ, Lellouch-Tubiana A, et al. Desmoplastic supratentorial neuroepithelial tumours of childhood: imaging in 5 patients. Neuroradiology 1996;38(Suppl 1):S165–8.

31. Tenreiro-Picon OR, Kamath SV, Knorr JR, et al. Desmoplastic infantile ganglioglioma: CT and MRI features. Pediatr Radiol 1995;25(7):540–3.

# Pineal Region Masses in Pediatric Patients

Benita Tamrazi, MD*, Marvin Nelson, MD, MBA, Stefan Blüml, PhD

## KEYWORDS

- Germ cell tumor • Pineoblastoma • Pineal parenchymal tumor of intermediate differentiation
- MR Spectroscopy • Arterial spin labeling • Dynamic susceptibility contrast enhanced perfusion

## KEY POINTS

- Diffusion-weighted imaging is a tool to identify hypercellular pineal region tumors, including germ cell tumors and pineoblastomas.
- MR spectroscopy can help differentiate germ cell tumors, pineoblastomas, and tectal astrocytomas based on differing metabolic profiles.
- Response to therapy of germ cell tumors as well as pineoblastomas can be evaluated using diffusion- and perfusion-weighted imaging.

## INTRODUCTION

Brain tumors are the second most common malignancy in the pediatric population and the leading cause of death from solid tumors.[1] Neoplasms arising from the pineal region account for approximately 4% of childhood intracranial tumors in the United States, with higher occurrence reported in Asia of up to 9%.[2] These tumors of the pineal region are classified into 3 categories as follows: germ cell tumors, tumors that arise from the pineal parenchyma, and tumors that arise from adjacent structures such as astrocytomas (Fig. 1). Understanding the imaging characteristics, including advanced imaging techniques, in conjunction with the clinical/laboratory findings, can help to differentiate among pineal brain tumors.

The clinical presentation of children with pineal region lesions is variable and is often related to mass effect on the adjacent structures. The clinical signs and symptoms can include precocious puberty, Perinaud syndrome secondary to mass effect on the tectum, headache, and nausea/vomiting.[3] In addition to the clinical presentation, it is important to recognize that some of the tumors arising in the pineal region have associated oncologic markers that can be identified with both serologic and cerebrospinal fluid (CSF) sampling, including alpha fetoprotein, beta human chorionic gonadotropin, and placental alkaline phosphatase (Table 1).[3]

In this article, we review the normal anatomy of the pineal region, discuss the differential diagnosis of pineal region masses, and present the imaging findings for these tumors with an emphasis on advanced imaging techniques, such as diffusion, perfusion, and spectroscopy.

## NORMAL ANATOMY AND IMAGING TECHNIQUE

The pineal gland is a small structure located midline, above the tentorium and superior colliculi and below the splenium of the corpus callosum and the vein of Galen, attached to the posterior border of the third ventricle.[2] The pineal region includes the pineal gland, the surrounding cisterns of the quadrigeminal plate and velum interpositum, posterior third ventricle, and adjacent tissue of the brainstem, thalami, and splenium of the corpus callosum as seen in Fig. 2.[2] The pineal gland normally measures less than 8 mm in greatest

The authors have no disclosures.
Department of Radiology, Children's Hospital Los Angeles, 4650 Sunset Boulevard, Los Angeles, CA 90027, USA
* Corresponding author. 4650 Sunset Boulevard, MS #81, Los Angeles, CA 90027.
*E-mail address:* btamrazi@chla.usc.edu

Neuroimag Clin N Am 27 (2017) 85–97
http://dx.doi.org/10.1016/j.nic.2016.08.002

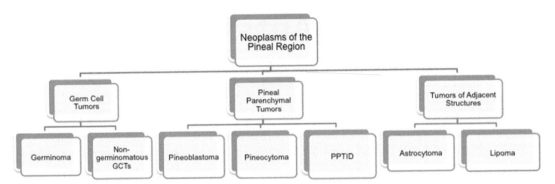

**Fig. 1.** Categories of pineal region tumors. GCTs, germ cell tumors; PPTID, pineal parenchymal tumors of intermediate differentiation.

dimension and can be commonly calcified. However, calcification is rare under the age of 10 years.[2]

Imaging protocols for the evaluation of pineal region masses include both conventional and advanced MR techniques. Although computed tomography (CT) may be the method most commonly used for the initial presentation of the patient, MR is the study of choice for the evaluation and characterization of brain tumors, including pineal region masses. A summary of both conventional and advanced imaging sequences is presented in **Table 2**. Conventional sequences, which can be obtained on 1.5 or 3 T magnets, include T1-weighted, T2-weighted, and Fluid-attenuated inversion recovery (FLAIR) imaging. These sequences should be acquired in multiple planes. For midline lesions such as pineal region masses, sagittal plane is a necessity. Sagittal T1 sequence should preferably be acquired using a 3-dimensional gradient echo sequence to generate reformations of additional planes for

detailed analysis. Intravenous gadolinium compounds are used to assess the degree of permeability of the blood–tumor barrier and to assess for CSF dissemination of tumor.[4]

Advanced imaging techniques such as diffusion-weighted imaging (DWI), perfusion imaging, and spectroscopy are used to assess tumor cellularity, vascular density, and metabolic profile, respectively. DWI is used routinely for the evaluation of brain tumors to distinguish hypercellular from hypocellular tumor.[4] Perfusion imaging can be acquired both with gadolinium intravenous contrast agents as well as without gadolinium using arterial spin labeling. The techniques used for perfusion imaging include T2*-weighted dynamic susceptibility, arterial spin labeling, and T1-weighted dynamic contrast-enhanced

| Table 1 Oncologic markers of germ cell tumors | | | |
|---|---|---|---|
| **Type of GCT** | **AFP** | **B-hCG** | **PLAP** |
| Pure germinoma | − | − | + or − |
| Syncytiotrophoblastic germinoma | − | + | + or − |
| Mature teratoma | − | − | − |
| Immature teratoma | + or − | + or − | − |
| Choriocarcinoma | − | + | + or − |
| Yolk sac | + | − | + or − |
| Embryonal | − | − | + |
| Mixed GCT | + or − | + or − | + or − |

*Abbreviations:* AFP, alpha fetoprotein; B-hCG, beta human chorionic gonadotropin; GCT, germ cell tumor; PLAP, placental alkaline phosphatase.

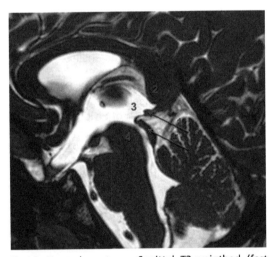

**Fig. 2.** Normal anatomy. Sagittal T2-weigthed (fast imaging employing steady-state acquisition) sequence demonstrating normal anatomy of the pineal region with labeled structures: (1) pineal gland, (2) splenium of the corpus callosum, (3) third ventricle, (4) tegmentum of the midbrain, and (5) tectum of the midbrain.

**Table 2**
Conventional and advanced imaging characteristics of pineal region tumors

| Sequence | GCT | Pineoblastoma | Astrocytoma |
|---|---|---|---|
| T1 | Isointense/hypointnese to GM | Heterogeneous | Hypointense to GM |
| T2 | Isointense/hypointense or slightly hyperintense to GM | Heterogeneous | Hyperintense to GM |
| GRE | ± Susceptibility secondary to hemorrhage | ± Susceptibility secondary to hemorrhage | ± Susceptibility secondary to hemorrhage |
| Contrast | Avid enhancement, heterogeneous | Moderate heterogeneous (may not enhance) | ± Enhancement |
| Diffusion-weighted imaging | Restricted | Restricted | Restricted in areas of higher grade (III/IV) |
| Dynamic susceptibility contrast perfusion | ↑ CBV (may be related to T2 effect) | Limited data | ↑ CBV in areas of higher grade (III/IV) |
| Arterial spin labeling perfusion | Limited data | Limited data | ↑ CBF in areas of higher grade (III/IV) |
| MRS | ↑ Cho, ↓ NAA, ± taurine | ↑ Cho, ↓ NAA, ± taurine (myoinositol may be seen) | ↑ Cho, ↓ NAA, absent taurine |

*Abbreviations:* CBF, cerebral blood flow; CBV, cerebral blood volume; Cho, choline; GCT, germ cell tumor; GM, gray matter; MRS, MR spectroscopy; NAA, *N*-acetylaspartate.

imaging. Perfusion imaging, both dynamic contrast-enhanced perfusion techniques using exogenous tracer agents such as gadolinium-based contrast or endogenous agents such as magnetically labeled blood, reflect tumor vascularity as well as tumor grade.[5] MR spectroscopy (MRS) is also a technique that has been shown to differentiate lower from higher grade tumors. The metabolic profile, including differences in key metabolites such as NAA, choline, myoinositol, and the presence of lipids and lactate, can help to narrow the differential diagnosis for pineal region tumors.

## IMAGING FINDINGS AND PATHOLOGY
### Germ Cell Tumors

The most common pineal region neoplasms are malignant germ cell tumors, often occurring in adolescent male patients.[2] These lesions account for greater than one-half of the pineal region neoplasms.[2] The World Health Organization (WHO) classifies germ cell tumors as germinomas and nongerminomatous germ cell tumors.[2] The nongerminomatous germ cell tumors include teratomas, embryonal carcinoma, yolk sac tumor, choriocarcinoma, and mixed germ cell tumors.

Germ cell tumors are derivatives of primordial ectoderm, mesoderm, or endoderm, with each tumor subtype representing the neoplastic correlate of a distinct stage of embryonic development.[3] Within the germ cell tumor group, there is a distinction between neoplasms that form embryonic tissue and those that form extraembryonic tissue.[2] Germinomas are the most common type of pineal tumors, accounting for more than 60% of germ cell tumors and approximately 40% of pineal region neoplasms.[2] These types of tumors affect male patients 2 to 17 times more often than female patients and are found predominantly in the pineal region, with approximately 20% of germinomas occurring outside of the pineal region in the suprasellar region or basal ganglia.[2] Germinomas may also compromise the corpus callosum as well as cranial nerves, mostly the trigeminal and optic nerves. Germinomas are not encapsulated tumors and therefore can invade adjacent structures of the brain and spread along the surface of the brain or through CSF.

Germ cell tumors are diagnosed by a combination of serum and CSF markers as well as imaging. These tumors result in elevated serum and CSF oncoproteins such as alphafetoprotein, beta human chorionic gonadotropin, and placental alkaline phosphatase (see **Table 1**). Germinomas are divided into 2 subgroups: pure germinomas and germinomas with syncytiotrophoblastic cells, which have a higher recurrence rate and decreased long-term survival, with increased CSF beta human chorionic gonadotropin.[3] Treatment regimens include chemotherapy, radiation, or a combination of both with a favorable prognosis and 5-year survival of at least 90%.[3,6]

On imaging, germinomas can have a heterogeneous appearance, often seen as a solid or solid/cystic mass with increased attenuation on CT. Often, the relationship between the tumor and the pattern of calcification within the pineal gland can help to distinguish germinomas from pineal parenchymal tumors, such as pineoblastomas. Calcification is typically engulfed by the tumor in germinomas, whereas in pineoblastomas, it is scattered in the periphery of the tumor (Fig. 3).[7,8] Other characteristic features differentiating germinomas from pineoblastomas are listed in Table 3, including multiplicity.[7] Additional conventional imaging characteristics of germinomas include decreased T2 signal as compared with gray matter and heterogeneous enhancement.[9]

The cellularity of germinomas is evaluated using advanced imaging techniques such as DWI. DWI is used in tumor imaging to assess the relative intracellular and extracellular volumes of the tissue based on molecular (Brownian) motion of water.[10] Multiple factors can contribute to overall restricted diffusion and lower apparent diffusion coefficient (ADC) values, including cellular compartmentalization, cell type and number, cell membrane density, and macromolecule size and type.[11] ADC values have often been used to determine the grade of a tumor, with a negative correlation reported between ADC values and a higher WHO grade of tumors.[12] Low ADC values have been reported in germinomas, and this is thought to reflect the underlying tumor cellularity.[3] Furthermore, the use of DWI and ADC values as an imaging tool to differentiate germinomas and pineoblastomas is debated in the neuroradiology literature, with mixed results. Although some studies have demonstrated higher ADC values in germinomas as compared with pineoblastomas, it is debated whether this difference truly reflects differences in cellularity or it is secondary to tissue heterogeneity with inclusion of cystic components of the tumor within the region of interest.[10] Some authors have also suggested using DWI and ADC values to monitor therapy, demonstrating increasing ADC values with response to therapy in tumors that are hypercellular as determined on the pretherapy DWI (Fig. 4).[13]

MR perfusion imaging provides an additional advanced imaging tool in the characterization of brain tumors. The techniques include T2*-weighted dynamic susceptibility contrast, T1-weighted dynamic contrast-enhanced method, as well as arterial spin labeling. The difference

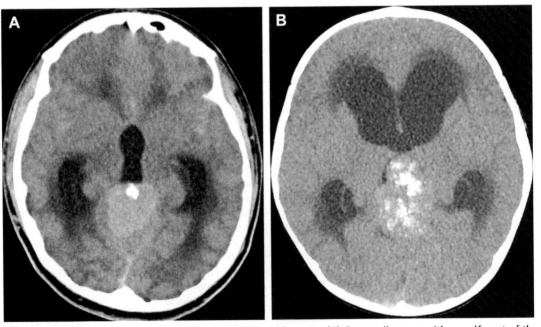

Fig. 3. Calcification pattern of germ cell tumor and pineoblastoma. (A) Germ cell tumor with engulfment of the calcification within the pineal gland by the tumor. (B) Pineoblastoma with exploded calcification along the periphery of the tumor.

**Table 3**
**Characteristic features differentiating GCT and pineoblastomas**

|  | GCT | Pineoblastoma |
|---|---|---|
| Location | Pineal, suprasellar cistern, basal ganglia, corpus callosum, cranial nerves | Pineal |
| Oncologic markers | + | − |
| Association with retinoblastoma | − | + |
| Gender | M >> F | M = F |
| Calcification | Engulfed (centrally) | Exploded (periphery) |

*Abbreviation:* GCT, germ cell tumor.

among these techniques is the use of either an exogenous tracer agent such as paramagnetic contrast material in dynamic susceptibility contrast and dynamic contrast-enhanced perfusion techniques or endogenous tracer agent, such as magnetically labeled blood in arterial spin labeling.[5] The degree of perfusion using these techniques is thought to reflect tumor vascularity in the presence or absence of the blood–brain barrier.[5] Both contrast-based and non–contrast-based techniques have demonstrated the advantages of perfusion imaging as a tool to predict tumor grade.[5,14] Specifically in pediatric brain tumors, high-grade regions have been shown to correlate with increased perfusion parameters, such as relative cerebral blood volume in contrast-based perfusion techniques as well as increased cerebral blood flow in arterial spin labeling techniques.[14,15] However, very little literature exists regarding the use of perfusion imaging in the evaluation of pineal region tumors. Vaghela and colleagues[16] reported increased relative cerebral blood volume in germinomas. At our

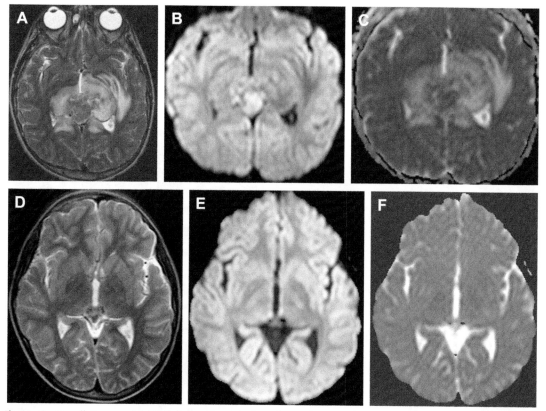

**Fig. 4.** Germ cell tumor at initial diagnosis and after chemotherapy. (*A*) Axial T2-weighted image, (*B*) axial diffusion-weighted image (DWI), (*C*) axial apparent diffusion coefficient (ADC) images before treatment at initial diagnosis demonstrating a T2 hypointense mass with restricted diffusion. (*D*) Axial T2-weighted, (*E*) axial DWI and (*F*) axial ADC demonstrating interval decrease in size with resolution of diffusion restriction after chemotherapy.

institution, we have seen similar findings of increased relative cerebral blood volume and cerebral blood flow in germinomas (Figs. 5 and 6).

In germinomas, perfusion may be elevated owing to an absence of blood–brain barrier and recirculation of contrast media, as seen with typical meningiomas (Lara A. Brandão, MD, personal communication, 2015). Interpolation of the perfusion curve for correction of T2 effects may demonstrate low cerebral blood volumes in these lesions.

MRS is an advanced imaging technique that is valuable in the assessment of pediatric brain tumors. Single voxel short TE MRS offers advantages over other spectroscopy techniques owing to the observation of more metabolites and an increased signal to noise ratio. MRS has been shown to help in characterizing tumors that occur in the pineal region, including germ cell tumors and pineal parenchymal tumors. Multiple prior studies reported significantly higher lipid and macromolecule concentrations in germ cell tumors as compared with other tumors of the pineal region.[17,18] Additional metabolic profiles seen in pure germinomas include elevated choline, decreased N-acetylaspartate, and decreased creatine.[19] Furthermore, Tzika and colleagues[14] demonstrated that choline is positively correlated with relative cerebral blood volume and inversely correlated with ADC, defining a multiparametric MR assessment of tumors. The presence of taurine is also reported as a distinguishing feature of germ cell tumors.

Panigrahy and colleagues[19] demonstrated that prominent lipid peak and a taurine peak could differentiate pure germinomas from pineal parenchymal tumors. However, other authors have demonstrated that pineal parenchymal tumors, specifically pineoblastomas, can also have metabolic profiles with increased lipids and the presence of taurine.[17] We have seen similar findings in patients with germinomas and pineoblastomas at our institution (Figs. 7 and 8). An interesting finding in pineoblastomas is elevation of the myoinositol peak.[20]

Nongerminomatous germ cell tumors include teratomas, embryonal carcinoma, yolk sac tumor, choriocarcinoma, and mixed germ cell tumors. Teratomas are the second most common pineal region tumors with a male predilection.[2] There are 3 histologic types of teratomas: the mature type, which is fully differentiated tissue; the immature type, which includes a complex mixture of fetal-type tissue elements, mature tissue elements, and tissue from all 3 germ layers; and teratomas, with malignant transformation, which includes malignant degeneration of mature tissue.[3] On imaging, teratomas can have foci of fat and calcification, as well as cystic regions.[3] On MR, these lesions appear as lobular, multiloculated, heterogeneously enhancing masses (Fig. 9).[2]

Other types of nongerminomatous germ cell tumors have imaging findings similar to other germ cell tumors. One distinguishing feature however is a propensity for intratumoral hemorrhage.[3]

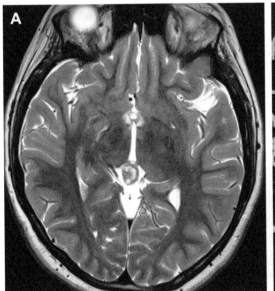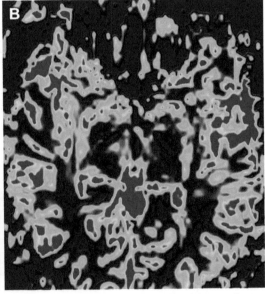

Fig. 5. Dynamic susceptibility contrast (DSC) perfusion germ cell tumor. (A) Axial T2-weighted image demonstrating a T2 hypointense mass within the pineal region with (B) elevated cerebral blood volume on DSC perfusion.

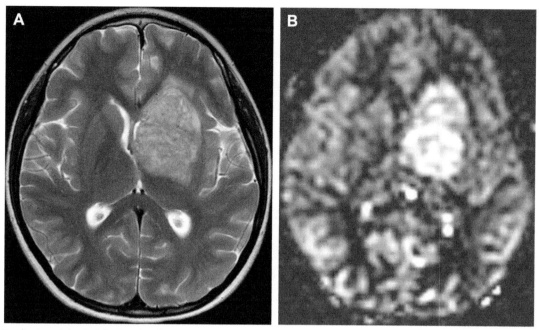

Fig. 6. Arterial spin labeling (ASL) perfusion of a germ cell tumor. (*A*) Axial T2-weighted image demonstrating a T2 hypointense mass in the left basal ganglia with (*B*) elevated cerebral blood flow on ASL perfusion.

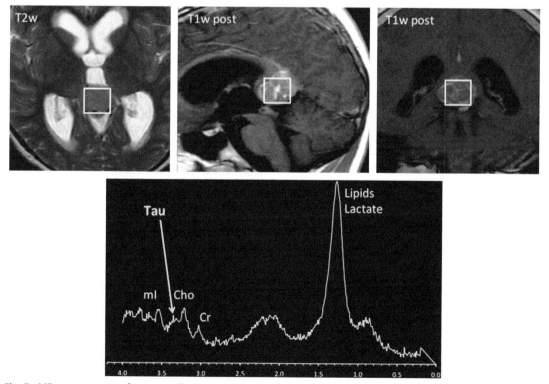

Fig. 7. MR spectroscopy of a germ cell tumor. Point-resolved spectroscopy sequence with a short TE of 35 ms demonstrates presence of taurine (Tau), elevated lipids/lactate with increased choline (Cho) relative to creatine (Cr).

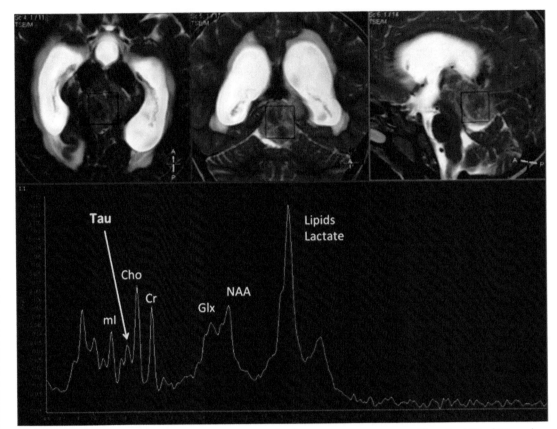

**Fig. 8.** MR spectroscopy of a pineoblastoma. Point-resolved spectroscopy sequence with a short TE of 35 ms demonstrates presence of taurine (Tau), elevated lipids/lactate, increased choline (Cho) relative to creatine (Cr), and decreased N-acetylaspartate (NAA). Additionally, there is presence of myoinositol (ml) and glutamine/glutamate (Glx).

Tumor markers in the serum and CSF better differentiate these tumors as seen in **Table 1**.

### Pineal Parenchymal Tumors

Tumors of pineal parenchymal origin are neuroepithelial tumors arising from pineocytes or their precursors.[3] These tumors represent approximately 15% to 30% of all pineal region masses.[3] Pineal parenchymal tumors vary in histologic grade and aggressiveness, with some tumors classified as benign and some as malignant. These tumors include pineocytomas, pineoblastomas, and pineal parenchymal tumors of intermediate differentiation (PPTID). Additionally, a recently recognized neoplasm in the WHO classification includes papillary tumor of pineal origin. This is a rare neuroepithelial neoplasm of pineal parenchymal origin.[3]

Pineoblastomas are malignant, WHO grade IV tumors that account for 40% of pineal parenchymal tumors and are often associated with CSF dissemination.[3] They are undifferentiated, embryonal tumors categorized as primitive neuroectodermal tumors. Similar to other primitive neuroectodermal tumors, these are highly aggressive tumors with a poor prognosis, often presenting with infiltration of adjacent structures and CSF dissemination. The 5-year survival is less than 60%.[3] Unlike germ cell tumors, there is no predilection by sex. These tumors are more commonly seen in children less than 2 years of age. Not only can pineoblastomas occur in isolation, but they can also occur in association with retinoblastoma, with the combined disease entity known as trilateral retinoblastoma.[21] Approximately 5% of children with retinoblastoma owing to mutation of the retinoblastoma gene will develop trilateral disease.[21] These patients often have a poor prognosis and require aggressive therapy, including chemotherapy and radiation.

On conventional imaging techniques, including CT, key features can be identified to help differentiate pineoblastomas from other tumors of the pineal region. The calcification pattern in the pineal region is a key finding in differentiating

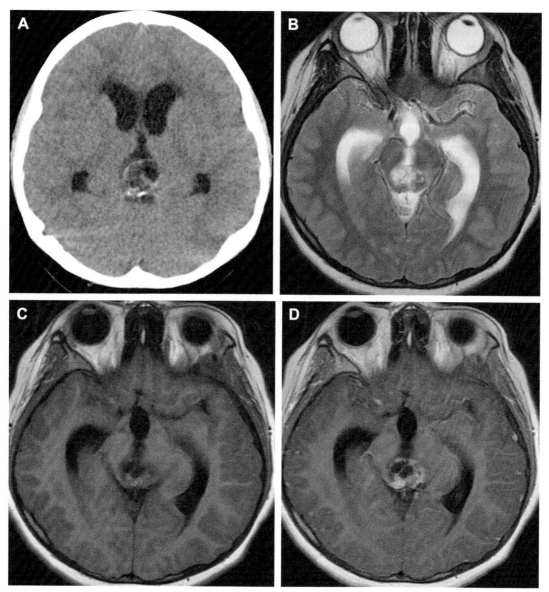

Fig. 9. Mature teratoma. (A) Axial computed tomography image demonstrates a pineal mass containing focal fat. (B) Axial T2-weighted, (C) axial T1-weighted and (D) axial T1-weighted image post contrast demonstrate a cystic and solid, lobulated mass with heterogeneous enhancement.

pineoblastomas from germ cell tumors. The calcification of the pineal gland will be seen dispersed peripherally with pineoblastomas, as opposed to engulfed centrally by the tumor as demonstrated with germ cell tumors (see Fig. 3).[3,7] Additionally, some reports of PET-CT imaging with with fludeoxyglucose have indicated that pineoblastomas and germ cell tumors can be differentiated based on differences in fludeoxyglucose uptake, with high uptake seen in pineoblastomas and little uptake in germ cell tumors.[6] On conventional MR imaging, pineoblastomas appear as heterogeneous masses with predominantly low signal on T2-

weighted sequences and heterogeneous or no enhancement.[18] Foci of necrosis and hemorrhage can also be seen.

MRS is a useful tool for the evaluation of pineoblastomas. Similar to germinomas, a metabolic profile with elevated choline, reduced N-acetylaspartate, and presence of taurine can be seen, and this combination is thought to be reflective of the underlying aggressiveness of these types of tumors (see Fig. 8).[17] Some pineoblastomas may demonstrate elevation of the myoinositol peak.[20] On the other hand, a combination of guanidinoacetate and taurine is often consistently observed in germ cell tumors and not pineal parenchymal tumors.[19] Additional advanced imaging techniques such as diffusion and perfusion imaging help to assess the cellularity and vascularity of pineoblastomas; however, they are not helpful in clearly differentiating these tumors from germ cell tumors. Diffusion weighted imaging demonstrates restricted diffusion with low ADC values in pineoblastomas, reflecting the highly cellular nature of these tumors (Fig. 10).[11] Although limited literature exists regarding the characteristics of pineal parenchymal tumors on perfusion weighted imaging, Vaghela and colleagues[16] reported increased relative cerebral blood volume in these tumors, corresponding with higher grade, but this may also be seen in germ cell tumors.

PPTID are subdivided into 2 groups based on mitotic activity and degree of differentiation.[22] These tumors can be classified as WHO grade II or III. A set therapeutic strategy for these tumors is not well-established, and histologic as well as imaging markers can be used to differentiate between the 2 groups. The proliferative marker, MIB-1 labeling index, has been reported as a useful tool to identify the higher grade subgroup of PPTIDs.[22] Clinically this distinction is critical, because grade III PPTIDs are often treated with aggressive therapy, including craniospinal radiation, surgery, and chemotherapy.[10,22] Although there is no literature regarding the perfusion and diffusion findings of PPTID, these techniques can be applied to help differentiate between grade II and III tumors, which in our limited experience demonstrated increased perfusion with restricted diffusion and low ADC values in grade III tumors (Fig. 11).

The benign type of pineal parenchymal tumor is the pineocytoma. These tumors are composed of well-differentiated mature cells that are nearly

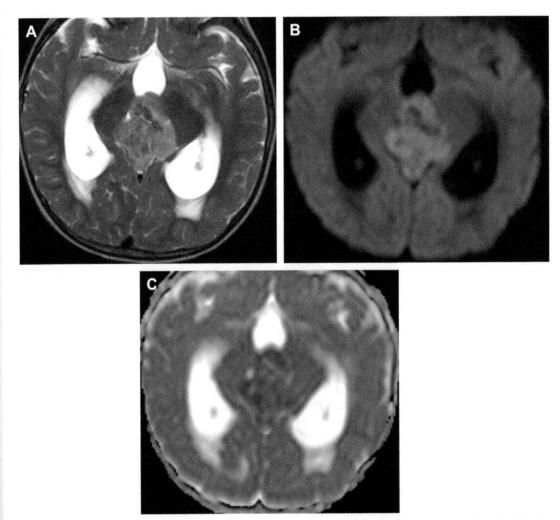

Fig. 10. Pineoblastoma. (A) Axial T2-weighted image demonstrates a large T2 hypointense mass in the pineal region with restricted diffusion as seen on (B) diffusion-weighted imaging and (C) apparent diffusion coefficient mapping.

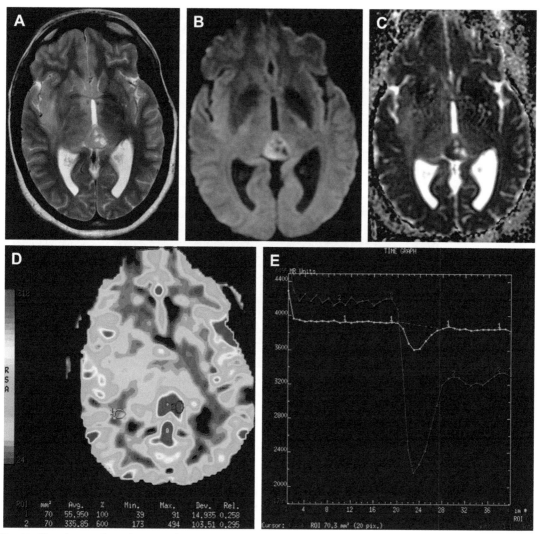

**Fig. 11.** Pineal parenchymal tumor of intermediate differentiation grade III. (*A*) Axial T2-weighted image demonstrating a cystic/solid mass in the pineal region with restricted diffusion as seen on (*B*) diffusion-weighted imaging and (*C*) apparent diffusion coefficient mapping. (*D*) There is elevated cerebral blood volume within the tumor (*E*) with the perfusion curves (relaxivity in the vertical axis, time in the horizontal axis) demonstrating decreased signal in the tumor (corresponding to increased blood volume, labeled as 2) as compared with normal white matter (labeled as 1).

indistinguishable histologically from normal pineal parenchyma.[2] These can appear as locally confined lesions and are classified as WHO grade I neoplasms.[3] Pineocytomas constitute approximately 14% to 30% of all pineal parenchymal tumors and present in all ages but are more common in adults from the third to sixth decades.[10] On MR imaging, they can appear as T2 hyperintense lesions with variable enhancement without associated restricted diffusion or increased perfusion.[3] Furthermore, cysts and hemorrhage can be seen within these lesions. The lesion may be entirely cystic, with a fluid–fluid level.

Papillary tumor of the pineal region is a rare tumor recognized in the WHO 2007 classification. This tumor is thought to arise from specialized ependymocytes of the subcommissural organ located in the lining of the posterior commissure.[16] They can vary in terms of grade, classified as either WHO grade II or III.[3] These tumors often recur locally and treatment options include radiotherapy.[16] Owing to inherent glycopeptide, there is associated intrinsic T1 shortening on MR imaging, which is reported with these tumors.[23] The diagnosis of a papillary tumor of the pineal region can be suggested if a solid mass with intrinsic T1

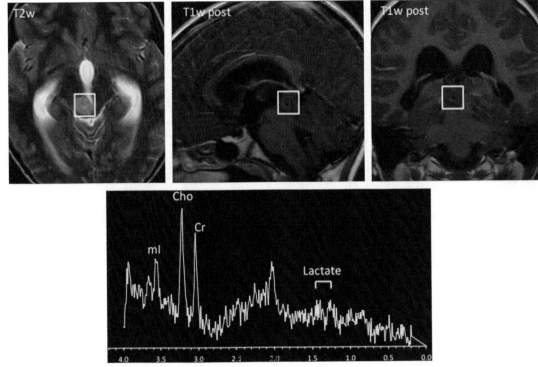

Fig. 12. MR spectroscopy of a tectal glioma. Point-resolved spectroscopy sequence with a short TE of 35 ms demonstrates increase choline (Cho) relative to creatine (Cr) and presence of myoinositol (ml) and minimal lactate peak. There is no taurine peak.

shortening is identified in the pineal region, especially if within the posterior commissure.[23]

Other pineal region neoplasms that arise from adjacent structures such as the thalamus, corpus callosum, third ventricle, subarachnoid space, and meninges include astrocytomas, ependymomas, lipomas, and meningiomas (see Fig. 1). Astrocytomas in this region often originate from the thalami, brainstem, or corpus callosum and contiguity with these structures can help to distinguish the mass as an astrocytoma. Additionally, MRS can be used to differentiate astrocytomas involving the pineal region from germ cell tumors and pineal parenchymal tumors. Low-grade astrocytoma of the tectum demonstrate a metabolic profile that is easily distinguishable from germ cell tumors and pineoblastomas with the absence of taurine and the absence of a high lipid peak, as well as lower levels of total choline concentration (Fig. 12).[19] Lipomas are congenital lesions that develop within the subararachnoid space as a result of abnormal differentiation from the embryologic structure, the meninx primitiva.[2] These lesions can be easily distinguished from other tumors of this region by T1 and T1 fat saturation techniques to identify fat within the lesion.

Pineal cysts are common lesions that are often seen incidentally on imaging. They are reported in 25% to 40% of autopsy cases and 23% of patients on imaging studies of normal, healthy volunteers.[3] On imaging, these are seen as T2 hyperintense, peripherally enhancing lesions in the pineal region. They can have foci of hemorrhage with susceptibility artifact on iron sensitive sequences. Histologically, pineal cysts have walls composed of 3 layers: an inner layer of gliotic tissue, a middle layer of pineal parenchymal tissue, and an outer layer of connective tissue.[3] The management of pineal cysts is controversial. Cysts that should be followed with MR imaging are those larger than 15 mm, and those that present with a thick enhancing wall.

## SUMMARY

Pineal region neoplasms are a heterogeneous group of tumors with variable histologic and radiologic features. With the use of conventional and advanced imaging techniques in conjunction with clinical and serologic markers, these tumors can be better classified and differentiated to ultimately help with the management of the patient.

# REFERENCES

1. Gurney J, Smith M, Bunin G. CNS and miscellaneous intracranial and intraspinal neoplasms. In: Reis L, Smith M, Gurney J, editors. Cancer incidence and survival among children and adolescents: United States SEER Program 1975-1995. Bethesda (MD): National Cancer Institute SEER Program; 1999. p. 51–63. NIH Publication No. 99-4649.

2. Smirniotopoulos JG, Rushing EJ, Mena H. From the archives of the AFIP. Pineal region masses: differential diagnosis. Radiographics 1992;12:577–96.

3. Smith AB, Rushing EJ, Smirniotopoulos JG. From the archives of the AFIP. Lesions of the pineal region: radiologic-pathologic correlation. Radiographics 2010;30:2001–20.

4. Barkovich AJ, Raybaud C. Pediatric neuroimaging. 5th edition. Philadelphia: Lippincott Williams & Wilkins; 2012.

5. Poussaint TY, Rodriguez D. Advanced neuroimaging of pediatric brain tumors: MR diffusion, MR perfusion, and MR spectroscopy. Neuroimaging Clin N Am 2006;16:169–92.

6. Kakigi T, Okada T, Kanagaki M, et al. Quantitative imaging values of CT, MR, and FDG-PET to differentiate pineal parenchymal tumors and germinomas: are they useful. Neuroradiology 2014;56:297–303.

7. Awa R, Campos F, Arita K, et al. Neuroimaging diagnosis of pineal region tumors-quest for pathognomonic finding of germinoma. Neuroradiology 2014; 56:525–34.

8. Borja MJ, Plaza MK, Altman N, et al. Conventional and advanced MRI features of pediatric intracranial tumors: supratentorial tumors. AJR Am J Roentgenol 2013;200:483–503.

9. Reis F, Faria AV, Zanardi VA, et al. Neuroimaging in pineal tumors. J Neuroimaging 2006;16:52–8.

10. Dumrongpisutikul N, Intrapiromkul J, Yousem DM. Distinguishing between germinomas and pineal cell tumors on MR imaging. AJNR Am J Neuroradiol 2012;33:550–5.

11. Gasparetto EL, Hygino da Cruz C, Doring TM, et al. Diffusion weighted MR images and pineoblastoma. Arq Neuropsiquiatr 2008;66:64–8.

12. Yamasaki F, Kurisu K, Satoh K, et al. Apparent diffusion coefficient of human brain tumors at MR imaging. Radiology 2005;235:985–91.

13. Hein PA, Eskey CJ, Dunn JF, et al. Diffusion weighted imaging in the follow up of treated high grade gliomas: tumor recurrence vs radiation injury. AJNR Am J Neuroradiol 2004;25:201–9.

14. Tzika AA, Astrakas LG, Zarifi MK, et al. Multiparametric MR assessment of pediatric brain tumors. Neuroradiology 2003;45:1–10.

15. Yeom KW, Mitchell LA, Lober RM, et al. Arterial spin-labeled perfusion of pediatric brain tumors. AJNR Am J Neuroradiol 2014;35:395–401.

16. Vaghela V, Radhakrishnan N, Radhakrishnan VV, et al. Advanced magnetic resonance imaging with histopathological correlation in papillary tumor of pineal region: report of a case and review of literature. Neurol India 2010;58:928–32.

17. Harris LM, Davies NP, Wilson S, et al. Short echo time single voxel H-Magnetic resonance spectroscopy in the diagnosis and characterization of pineal tumors in children. Pediatr Blood Cancer 2011;57: 972–7.

18. Tong T, Zhenwei Y, Xiaoyuan F. MRI and H-MRS on diagnosis of pineal region tumors. Clin Imaging 2012;36:702–9.

19. Panigrahy A, Krieger MD, Gonzalez-Gomez I, et al. Quantitative short echo time H-MR spectroscopy of untreated pediatric brain tumors: preoperative diagnosis and characterization. AJNR Am J Neuroradiol 2006;27:560–672.

20. Brandão L, Poussaint T. Pediatric brain tumors. Neuroimaging Clin N Am 2013;23:499–525.

21. de Jong MC, Kors WA, de Graaf P, et al. Trilateral retinoblastoma: a systemic review and meta-analysis. Lancet Oncol 2014;15:1157–67.

22. Fukuoka K, Sasaki A, Yanagisawa T, et al. Pineal parenchymal tumor of intermediate differentiation with marked elevation of MIB-1 labeling index. Brain Tumor Pathol 2012;29:229–34.

23. Junior MR, da Rocha AJ, da Silva AZ, et al. Papillary tumor of the pineal region: MR signal intensity correlated to histopathology. Case Rep Neurol Med 2015; 2015:4. Article ID 315095.

# Imaging of the Sella and Parasellar Region in the Pediatric Population

Daniel P. Seeburg, MD, PhD[a,b],
Marjolein H.G. Dremmen, MD[c],
Thierry A.G.M. Huisman, MD[a,d],*

## KEYWORDS

• Sella • Suprasellar mass • Parasellar mass • Infundibulum

## KEY POINTS

• Sellar and parasellar masses are not infrequent in the pediatric population, comprising about 10% of all pediatric brain tumors.
• Key features that help to distinguish between these lesions include the primary site of origin (eg, sellar, suprasellar, infundibular), the intrinsic signal and enhancement pattern, and the age and clinical presentation of the patient.
• There are many important differences between children and adults with respect to the type and frequency of sellar and suprasellar masses.

## INTRODUCTION

Masses arising in the sella and parasellar region are not infrequent in the pediatric population, comprising about 10% of all pediatric brain tumors.[1] Imaging, especially Magnetic resonance (MR) imaging, which renders high soft tissue contrast and great anatomic detail, remains a critical component in diagnosis and characterization of these lesions, helping suggest whether lesions are most likely benign or malignant.

Some of the key features on MR imaging that allow one to distinguish 1 type of lesion from another in the sellar and suprasellar regions include primary location and extension, the intrinsic signal and contrast enhancement patterns, and the presence or absence of distinguishing features, such as cysts and calcifications. Based on location, lesions are classified as either entirely intrasellar, sellar and suprasellar, infundibular, or entirely suprasellar. Lesions can be further characterized as being entirely solid, entirely cystic, or partially solid and partially cystic. This article summarizes the characteristic imaging features of the most frequent pediatric tumors and tumor-mimicking lesions in this region.

Historically, intrasellar lesions were indirectly imaged or diagnosed with plain skull radiographs and polytomography based on widening of the sella and the presence of calcifications in the sella and suprasellar region. Pneumoencephalography was

---

The authors have nothing to disclose.
[a] Division of Pediatric Radiology, Russell H. Morgan Department of Radiology and Radiological Science, The Johns Hopkins Medical Institutions, 1800 Orleans Street, Baltimore, MD 21287, USA; [b] Division of Neuroradiology, Russel H. Morgan Department of Radiology and Radiologic Science, The Johns Hopkins Hospital, The Johns Hopkins Medical Institutions, Phipps B-100, 600 North Wolfe Street, Baltimore, MD 21287, USA; [c] Division of Pediatric Radiology, Department of Radiology, Erasmus MC – University Medical Center, 's-Gravendijkwal 230, 3015 CE Rotterdam, Netherlands; [d] Division of Neuroradiology, Russell H. Morgan Department of Radiology and Radiological Science, The Johns Hopkins Medical Institutions, 600 North Wolfe Street, Baltimore, MD 21287, USA
* Corresponding author.
E-mail address: thuisma1@jhmi.edu

Neuroimag Clin N Am 27 (2017) 99–121
http://dx.doi.org/10.1016/j.nic.2016.08.004

used to outline sellar and suprasellar tumors.[2] Currently, MR imaging is the primary imaging modality for sellar and suprasellar lesions, especially in the pediatric age group. Computed tomography (CT) may occasionally provide complementary information when more definitive assessment for the presence of calcifications is desired. Magnetic resonance (MR) imaging of the pituitary and suprasellar region is performed on a 1.5 T or 3 T MR scanner with conventional T1-weighted and T2-weighted, multiplanar, thin-slice, noncontrast, and gadolinium-enhanced MR sequences. In general, sagittal and coronal planes are most advantageous in evaluating this region. Additional sequences may be added in specific situations, such as when hemorrhage (susceptibility weighted imaging [SWI]) or a microadenoma (dynamic contrast-enhanced imaging) is suspected. High-resolution T2-weighted isotropic sequences may also occasionally be helpful when exact anatomic relationships need to be assessed, such as when trying to determine if a cystic mass arises from the third ventricle or is extending into it or where important functional structures, such as the optic chiasm, are located in relation to the lesion. The standard pituitary protocol performed at the corresponding author's institution listed in **Table 1**. Finally, advanced imaging sequences such as diffusion-weighted imaging (DWI), diffusion tensor imaging, perfusion-weighted imaging, or hydrogen proton ($^{1}$H) MR spectroscopy are progressively used to further narrow down the differential diagnosis.

In addition to the imaging findings, the clinical presentation can offer important clues regarding the diagnosis and primary location of the tumor. Depending on the size and location of the lesion, the clinical presentation can vary from nonspecific symptoms caused by increased intracranial pressure to more specific symptoms related to pituitary hormone deficiencies or excesses. Vision changes are also not uncommon and occur secondary to mass effect on the optic apparatus.[3] Some lesions are asymptomatic and are incidentally found during imaging of the brain for other indications.

There are many differences between children and adults with respect to sellar and suprasellar tumors. For example, the type and frequency of tumors seen is quite different. Thus, macroadenomas are common in adults but rare in children. Similarly, optic gliomas are common childhood tumors but do not typically arise de novo in adults.[4] There are also different challenges when it comes to imaging the pediatric sellar and suprasellar region. Compared with adults, pediatric imaging requires a smaller field of view and thinner slices because of the smaller anatomic structures involved. Finally, the response to increased intracranial pressure is different in young children compared with adults. The presence of open sutures allows sutural diastasis in the setting of increasing intracranial pressure, sometimes accommodating very large intracranial masses before the patient becomes symptomatic.

## Normal Anatomy and Pituitary Embryology

Identification of abnormalities in the sellar and parasellar regions requires a basic familiarity with both the normal anatomy and embryologic development of the pituitary gland. The pituitary gland is composed of 2 different parts with embryonically distinct development: the anteriorly located adenohypophysis and the posteriorly located neurohypophysis. The adenohypophysis is thought to derive from Rathke pouch, which separates during embryologic development from the oral ectoderm, then migrates upwards toward the infundibulum, a downward extension from the hypothalamus. The infundibulum represents the budding neurohypophysis that eventually extends inferiorly to the sella to form the posterior pituitary proper.[5] The adenohypophysis is made up of 3 parts: the pars tuberalis, the pars intermedia, and the pars distalis. The pars tuberalis is located in the pituitary stalk where it surrounds the neurohypophyseal axons extending from the hypothalamus to the posterior pituitary proper. The pars distalis is the largest, most anterior portion of the adenohypophysis, and the pars intermedia is the portion located directly in contact with the neurohypophysis.

In both preterm and term newborns, the anterior lobe of the pituitary (adenohypophysis) is characteristically T1 hyperintense, and gradually

| Table 1 |
| :--- |
| Pituitary protocol used for imaging of the sella and parasellar region |

| Plane | Sequence Name |
| :--- | :--- |
| Sagittal | T1 3D sagittal |
| Axial | T2 fluid-attenuated inversion recovery (FLAIR) axial |
| Axial | T2 axial (no fat saturation) |
| Axial | Diffusion tensor imaging |
| Coronal | T1 coronal thin (pituitary) |
| Sagittal | T1 sagittal thin (pituitary) |
| Contrast bolus 1× dose (0.1 mmol/kg): 1 cc/sec, dynamic pituitary if ordered | |
| Coronal | T1 postcoronal thin (pituitary) |
| Sagittal | T1 postsagittal thin (pituitary) |
| Axial | T1 axial post |

becomes T1 isointense to the pons by 6 to 8 weeks of life.[6] The normal craniocaudal dimension in children younger than 12 years of age is less than 6 mm and the upper surface should be flat or slightly concave. In pregnancy, during lactation, and during puberty, the upper margin can become convex superiorly and pituitary heights up to 12 mm can be normal. In men and postmenopausal women, the normal pituitary craniocaudal dimension is less than 8 mm and, in young menstruating girls and women, less than 10 mm.[7,8] The anterior pituitary takes up about 70% of the volume of the gland and has a homogenous appearance on both precontrast and postcontrast sequences. The posterior pituitary has a characteristic intrinsic T1 hyperintensity, which is also known as the posterior pituitary bright spot. The infundibulum (or pituitary stalk) is widest at its origin at the hypothalamus and tapers to its distal attachment at the level of the pituitary gland. Both the adenohypophysis and neurohypophysis, including pituitary stalk, show strong contrast enhancement. At the insertion of the pituitary stalk, a focal hyperenhancement may be seen that matches the distal component of the portal venous system that connects the adenohypophysis with the hypothalamus.

## INTRASELLAR LESIONS
### Rathke Cleft Cyst

Rathke cleft cysts are benign cysts arising from remnants of Rathke cleft (lumen between anterior and posterior walls of Rathke pouch) that fails to involute during development. The walls of the cysts are lined by columnar or cuboidal epithelium.[9] They are not uncommon in the general population and found in about 4% of routine autopsies.[10] Compared with the adult population, they are less common and smaller in size in children, typically measuring less than 2 mm in children younger than 9 years of age, likely due to their natural history of slow expansion over time.[11,12] They are often asymptomatic and found incidentally, especially when small. When larger, they may cause symptoms from mass effect, including headache, visual symptoms, and pituitary dysfunction. They may rarely bleed and cause pituitary apoplexy-like symptoms.

On imaging, Rathke cleft cysts are centered between the anterior and posterior lobes of the pituitary gland and are either entirely intrasellar; intrasellar with suprasellar extension; and, uncommonly, entirely suprasellar (**Fig. 1**). With suprasellar extension, they are located along the anterior aspect of the infundibulum. Their T1 signal intensity varies from hypointense (serous cystic contents) to more hyperintense with increasing proteinaceous or mucoid contents of the cyst.[1] There is no solid enhancing tissue and the walls of the cyst do not enhance but there may be pseudoenhancement of the walls when enhancing pituitary gland is stretched over the cyst walls (claw sign). A characteristic nonenhancing T1 hyperintense nodule is present in 44% to 77% of Rathke cleft cysts.[13,14]

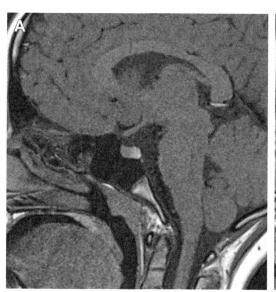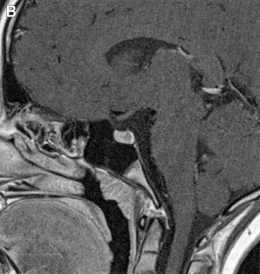

**Fig. 1.** Rathke cleft cyst. Sagittal noncontrast T1-weighted image (A) demonstrates a slightly T1 hyperintense cystic lesion centered between the anterior and posterior lobes of the pituitary gland, which does not enhance and becomes hypointense to the normally enhancing surrounding pituitary gland after contrast administration (B).

Features differentiating Rathke cleft cysts from other cystic pituitary lesions, in particular craniopharyngiomas (CPs) and cystic adenomas, include its sharply demarcated appearance with homogenous signal intensity, lack of a solidly enhancing component, and characteristic location between the anterior and posterior lobes of the pituitary. In the setting of a CP, normal pituitary gland can often be identified inferior to the tumor, and there is often calcification as well as tumor wall enhancement. Pituitary adenomas are centered within the adenohypophysis and cystic components have thick, irregular, enhancing walls. Finally, the cytokeratin expression pattern from pathologic specimens can differentiate Rathke cleft cysts from CPs because the former express cytokeratins 8 and 20, whereas the latter do not.[15]

In young children, small cysts (<3 mm) are sometimes seen incidentally in the pars intermedia region and often referred to as pars intermedia cysts. These are also derived from embryologic remnants of the Rathke cleft[9] and do not require follow-up imaging in asymptomatic individuals.[1,11]

## Craniopharyngioma

CPs are the most common pediatric intracranial tumor of nonglial origin. They account for about 5% of intracranial tumors in children[16,17] and up to 50% of pediatric suprasellar tumors.[18,19] There are 2 main histologic subtypes: the adamantinomatous and the squamous-papillary. Adamantinomatous CP has a bimodal age distribution, with most cases arising in the pediatric age group and a smaller peak in older adults (>65 years), whereas papillary CP occurs mostly in adults older than 50 years of age.[17,20] The prevailing theory for pathogenesis of CPs is the embryogenetic theory, whereby adamantinomatous CPs arise from epithelial remnants of Rathke pouch along the craniopharyngeal duct, which is the pathway of migration of Rathke pouch from the stomodeum (embryologic precursor of the mouth) to the infundibulum.[19] The squamous papillary subtype is thought to occur by squamous metaplasia of cells derived from the pars tuberalis of the adenohypophysis.[1] Clinical symptoms arise from either local mass effect or increased intracranial pressure, and include headache, visual disturbance, and endocrine abnormalities, including decreased growth rate and polydipsia or polyuria.[17]

CPs are most commonly both intrasellar and suprasellar in location (53%–75%), followed by purely suprasellar (20%–41%), and least commonly purely intrasellar (5%–6%).[16] Although characteristic imaging features have been described for adamantinomatous and squamous-papillary CP subtypes, some investigators maintain that there are no reliable distinguishing features between them.[21,22] In general, adamantinomatous CPs are described as lobulated multicystic tumors with enhancing walls and calcifications, typically with a solid enhancing portion also present (Fig. 2).[1,12,20,23,24] The cyst contents are T1 hyperintense in about 33% of cases due to high protein content or methemoglobin.[25] The squamous-papillary subtype, in contrast, is described as more spherical and predominantly solid. If cystic components are present, they are typically T1 hypointense and calcifications are atypical. This subtype can sometimes arise in ectopic locations, such as the floor of the third ventricle, the posterior fossa, or the nasopharynx.[12] For presurgical planning, CPs can be classified into groups based on their relationship to the optic chiasm as either sellar (sellar ± suprasellar extension without mass effect on the chiasm), prechiasmatic (centered anterior to the optic chiasm with posterior or superior displacement of the optic chiasm), or retrochiasmatic (centered posteriorly with anterior displacement of the optic chiasm). In addition, their relationship to the hypothalamus, third ventricle, and vessels of the circle of Willis is important to document in the report.[1]

Although these tumors are benign, malignant transformation can rarely occur after irradiation.[12] Rarely, CPs may spread along the surgical path or more distantly through leptomeningeal spread.[26] Adamantinomatous CPs are histologically benign but biologically aggressive and have a tendency to invade surrounding structures, which often prevents gross total resection.[12] For squamous-papillary CPs, gross total resection is typically curative.

## Pituitary Adenoma

Although common in the adult population, pituitary adenomas are rare in children, and comprise less than 3% of supratentorial tumors in this age group.[27] On the other hand, pituitary adenomas are quite common in the setting of a purely intrasellar enhancing lesion, so should probably be considered as a diagnostic possibility, even in the pediatric age group.[21] In children, most are of the functional variety, with prolactinomas accounting for about half of those, followed by corticotropin-secreting tumors and growth hormone–secreting tumors.[1,19] Prolactinomas are seen most commonly in female patients and tend to present with galactorrhea and amenorrhea.[19] Nonfunctioning adenomas tend to present when they are larger and produce mass effect on

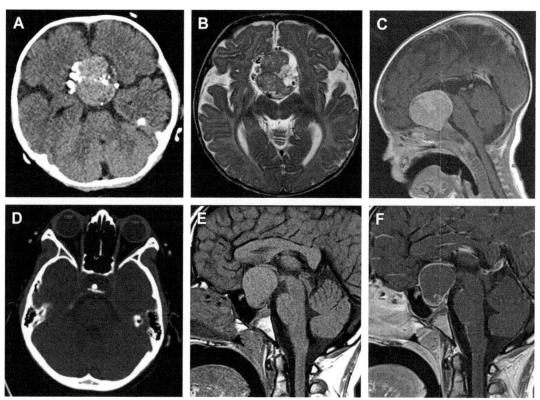

**Fig. 2.** Two patients with CP. The first patient (*A–C*) has a predominantly solid sellar-suprasellar mass with internal calcifications, which are seen best on the axial CT image (*A*). The mass is predominantly T2 isointense to hypointense and there are few T2 hyperintense cystic components along the left aspect of the mass (*B*). The solid components show enhancement (*C*). The second patient (*D–F*) has a predominantly cystic sellar-suprasellar mass with internal calcification (*D*), intrinsic T1 hyperintensity of the cyst contents (*E*), and a thin rim of postcontrast enhancement (*F*). Both lesions result in posterior and superior displacement of the optic chiasm.

adjacent structures, which can result in headache and visual disturbances.

Imaging appearance of microadenomas (<10 mm in size) and macroadenomas (>10 mm in size) is identical to that of the adult population. Prolactin and growth hormone–secreting microadenomas tend to be located more laterally in the adenohypophysis, whereas corticotropin, thyroid-stimulating hormone, and gonadotropin-secreting microadenomas tend to be located more medially. Microadenomas often show delayed enhancement relative to the normal adjacent pituitary gland, with peak enhancement occurring after about 1 to 4 minutes. This differential enhancement pattern can be taken advantage of in detection of otherwise difficult to identify microadenomas by using thin section coronal T1-weighted dynamic precontrast and postcontrast imaging. On unenhanced sequences, microadenomas are typically isointense or hypointense on T1-weighted images compared with the normal surrounding gland (**Fig. 3**). On T2-weighted imaging, their appearance is more variable but tends to be bright (80% of prolactinomas) and those

tend to be softer tumors that are easier to resect than those that are T2 dark.[12] Macroadenomas often extend beyond the confines of the pituitary gland, most commonly into the suprasellar cistern (80%), with less common extension into the cavernous sinus, sphenoid sinus, or dorsum sella (see **Fig. 3**).[12] Their signal is often more heterogeneous than that of microadenomas and is related to cystic, necrotic, and hemorrhagic components (see **Fig. 3**). If possible, it is important to try to identify any normal-appearing remaining pituitary tissue because its preservation is the goal during surgery to prevent pituitary insufficiency.[12]

## Pituitary Hyperplasia

Pituitary hyperplasia is defined as a nonneoplastic polyclonal absolute increase in the number of 1 or more adenohypophyseal cell subtypes, which results in enlargement of the gland. This may be physiologic as, for example, during puberty, pregnancy, or during lactation. Pathologic pituitary hyperplasia, on the other hand, is present when the

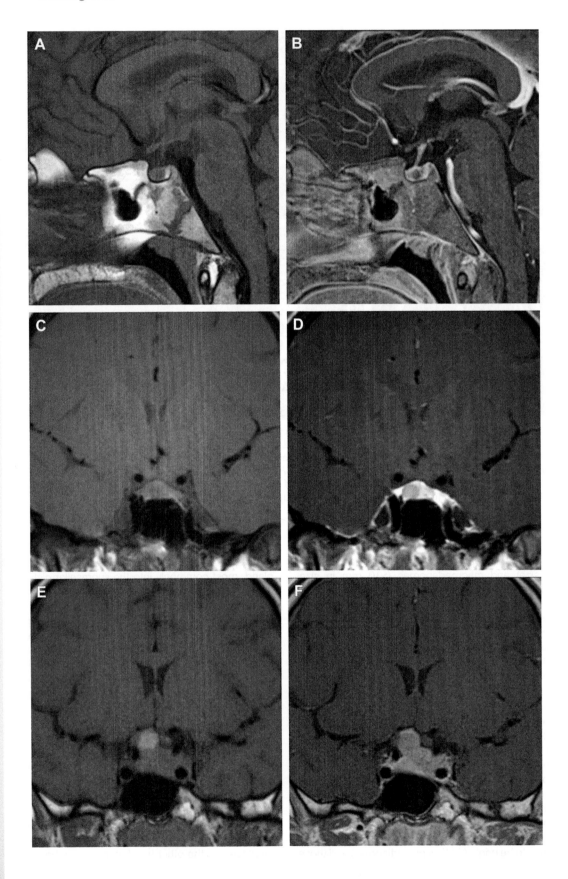

gland enlarges beyond what is considered normal as predicted by the patient's age, gender, and physiologic state.[7,12] In pregnancy and in the postpartum state, for example, it is normal to see physiologic enlargement of the pituitary gland height to up to approximately 12 mm.[28] Pathologic pituitary hyperplasia is most commonly encountered in the setting of end-organ deficiency, including thyroid insufficiency and primary hypogonadism.[7] Thyroid insufficiency and lack of thyroxine hormone results in overproduction of hypothalamic thyrotropin-releasing hormone, which in turn leads to thyrotroph hyperplasia in the pituitary gland and increased thyroid-stimulating hormone production. In addition, prolactin releasing cells may be stimulated and these patients may present clinically due to symptoms related to hyperprolactinemia.[7,12]

On imaging, the normal pituitary gland in children should be less than 6 mm in height and in young menstruating female patients less than 10 mm in height. During puberty, and in pregnant as well as lactating patients, pituitary heights up to 12 mm can be normal (Fig. 4).[7,8] In both physiologic and pathologic pituitary hyperplasia, the pituitary gland demonstrates diffuse symmetric enlargement and, especially in pathologic cases, the gland can extend far into the suprasellar cistern, even causing mass effect on the prechiasmatic optic nerves and optic chiasm.[1,7,12] In contrast to macroadenomas, there is no remodeling of the sella, and the gland will always show homogenous postcontrast enhancement.[12] On precontrast and postcontrast T1-weighted images, as well as on T2-weighted images, the gland will be homogenous in signal (see Fig. 4).[12]

### Empty Sella

The empty sella, defined as a pituitary gland measuring 2 mm or less in height with cerebrospinal fluid (CSF) occupying greater than half of the sella (see Fig. 4),[1] is rare in children, with an incidence of about 1% in patients with a normal hypothalamic-pituitary axis.[29,30] Primary empty sella occurs when CSF enters the sella through a rent in the sellar diaphragm and may or may not be associated with increased intracranial pressure. Secondary empty sella occurs as a result of injury to the pituitary itself, for example, in the setting of pituitary apoplexy, or following surgery or radiation treatment. In adults, the empty sella is commonly seen in older, obese, or hypertensive patients, and may often be asymptomatic. In children, conversely, an empty sella is more likely associated with clinical symptoms and endocrinopathies, especially growth hormone deficiency, hypogonadism, or multiple pituitary hormone deficiency. In children with known endocrinopathy, empty sella may be seen in up to 68% of patients.[29,30] Thus, the presence of an empty sella in the pediatric population should prompt endocrinologic and ophthalmologic evaluation.[30]

### INFUNDIBULAR LESIONS

Pediatric patients with central diabetes insipidus typically have absence of the posterior pituitary T1-bright spot and about one-third of them also show thickening of the infundibulum.[31] The most common causes in these cases are Langerhans cell histiocytosis (LCH) and germinoma (see later discussion).[12,32] If the infundibulum is initially normal on imaging, follow-up imaging in these patients with so-called idiopathic central diabetes insipidus is warranted because a time lag of up to 14 months has been reported in detecting an infundibular lesion.[33] Other differential considerations for infundibular lesions in the pediatric age group include granulomatous disease (eg, sarcoid and tuberculosis [TB]) and lymphocytic hypophysitis.

### Langerhans Cell Histiocytosis

LCH is a rare idiopathic disorder characterized by proliferation of Langerhans cell histiocytes, resulting in the formation of granulomas and can be found in any organ system.[34] The clinical course of LCH is variable, ranging from a solitary lytic bone or skin lesions with complete remission to a multisystem disorder with potentially lethal outcome.[34] The peak incidence is between the ages of 1 to 4 years but LCH can present at any age from the newborn period to the geriatric age group.[12,35] Intracranial involvement most

Fig. 3. Microadenoma in 2 patients (A–D) and macroadenoma in a third patient (E–F). The microadenomas demonstrate slight intrinsic T1 hypointensity on the T1 precontrast images (A, C), and are hypoenhancing relative to the normal surrounding pituitary enhancement on the T1 postcontrast images (B, D). The macroadenoma extends into the suprasellar cistern and exerts mass effect on the optic chiasm (E, F); is heterogeneous in signal intensity, with a focal area of intrinsic T1 hyperintensity superiorly compatible with proteinaceous or hemorrhagic contents (E); and demonstrates extension into the patient's left cavernous sinus, best seen on the postcontrast sequence (F). Normal-appearing pituitary gland is seen along the floor of the sella to the patient's right (F).

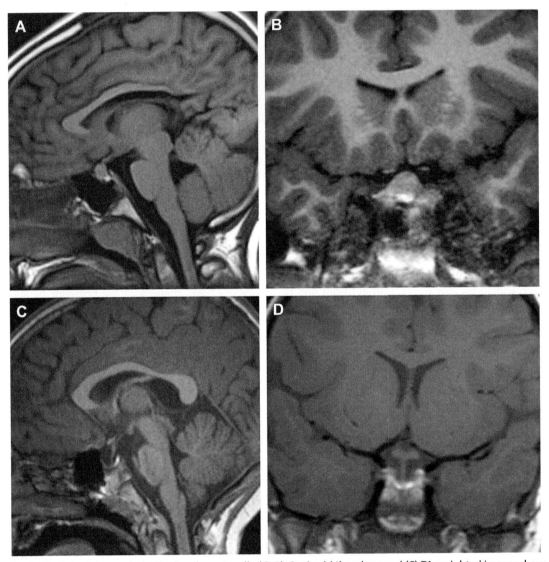

**Fig. 4.** Physiologic hyperplasia (*A, B*) and empty sella (*C, D*). Sagittal (*A*) and coronal (*B*) T1-weighted images show homogenous T1 isointense enlargement of the pituitary gland, with extension into the suprasellar cistern in this 12-year-old adolescent. Sagittal (*C*) and coronal (*D*) T1-weighted images in another patient show thinned pituitary gland along the floor of the sella with CSF signal occupying the remainder of the sella.

commonly occurs in the form of a lytic bone mass or diabetes insipidus. In multicentric LCH, the hypothalamus and infundibulum are involved in up to 20% of patients[12,34] and, in those cases, diabetes insipidus and absence of the posterior pituitary bright spot are also typically present.[34] When involved, the infundibulum becomes focally or diffusely thickened (typically > 3.5 mm if proximal, or >2 mm if distal) and enhances avidly.[34] The pituitary gland itself may also be involved in up to about 10% of patients with central nervous system (CNS) involvement, with imaging demonstrating infiltration and enlargement of the gland.[34]

Neither absence of the posterior pituitary bright spot nor thickening of the infundibulum is specific to LCH, and there is significant imaging overlap with germinomas and the other entities discussed in this section (**Fig. 5**). However, there may often be additional findings to suggest the diagnosis of LCH. For example, calvarial involvement with lytic punched-out bone lesions in the skull, including the frontal, parietal, and mastoid portion of the temporal bones, is common, as are involvement of the orbit and facial bones.[12,34] Additional findings that may be encountered include prominent Virchow-Robin spaces, white matter parenchymal changes with a leukoencephalopathy-like pattern,

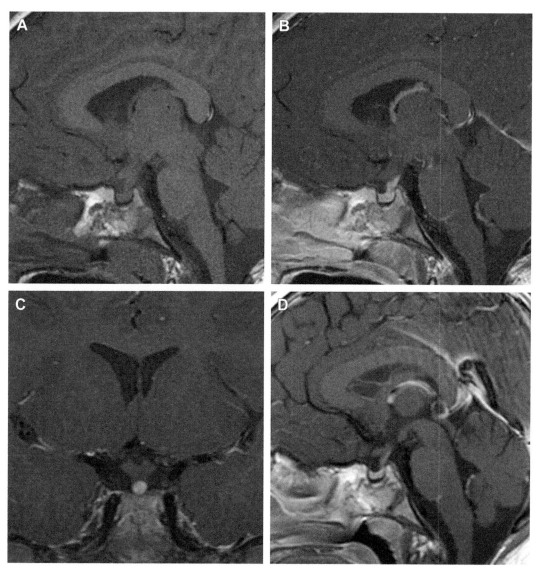

**Fig. 5.** Lymphocytic hypophysitis. The patient initially presented at 5 years of age with panhypopituitarism, central diabetes insipidus, and growth restriction. Sagittal T1-weighted precontrast (*A*) and postcontrast (*B*), as well as coronal postcontrast (*C*) images show absence of the posterior pituitary bright spot (*A*) and a thickened nodular enhancing infundibulum (*B*, *C*). Initial imaging findings were thought to be due to LCH. However, no other lesions were found elsewhere in the body and thickening of the infundibulum gradually resolved on follow-up imaging. Five years after the images obtained in *A–C*, a sagittal T1-weighted postcontrast image shows interval near complete resolution of the infundibular thickening (*D*). The final diagnosis was presumed to be lymphocytic hypophysitis.

and gray matter signal changes in the cerebellar dentate nucleus and basal ganglia.[36]

## Lymphocytic Hypophysitis

Lymphocytic hypophysitis is a rare, most likely autoimmune, inflammatory disease of the pituitary gland that typically affects women in their ante-postpartum or immediate postpartum period.[37] Based on the anatomic location involved, it may be classified as primarily affecting the adenohypophysis, the infundibulum plus neurohypophysis, or the entire gland.[1,38] Symptoms reflect the site of disease and are due to anterior or posterior pituitary dysfunction, as well as mass effect on adjacent structures. When the infundibulum and neurohypophysis are involved, diabetes insipidus is the most common presenting symptom.[38,39] Lymphocytic hypophysitis is rare in children but, when present, about 50% of these patients present with involvement of both the adenohypophysis and neurohypophysis,[38] and central diabetes insipidus is commonly present. In adults, by comparison, the adenohypophysis is typically the primary site of involvement.[39]

Imaging depends on which part of the pituitary is primarily involved. With primary adenohypophyseal involvement, as characteristically seen in adults in the peripartum period, typical findings include an enhancing mass centered in the anterior lobe of the pituitary, which may demonstrate triangular extension toward the infundibulum, along with a dural tail, which is from enhancement and inflammation of the diaphragm sella.[40] In some cases, there may be more prominent suprasellar extension toward the hypothalamus.[40] Unlike pituitary adenomas, the pituitary stalk typically remains midline, which may help differentiate between these 2 entities. With involvement of the infundibulum and neurohypophysis, there is thickening of the pituitary stalk (>3.5 mm at the median eminence), with loss of the normal smooth infundibular tapering (see Fig. 5). In addition, there is absence of the posterior pituitary bright spot (see Fig. 5). If the entire gland is involved, there will typically be diffuse inflammatory change in and around the sella, with involvement of the optic chiasm and cavernous sinuses.[1]

*Granulomatous Hypophysitis*

Granulomatous hypophysitis represents a histologically distinct variant of hypophysitis that may be idiopathic, associated with infection (eg, fungal, TB, or syphilis), or systemic processes (eg, sarcoidosis, granulomatosis with polyangiitis [Wegener], LCH, or Erdheim-Chester disease).[39] Granulomatous inflammation can also occur as a result of rupture of a Rathke cleft cyst.[12] The imaging is typically nonspecific and overlaps with that of lymphocytic hypophysitis. Clues to the correct diagnosis may come from ancillary imaging findings outside of the sellar region, CNS analysis, and clinical presentation. See later discussion of imaging findings typically seen with TB and sarcoidosis.

Infection with *Mycobacterium tuberculosis* continues to be of major international concern, with about 9 million cases detected in 2013, 1.5 million of which resulted in death.[41] Of these cases, 15% present with extrapulmonary TB with higher associated mortality and morbidity. Tuberculous meningitis, to which young children in particular are highly susceptible, is the most frequently observed form of tuberculous CNS involvement.[42,43] In tuberculous meningitis, thick nodular leptomeningeal enhancement in the basal cisterns,

perivascular spaces, or along cranial nerves is typical (Fig. 6). When the sella and parasellar structures are involved, patients may present with diabetes insipidus, hypopituitarism, or hyperprolactinemia from stalk compression. The pituitary stalk may show enlargement with nodular enhancement (see Fig. 6).[37] The presence of parenchymal tuberculomas, which may be centrally T2 hypointense (see Fig. 6), as well as pulmonary findings consistent with TB, may help suggest the correct diagnosis.

Sarcoidosis is an idiopathic systemic disease characterized histologically by the formation of noncaseating granulomas. It is rare in children and, compared with adults, children with neurosarcoidosis more commonly present with seizures and are less likely to have cranial nerve involvement.[44] On imaging, there is significant overlap with tuberculous meningitis, with nodular leptomeningeal enhancement predominantly in the basal cisterns. Similar to TB, the infundibulum may have a nodular thickened appearance.[45] Sarcoidosis is less likely than TB to show parenchymal nodules but is more likely to demonstrate focal pachymeningeal masses and dural thickening.

## SUPRASELLAR LESIONS

The superior aspect of the pituitary gland is delineated by the diaphragm sella above which the suprasellar cistern is located. The pituitary stalk or infundibulum traverses the diaphragm sella via an opening in the diaphragm. The suprasellar cistern contains the optic chiasm, the A1 segments of the anterior cerebral arteries, and the anterior communicating artery.[46] The superior border of the suprasellar cistern is formed by the hypothalamus and mammillary bodies. The median eminence and the tuber cinereum as parts of the hypothalamus lack a blood-brain barrier and enhance on postcontrast sequences. The anterior part of the mesencephalon forms the posterior border of the suprasellar cistern.

*Germ Cell Tumors*

Germ cell tumors are classified as germinomatous germ cell tumors (GCTs) or nongerminomatous GCTs (NGGCTs) and account for 4% to 11% of intracranial tumors.[1] These tumors are located in the pineal region, suprasellar region, or third ventricle. Suprasellar germ cell tumors encompass 75% of germ cell tumors in female patients, whereas pineal germ cell tumors comprise 70% of germ cell tumors in male patients. Bifocal germ cell tumors, with simultaneous involvement of the suprasellar and pineal region, are reported in 15% of cases.[1] The characteristic MR imaging

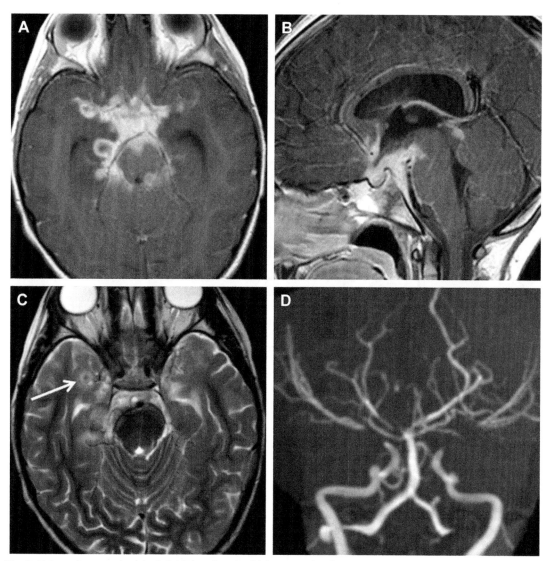

**Fig. 6.** Tuberculous meningitis. Axial (*A*) and sagittal (*B*) T1-weighted postcontrast enhanced images demonstrate thick, nodular leptomeningeal enhancement in the basal cisterns, with involvement of the suprasellar cistern and encasement of the infundibulum (*B*). A parenchymal tuberculoma with T2 hypointensity (*arrow*) is seen in the anterior right temporal lobe on the axial T2-weighted image (*C*). On the maximum intensity projection from the time-of-flight MR angiogram (*D*), marked narrowing of the distal internal carotid arteries, as well as the proximal middle and anterior cerebral arteries is present, caused by tuberculous vasculitis.

features include a small homogeneous lesion centered in the pituitary stalk or in the region of the infundibular recess. Thickening of the pituitary stalk associated with absence of the normal T1 hyperintense neurohypophysis bright spot may be seen (**Fig. 7**). The larger germ cell tumors have solid and cystic components. The solid components tend to show isointense to hypointense T2 signal intensity compared with gray matter and usually demonstrate significant contrast enhancement. Furthermore, the larger germ cell tumors typically have a tendency to infiltrate the

basal ganglia. These tumors show relatively mild peritumoral edema. The risk of leptomeningeal dissemination emphasizes the importance of imaging of the entire craniospinal axis (see **Fig. 7**).[46] In general, germinomas tend to have a better prognosis compared with NGGCTs.

Germinomas comprise 70% of all germ cell tumors with a peak incidence in patients between 10 and 14 years of age.[1,47] The clinical presentation often includes central diabetes insipidus, similar to LCH, and, as mentioned, in children presenting with central diabetes insipidus, the

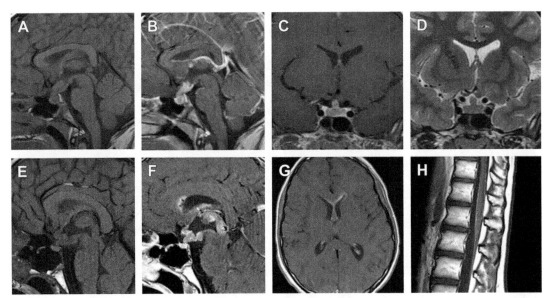

Fig. 7. Germinoma in 2 patients. In the first patient (A–D), absence of the posterior pituitary bright spot is seen on the sagittal T1 precontrast image (A). On the sagittal (B) and coronal (C) T1-weighted postcontrast images, marked nodular thickening of the infundibulum is demonstrated. The thickened infundibulum shows T2 hypointensity compatible with hypercellularity (D). In the second patient (E–H), precontrast (E) and postcontrast (F) T1-weighted images show nodular enhancing soft tissue masses centered in the infundibulum and floor of the third ventricle, as well as in the pineal region. Subependymal and leptomeningeal spread is evident both on the axial T1-weighted postcontrast image at the level of the lateral ventricles (G), as well as on the sagittal T1-weighted postcontrast image of the lower thoracic cord and conus medullaris (H).

appearance of an infundibular mass on imaging may lag symptomatic presentation by up to 14 months.[33] Suprasellar germinomas often involve the pituitary stalk and/or the hypothalamus, and may present with infundibular thickening and absence of the normal posterior pituitary bright spot; therefore, they may be difficult to distinguish from LCH or lymphocytic hypophysitis (see Fig. 7, compare to Fig. 5). The presence of basal ganglia and hypothalamus infiltration may help in those cases to suggest the diagnosis of a GCT. Due to their high cellularity, germinomas may demonstrate CT hyperdensity, hypointense T2 signal intensity, and restricted diffusion (see Fig. 7),[12] which helps distinguish them from pilocytic astrocytomas, which are characteristically T2 hyperintense.

NGGCTs are subdivided into teratomas, yolk sac tumors, embryonal carcinomas, and choriocarcinomas. NGGCTs may demonstrate elevated levels of tumor markers such as α- fetoprotein and β-human chorionic gonadotrophin in serum or CSF, which may be useful in distinguishing NGGCTs from germinomas.[12] Teratomas are often considered as a separate category from the other NGGCTs subtypes. Teratomas are composed of ectodermal, mesodermal, and/or endodermal elements, and may be benign or malignant. They are

the second most common type of germ cell tumors and are more common in male patients. Teratomas account for more than 50% of intracranial tumors in infants younger than 2 months of age.[47] In addition to the characteristic MR imaging features of germ cell tumors, teratomas often contain fat elements and may show signal suppression on fat-saturated sequences. They may also contain calcifications. Mature teratomas have capsules and do not damage the blood-brain barrier. Therefore, perilesional edema and enhancing solid components indicate immaturity of the teratoma.[46,47]

## Hypothalamic-Chiasmatic or Optic Pathway Glioma

Gliomas of the optic chiasm and hypothalamus account for 25% to 30% of suprasellar neoplasms in the pediatric population and 4% of all intracranial pediatric tumors.[1,47] Approximately 85% of optic pathway gliomas involve the hypothalamus or optic chiasm. Median age at diagnosis is 5 to 9 years. Vision loss, hydrocephalus, and hypothalamic dysfunction are common presenting symptoms. Almost all hypothalamic-chiasmatic gliomas in the pediatric population are low-grade, slow-growing World Health

Organization (WHO) grade I-II astrocytomas.[1,4,46,47] Distinguishing hypothalamic gliomas from optic chiasm gliomas is challenging, and is typically determined by locating the epicenter of the lesion and assessing for the presence or absence of optic nerve involvement. Large gliomas involve both the optic chiasm and hypothalamus, and the site of origin often cannot be determined (Fig. 8).[1,25]

Of patients with hypothalamic-chiasmatic gliomas, 20% to 50% have neurofibromatosis (NF)-type I.[25] NF1-associated hypothalamic-chiasmatic gliomas are almost always pilocytic astrocytomas (biopsy is rarely indicated), show a high degree of prechiasmatic optic nerve involvement, and present at a younger age. Sporadic, non-NF1–associated hypothalamic-chiasmatic gliomas more frequently show chiasmatic involvement and posterior extension beyond the optic pathways, and are associated with more aggressive astrocytomas.[1,46] Development of obstructive hydrocephalus is more common in sporadic hypothalamic-chiasmatic gliomas.[1]

The MR imaging features of pilocytic astrocytomas (WHO grade 1) include fusiform and/or nodular enlargement of the hypothalamus and/or optic chiasm with moderate T2 hyperintensity and hypointense or isointense T1 signal (see Fig. 8). Approximately 50% of lesions show contrast enhancement in a homogenous or, less commonly, in a rim-like pattern. Large lesions can demonstrate areas of cystic degeneration and sometimes grow into the pituitary stalk (see Fig. 8).[25,47] In these patients, it is important to assess for extension anteriorly along the optic nerves and/or posteriorly along the optic radiations.

The fourth (most recent) edition of the WHO *Classification of Tumors of the Central Nervous Systems* formally considers pilomyxoid astrocytoma as a distinct, more aggressive variant of pilocytic astrocytoma.[48] Pilomyxoid astrocytomas are considered WHO grade II neoplasms. These lesions have a strong predilection for the hypothalamus and chiasmatic region, tend to occur at an earlier mean age, and demonstrate more aggressive behavior (including CSF dissemination) and higher local recurrence rates compared with pilocytic astrocytomas.[1,47,48] MR imaging features include a large bulky U-shaped or H-shaped suprasellar lesion, T2 hyperintensity, and hypointense or isointense T1 signal. They typically extend toward or into the adjacent temporal lobes. Demonstration of intralesional hemorrhage favors pilomyxoid astrocytoma instead of pilocytic astrocytoma. More than 90% of lesions show contrast enhancement in a homogenous or, less likely, a heterogeneous or rim-like pattern.[48]

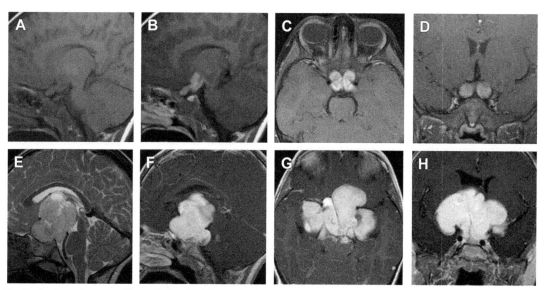

**Fig. 8.** Optic pathway and hypothalamic-chiasmatic glioma in 2 patients. In the first patient (*A–D*), precontrast (*A*) and postcontrast sagittal (*B*), axial (*C*), and coronal (*D*) T1-weighted images show an avidly enhancing mass centered in the prechiasmatic optic nerves and optic chiasm, with extension into the hypothalamus. In the second patient (*E–H*), a large multilobulated mass is seen in the region of the hypothalamus and optic chiasm. The mass is T2 hyperintense and has regions of cystic degeneration superiorly (*E*). The mass extends inferiorly toward the sella and compresses the upper margin of the pituitary (*E, H*). Solid portions show avid enhancement (*F–H*). Due to its large size, it is difficult to precisely localize the origin of this mass to the hypothalamus or optic chiasm.

## Hypothalamic Hamartoma

Hamartomas of the hypothalamus (tuber cinereum hamartomas) consist of disorganized heterotopic neural tissue arising in the hypothalamic region involving the inferior hypothalamus, tuber cinereum, and/or mammillary bodies. Because they are made up of heterotopic foci of neural tissue similar to hypothalamic neural tissue, they are largely composed of gray matter.[1,20] They are non-neoplastic and are considered congenital malformations. They increase in size over time in proportion to normal brain growth. The estimated incidence of hypothalamic hamartomas varies widely from 1 in 50,000 to 1 in 1,000,000 because not all lesions cause symptoms and the malformation can be an incidental finding.[1] They are more common in male patients and the clinical presentation depends on the type and location of the hamartoma.

Pedunculated parahypothalamic hamartomas are attached to the floor of the third ventricle (inferior hypothalamus, tuber cinereum, and/or mammillary bodies) by a stalk or narrow base and extend into the suprasellar cistern posterior to the pituitary stalk.[46] The presenting symptoms include isosexual central precocious puberty and seizures.[1,25] Sessile intrahypothalamic hamartomas are encased in the hypothalamus, have a broad attachment to the hypothalamus, and typically deform the third ventricle.[46] Presenting symptoms include the characteristic gelastic seizures.[1] Hypothalamic hamartomas may be associated with holoprosencephaly, midline facial, and cardiac and renal anomalies.[1,47]

The MR imaging features include a pedunculated or sessile lesion with T1 signal intensity isointense to gray matter (Fig. 9). The T2 signal intensity depends on the glial component of the hamartoma resulting in signal intensity, which may be similar to or slightly hyperintense or hypointense to gray matter. The lesion shows no contrast enhancement (see Fig. 9).[1] Intralesional cystic or fatty elements may occasionally be seen. MR spectroscopy of the lesion can demonstrate elevated myoinositol values.[46,47] The lack of contrast enhancement and stable interval size and signal intensity allow differentiation of hypothalamic hamartomas from gliomas.

## Lipomas

Intracranial lipomas are thought to derive from abnormal persistence of the primitive meninges (meninx primitiva) with differentiation into mature adipose tissue[1,20,46] and are, therefore, considered congenital malformations rather than intracranial benign tumors. The persistence of the primitive meninges may influence development of adjacent intracranial structures. Thus, hypoplasia of the mammillary bodies and hypothalamic hamartoma are developmental anomalies associated with intracranial lipomas.[1,46] Intracranial lipomas are typically located in or just off midline. About 11% arise in the suprasellar region[1] and common locations are along the surface of the infundibulum, along the floor of the third ventricle, or adjacent to cranial nerves.[47] Typically, they are incidental findings, although in some cases there is mass effect from enlargement, which can make them symptomatic.

On imaging, lipomas are homogenous in appearance with signal intensity similar to subcutaneous fat on all imaging sequences and show no enhancement. Within the cisternal spaces, traversing vessels are encircled rather than displaced, which, along with their greater homogeneity, helps distinguish lipomas from dermoids.[1,20,47] Fat-suppressed T1-weighted images are also useful to differentiate lipomas from lesions with hemorrhagic or proteinaceous contents.

Osteolipomas are rare intracranial lipomatous lesions. They are consistently located between the infundibular stalk and the mammillary bodies. The MR imaging features include 1 or more lesions with central fatty elements and peripheral osseous tissue or rim calcifications.[49]

## Dermoids and Epidermoids

Dermoid and epidermoid cysts are congenital inclusion cysts resulting from inclusion of epithelial elements during embryonic closure of the neural tube. The cysts are lined by squamous epithelium[46,50] and are commonly located in the sellar and suprasellar region. Intracranial epidermoid cysts are 4 to 10 times more common than intracranial dermoid cysts.[12] Both types of inclusion cyst show a slight male predilection and both have the potential to increase in volume due to accumulation of desquamated cell debris originating from the capsule of the cyst.[49]

Dermoid cysts are extra-axial lesions and almost always located in the midline. The cysts contain variable amounts of dermal derivates, such as fluid, lipid material, cholesterol, keratinaceous debris, calcification, and hair. Depending on the content of the cyst, MR imaging features consist of a well-circumscribed spherical or multilobulated lesion with T1 hyperintense signal (if fat is present) intermixed with T1 hypointense foci and heterogeneous T2 signal intensity, and no contrast enhancement.[1,12,20] On fat-saturated sequences, the fatty elements show signal dropout. The lesion may demonstrate fluid-fluid

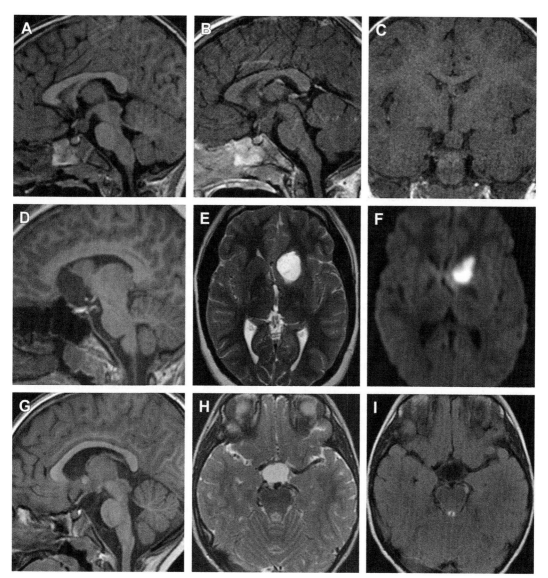

**Fig. 9.** Hamartoma (*A–C*), epidermoid cyst (*D–F*), and arachnoid cyst (*G–I*). Sagittal T1 precontrast (*A*), postcontrast (*B*), and coronal precontrast (*C*) images show a nonenhancing soft tissue mass centered between the mammillary bodies and the infundibulum, with signal characteristics similar to gray matter, compatible with a tuber cinereum hamartoma. Sagittal T1 precontrast (*D*), axial T2 (*E*), and axial DWIs (*F*) show an extra-axial lesion centered in the left paramedian suprasellar cistern with signal characteristics similar to CSF and with evidence of restricted diffusion, compatible with an epidermoid inclusion cyst. Sagittal T1 precontrast (*G*), axial T2-weighted (*H*), and axial fluid-attenuated inversion recovery (FLAIR) (*I*) images show a suprasellar lesion that has signal characteristics identical to CSF, including complete FLAIR suppression. In contrast, the epidermoid depicted in (*D–F*) lacked FLAIR suppression (not shown).

or fluid-debris levels, and local mass effect can be seen.[46] In case of rupture of a dermoid cyst, numerous T1 hyperintense foci are spread in the subarachnoid spaces. Lack of enhancement differentiates these lesions from teratomas.

Epidermoid cysts are typically extra-axial lesions located off-midline or asymmetric to 1 side of the midline. The degree of proteinaceous fluid

in the cysts varies. On MR imaging, they are relatively well circumscribed lesions with subtle surface irregularity and may be either subtly T1 hypointense or hyperintense depending on their protein content. When the protein content is low, the signal intensity is similar to CSF on conventional sequences, although there is typically subtle lack of fluid-attenuated inversion recovery (FLAIR) suppression present (see Fig. 9). DWI typically shows restricted diffusion and there is no contrast enhancement (see Fig. 9).[1,12] Epidermoids commonly insinuate within cisterns and encase neurovascular structures.[12]

The location (midline or off-midline) and the MR signal characteristics of the lesion often suggest the diagnosis of either dermoid or epidermoid cyst. However, both lesions may demonstrate significant overlap in imaging features and, to a lesser degree, in location.[50] The presence of restricted diffusion; the subtle surface irregularity of the lesion; the encasement, rather than displacement of neurovascular structures; and the lack of complete FLAIR suppression are helpful features to differentiate epidermoid cysts from arachnoid cysts.

## Arachnoid Cyst

Arachnoid cysts are developmental in origin and arise either from an obstructed arachnoid diverticulum, from failure of merging of the embryonic meninges or de novo from subarachnoid rests. Secondary arachnoid cysts may result from trauma, hemorrhage, infection, or iatrogenic causes.[47] Arachnoid cysts comprise 1% of all intracranial masses and approximately 9% to 15% of supratentorial arachnoid cysts occur in the suprasellar region.[1,25] When large, they may become symptomatic with varied presentations, including signs and symptoms of obstructive hydrocephalus, visual deficits, endocrine dysfunction, gait ataxia, and rarely may cause bobble-head doll syndrome.[51] The MR imaging features consist of a homogenous cystic lesion with or without visible cyst wall and signal intensity similar to CSF on all sequences (see Fig. 9). The lesion shows no restricted diffusion and no contrast enhancement. The presence of chronic CSF pulsation within the arachnoid cyst may result in remodeling or thinning of the adjacent calvarium.[46]

## Other Suprasellar Masses

Gangliogliomas are benign tumors composed of neurons and glial cells. These are rare tumors, responsible for 0.4% to 1.3% of brain tumors, and suprasellar gangliogliomas involving the hypothalamus and/or optic chiasm are even less common.[49] These lesions are typically found in adolescents or young adults. The clinical presentation often consists of visual impairment and pituitary dysfunction. The MR imaging features are nonspecific with demonstration of a solid or partially cystic lesion with isointense to hypointense T1 signal intensity and hyperintense T2 signal intensity. The lesions show solid or nodular rim enhancement.[49]

Hemangioblastomas are benign vascular tumors and when associated with von Hippel-Lindau disease, they typically occur in the pediatric population. A few cases arising from the hypothalamic-pituitary axis have been reported and these are strongly correlated with von Hippel-Lindau disease.[49] The MR imaging features include a complex cystic lesion with intensely enhancing mural nodule. Flow voids may be identified.

Heterotopic cerebellar masses are organized dysplastic collections of cerebellar cells localized at inappropriate locations in the cerebellum and, less commonly, in the orbits, spine, and suprasellar region. Isolated normal cerebellar tissue in various anatomic locations is hypothesized to be due to maldifferentiation of pluripotent cells. The heterotopic cerebellar tissue can cause clinical symptoms, depending on the size and location of the mass. The MR imaging features are similar to hypothalamic hamartoma and the diagnosis has to be established based on histology.[52]

Ecchordosis physaliphora is a rare congenital hamartoma of ectopic notochordal remnant tissue. Typically, the lesion is intradural and projecting off the clivus in the prepontine cistern but may rarely extend into the suprasellar cistern or present as a solitary lesion in the suprasellar cistern.[46]

## Third Ventricular Lesions

The lamina terminalis forms the anterior wall of the third ventricle toward the optic chiasm. The contour of the inferior anterior wall of the third ventricle is formed by the optic recess and the infundibular recess of the proximal hypothalamic infundibulum. The median eminence created by focal thickening of the hypothalamic gray matter forms the base of the infundibulum. The median eminence and the tuber cinereum together shape the floor of the third ventricle. The subthalamus forms the posterior part of the floor of the third ventricle.[53] Third ventricular lesions may cause expansion of the third ventricle into the suprasellar region.

## Intraventricular Cyst

Congenital intraventricular cysts of the third ventricle are rare. The different subtypes include arachnoidal, neuroepithelial, and ependymal. The clinical presentation is typically related to (intermittent) hydrocephalus due to obstruction of the sylvian aqueduct or foramina of Monro. MR imaging features consist of a thin-walled intraventricular cyst with signal intensity similar to CSF on all sequences. High-resolution, thin-slice, T2-weighted imaging is indicated to delineate the cyst and to not misinterpret the imaging appearance as a dilated third ventricle.[53]

## Choroid Plexus Papilloma and Carcinoma

Choroid plexus papillomas are low-grade WHO grade 1 neoplasms. The tumors originate from the epithelium of the choroid plexus. The fewest, approximately 5% to 10%, arise in the third ventricle.[1,53] Choroid plexus papillomas cause overproduction of CSF, mechanical obstruction, and impaired CSF resorption due to hemorrhage. As a consequence, hydrocephalus typically develops (Fig. 10). The characteristic imaging features include a multilobulated lesion in the third ventricle with CT isodensity to hyperdensity and variable T1 and T2 signal intensities. The lesion demonstrates flow voids and strong enhancement and may show calcifications (see Fig. 10).[1]

Atypical choroid plexus papilloma (aCPP) is a recently identified entity added to the fourth edition of the WHO *Classification of Tumors of the Central Nervous Systems*. aCPPs are intermediate WHO grade II neoplasms. They demonstrate younger age at presentation, earlier metastases, and a higher recurrence rate compared with choroid plexus papillomas.[48] The MR imaging features are identical to those of choroid plexus papillomas, except for the more prevalent bleeding. The only potential discriminating feature is presentation in a child younger than 5 years of age.[48]

Choroid plexus carcinomas are rare neoplasms in the pediatric populations. The overall features are similar to (atypical) choroid plexus papillomas, although these tumors may show more aggressive features with extension into the adjacent brain parenchyma.[53]

## Ependymoma

Ependymomas are glial tumors originating from differentiated ependymal cells lining the ventricular wall. Few supratentorial ependymomas are intraventricular and they rarely involve the third ventricle. In the pediatric population, these tumors most commonly arise in the adolescent

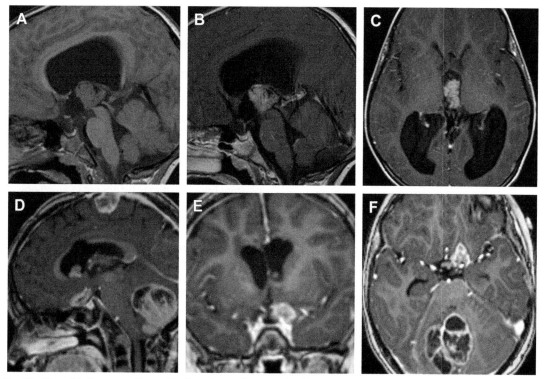

Fig. 10. Choroid plexus papilloma (*A–C*) and ependymoma (*D–F*). Sagittal T1 precontrast (*A*), as well as sagittal (*B*) and axial (*C*) postcontrast images, demonstrate an avidly enhancing mass centered in the third ventricle. The ventricles are enlarged, a common finding in patients with choroid plexus papilloma. Sagittal (*D*), coronal (*E*), and axial (*F*) T1 postcontrast images show a heterogeneous partially solid and partially cystic-necrotic posterior fossa mass, representing the patient's known recurrent ependymoma. There is evidence of leptomeningeal spread, including to the left parasellar region (*D–F*), left lateral ventricle (*D*), and left paracentral lobule (enhancing mass in upper aspect of *D*).

age group.[1] Ependymomas may be predominantly solid or may be partially cystic and partially solid and may show intratumoral hemorrhage. The solid components shows intense contrast enhancement.[53] These tumors have a propensity for leptomeningeal spread (see **Fig. 10**).[47]

### Secondary Extension by Suprasellar or Infundibular Lesions

Suprasellar and infundibular masses may extend into the third ventricle. In particular, astrocytomas, germinomas, and CPs have a tendency to demonstrate mass effect on or involvement of the third ventricle.

## PARASELLAR AND OTHER LESIONS IN AND AROUND THE SELLA

The lateral margins of the sella turcica are formed by the thin medial dural walls of the cavernous sinuses. The cavernous sinuses are dural venous channel extending from the orbital apex to Meckel cave, draining venous blood dorsally into the superior and inferior petrosal sinuses. Contents of the cavernous sinuses include the cavernous segment of the internal carotid artery and the abducens nerve, which course centrally through the cavernous sinus. From superior to inferior, the oculomotor nerve, the trochlear nerve, and the ophthalmic and maxillary divisions of the trigeminal nerve course within the dura duplicature lining the lateral cavernous sinus.

### Schwannoma

Schwannomas in the region of the cavernous sinus are rare in the pediatric population and, if present, are often associated with NFII. Schwannomas of the trigeminal nerve are the most common type to involve the cavernous sinus and they have a tendency to extend into the Meckel cave (**Fig. 11**). On imaging, these are well-defined lobulated enhancing lesions with hyperintense T2 signal intensity and, sometimes, cystic components (see **Fig. 11**).[47,54]

### Plexiform Neurofibroma

Plexiform neurofibromas are predominantly seen in patients with NFI. Parasellar plexiform neurofibromas frequently involve the trigeminal nerve, particularly the ophthalmic and maxillary divisions. On imaging, these typically present as lobular, serpiginous, infiltrative masses, withT2 hyperintense lobulations containing central hypointense foci (target signs).[47,54]

### Meningioma

Meningiomas are rare tumors in the pediatric age group. Similar to schwannomas, the occurrence of pediatric meningiomas is related to NFII. Meningiomas are extra-axial dural-based lesions. Parasellar locations include the lateral wall of the cavernous sinus, the diaphragm sella, the tuberculum sella, the anterior clinoid and the planum sphenoidale. The characteristic MR imaging features consist of an avidly enhancing lesion demonstrating a dural tail with signal intensity similar to gray matter (see **Fig. 11**).[54]

### Ectopic Posterior Pituitary Gland

Ectopic location of the posterior pituitary gland results from congenital malpositioning of the neurohypophysis during embryogenesis. The downward extension of the diencephalon (infundibulum) is incomplete, with resulting high position of the posterior pituitary gland in the infundibular or hypothalamic region. Hypothalamic releasing factors cannot reach the anterior pituitary gland via the portal circulation and are released into the systemic circulation. There is a male predilection and clinical presentation ranges from growth hormone deficiency to panhypopituitarism.[47] Associated anomalies include various midline brain malformations, including septo-optic dysplasia, Chiari 1 malformation, agenesis of the corpus callosum, and vermian dysplasia.[55]

The characteristic MR imaging features consist of an abnormal location of the T1 hyperintense posterior pituitary bright spot in the upper portion of the infundibulum or undersurface of the hypothalamus and an associated small anterior pituitary gland (see **Fig. 11**).[47] It should be noted that the posterior pituitary bright spot may be absent in an otherwise normal posterior pituitary gland as a physiologic variation without any associated clinical symptoms in up to 10% to 30% of the normal population.[56] On the other hand, several pathologic entities present with absence of the normal posterior bright spot with or without additional associated abnormalities as characteristic imaging features. These entities include LCH, lymphocytic hypophysitis, and germ cell tumors (see previous discussion).

### Osseous Lesions

Osteosarcomas, Ewing sarcomas, chondrosarcomas, and chordomas are bone tumors occurring in the pediatric population. Fibrous dysplasia results from failure in the remodeling process of primitive bone to mature lamellar bone (associated with McCune-Albright syndrome). Lesions of these osseous entities can be localized in the skull

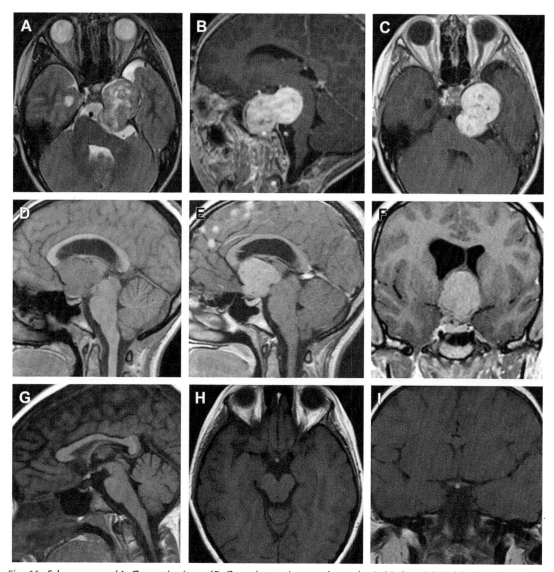

**Fig. 11.** Schwannoma (*A–C*), meningioma (*D–F*), and ectopic neurohypophysis (*G–I*). Axial T2 (*A*), sagittal oblique T1 postcontrast (*B*), and axial T1 postcontrast (*C*) images show a well-defined, lobulated, mildly T2 hyperintense mass containing small cysts (*A*) and involving the cisternal segment of the left trigeminal nerve root with extension into the left cavernous sinus and into left Meckel cave. Sagittal precontrast (*D*), as well as sagittal (*E*) and coronal (*F*) T1 postcontrast images, demonstrate an extra-axial enhancing mass centered in the suprasellar cistern, with additional dural-based masses seen along the falx (*E*) compatible with multiple meningiomas in this patient with NFII. Sagittal (*G*), axial (*H*), and coronal (*I*) precontrast T1-weighted images show an abnormal position of the posterior pituitary bright spot in the upper portion of the infundibulum and a small associated anterior pituitary gland in this patient with ectopic neurohypophysis.

base in the juxtasellar region (**Fig. 12**).[47] Rarely, extraosseous Ewing sarcoma can present as a primary extra-axial intracranial mass and may resemble a meningioma (see **Fig. 12**).[57]

## Persistent Embryonic Infundibular Recess

An abnormal contour of the anterior wall of the third ventricle is associated with malformations of the neurohypophysis. A persistent embryonic infundibular recess is a rare congenital malformation of the neurohypophysis, in which the distal aspect of the infundibular recess in not obliterated due to failure of cellular proliferation. The maldevelopment of the normal infundibular recess causes the anterior wall of the third ventricle to extend into the sella turcica. These patients may present with abnormal pituitary function.[53]

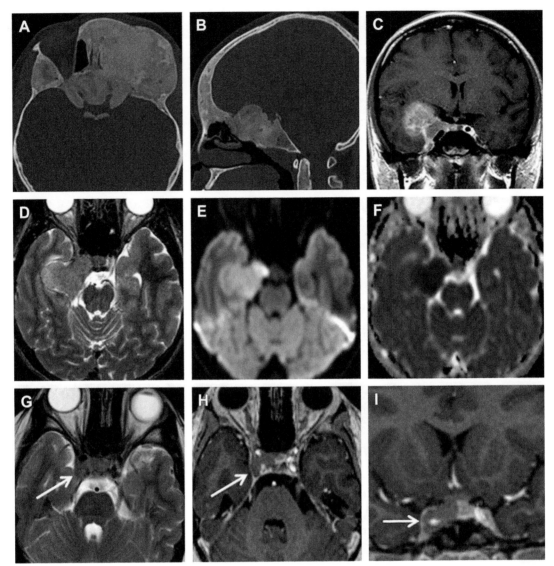

**Fig. 12.** Fibrous dysplasia (*A*, *B*), Ewing sarcoma (*C–F*), and Burkitt lymphoma (*G–I*). Axial (*A*) and sagittal (*B*) bone window CT images demonstrate expansile bony remodeling with ground glass opacity involving the skull base, including the sella, as well as the orbits and frontal bones, with imaging appearance characteristic for fibrous dysplasia. Coronal T1 postcontrast (*C*), axial T2-weighted (*D*), DWI (*E*), and apparent diffusion coefficient map (*F*) images show an extra-axial heterogeneously enhancing mass centered in the right cavernous sinus with extension into the right middle cranial fossa. The mass is T2 hypointense and demonstrates restricted diffusion compatible with a hypercellular tumor. Pathologic testing demonstrated rare intracranial extra-osseous Ewing sarcoma. Axial T2-weighted (*G*), T1 postcontrast (*H*), and coronal T1 postcontrast (*I*) images show a T2 hypointense mass expanding the right cavernous sinus (*arrows*), and showing relative hypoenhancement compared with the adjacent pituitary gland on which it exerts mass effect with compression and mild leftward displacement (*I*). Bone marrow biopsy demonstrated Burkitt lymphoma.

## Vascular Malformations

Various vascular anomalies can involve the juxtasellar region, including cavernous malformations, carotid cavernous fistulas, arterial aneurysms (saccular or giant aneurysms of the ophthalmic division of the internal carotid artery), arteriovenous malformations, and venous malformations.

Cavernous malformations (cavernomas) result from maldevelopment of vascular structures in the embryonic period and are the most common vascular lesion of the CNS in the pediatric population. In this age group, cavernous malformations demonstrate high growth rates and high risk of hemorrhage. These vascular malformations are occasionally identified in the hypothalamic region in the pediatric population.[49] On MR imaging, these present as T2 hyperintense lesions with a rim of hypointensity and associated susceptibility-related signal loss on SWI sequences secondary to recurrent hemorrhages. In the setting of recent hemorrhage, there will be surrounding vasogenic edema.[46,47]

## METASTASES

Metastatic dissemination can reach the sellar and suprasellar region via CSF dissemination or via hematogenous spread. CSF dissemination often involves subarachnoid metastatic dissemination to the third ventricle with the infundibular recess as a favored site for metastatic deposits. Hematogenous dissemination commonly affects the posterior pituitary gland and the pituitary stalk due to the systemic arterial supply of these regions.[20] In general, metastatic dissemination to the sellar and suprasellar region is rare in the pediatric population. Certain pediatric intracranial tumors have a high propensity for CSF dissemination, including ependymoma (see **Fig. 10**), medulloblastoma, germinoma (see **Fig. 7**), pineoblastoma, neuroblastoma of the skull base, lymphomatous tumors (see **Fig. 12**), or leukemia.[1,20,47] The MR imaging features of metastatic disease are varied and depend on the underlying pathologic condition but include focal sellar or parasellar lesions, multiple nodular lesions, and/or abnormal leptomeningeal enhancement.[20]

## SUMMARY

Sellar and parasellar masses are not infrequent in the pediatric population, comprising about 10% of all pediatric brain tumors; however, the type and frequency of tumors is quite different than what is encountered in adults. Imaging is a critical component in diagnosis and characterization of these lesions. By assessing the site of origin, signal, and contrast enhancement characteristics, the differential diagnosis can typically be narrowed down to 1 or a few possibilities. The clinical presentation is also important and often characteristic for a type of lesion, and should be taken into account when interpreting images.

## REFERENCES

1. Schroeder JW, Vezina LG. Pediatric sellar and suprasellar lesions. Pediatr Radiol 2011;41(3): 287–98.
2. Tindall GT, Hoffman JC Jr. Evaluation of the abnormal sella turcica. Arch Intern Med 1980; 140(8):1078–83.
3. Taylor M, Couto-Silva AC, Adan L, et al. Hypothalamic-pituitary lesions in pediatric patients: endocrine symptoms often precede neuro-ophthalmic presenting symptoms. J Pediatr 2012;161(5):855–63.
4. Nair AG, Pathak RS, Iyer VR, et al. Optic nerve glioma: an update. Int Ophthalmol 2014;34(4):999–1005.
5. Chambers TJ, Giles A, Brabant G, et al. Wnt signaling in pituitary development and tumorigenesis. Endocr Relat Cancer 2013;20(3):R101–11.
6. Kitamura E, Miki Y, Kawai M, et al. T1 signal intensity and height of the anterior pituitary in neonates: correlation with postnatal time. AJNR Am J Neuroradiol 2008;29(7):1257–60.
7. De Sousa SM, Earls P, McCormack AI. Pituitary hyperplasia: case series and literature review of an under-recognised and heterogenous condition. Endocrinol Diabetes Metab Case Rep 2015;2015: 150017.
8. Chanson P, Daujat F, Young J, et al. Normal pituitary hypertrophy as a frequent cause of pituitary incidentaloma: a follow-up study. J Clin Endocrinol Metab 2001;86(7):3009–15.
9. Spampinato MV, Castillo M. Congenital pathology of the pituitary gland and parasellar region. Top Magn Reson Imaging 2005;16(4):269–76.
10. Teramoto A, Hirakawa K, Sanno N, et al. Incidental pituitary lesions in 1,000 unselected autopsy specimens. Radiology 1994;193(1):161–4.
11. Takanashi J, Tadea H, Barkovich AJ, et al. Pituitary cysts in childhood evaluated by MR imaging. AJNR Am J Neuroradiol 2005;26(8):2144–7.
12. Hess CP, Dillon WP. Imaging the pituitary and parasellar region. Neurosurg Clin N Am 2012; 23(4):529–42.
13. Binning MJ, Gottfried ON, Osborn AG. Rathke cleft cyst intracystic nodule: a characteristic magnetic resonance imaging finding. J Neurosurg 2005; 103(5):837–40.
14. Byun WM, Kim OL, Kim D. MR imaging findings of Rathke's cleft cysts: significance of intracystic nodules. AJNR Am J Neuroradiol 2000;21(3):485–8.
15. Xin W, Rubin MA, McKeever PE. Differential expression of cytokeratins 8 and 20 distinguishes craniopharyngioma from rathke cleft cyst. Arch Pathol Lab Med 2002;126(10):1174–8.
16. Karavitaki N, Wass JA. Craniopharyngiomas. Endocrinol Metab Clin North Am 2008;37(1):173–93.
17. Muller HL. Childhood craniopharyngioma. Pituitary 2013;16(1):56–67.
18. Rossi A, Cama A, Consales A, et al. Neuroimaging of pediatric craniopharyngiomas: a pictorial essay. J Pediatr Endocrinol Metab 2006; 19(Suppl 1):299–319.
19. Harrington MH, Casella SJ. Pituitary tumors in childhood. Curr Opin Endocrinol Diabetes Obes 2012; 19(1):63–7.

20. Rao VJ, James RA, Mitra D. Imaging characteristics of common suprasellar lesions with emphasis on MRI findings. Clin Radiol 2008; 63(8):939–47.

21. Zimmer A, Reith W. Tumors of the sellar and pineal regions. Radiologe 2014;54(8):764–71.

22. Karavitaki N, Cudlip S, Adams CB, et al. Craniopharyngiomas. Endocr Rev 2006;27(4):371–97.

23. Sartoretti-Schefer S, Wichmann W, Aguzzi W, et al. MR differentiation of adamantinous and squamous-papillary craniopharyngiomas. AJNR Am J Neuroradiol 1997;18(1):77–87.

24. Zhang YQ, Wang CC, Ma ZY. Pediatric craniopharyngiomas: clinicomorphological study of 189 cases. Pediatr Neurosurg 2002;36(2):80–4.

25. Kumar J, Kumar A, Sharma R, et al. Magnetic resonance imaging of sellar and suprasellar pathology: a pictorial review. Curr Probl Diagn Radiol 2007;36(6): 227–36.

26. Frangou EM, Tynan JR, Robinson CA, et al. Metastatic craniopharyngioma: case report and literature review. Childs Nerv Syst 2009;25(9):1143–7.

27. Steele CA, MacFarlane IA, Blair J, et al. Pituitary adenomas in childhood, adolescence and young adulthood: presentation, management, endocrine and metabolic outcomes. Eur J Endocrinol 2010; 163(4):515–22.

28. Elster AD, Sanders TG, Vines FS, et al. Size and shape of the pituitary gland during pregnancy and post partum: measurement with MR imaging. Radiology 1991;181(2):531–5.

29. Rath D, Sahoo RK, Choudhury J. Empty sella syndrome in a male child with failure to thrive. J Pediatr Neurosci 2015;10(1):45–7.

30. Lenz AM, Root AW. Empty sella syndrome. Pediatr Endocrinol Rev 2012;9(4):710–5.

31. Maghnie M, Cosi G, Genovese E, et al. Central diabetes insipidus in children and young adults. N Engl J Med 2000;343(14):998–1007.

32. Czernichow P, Garel C, Leger J. Thickened pituitary stalk on magnetic resonance imaging in children with central diabetes insipidus. Horm Res 2000; 53(Suppl 3):61–4.

33. Mootha SL, Barkovich AJ, Grumbach MM, et al. Idiopathic hypothalamic diabetes insipidus, pituitary stalk thickening, and the occult intracranial germinoma in children and adolescents. J Clin Endocrinol Metab 1997;82(5):1362–7.

34. Demaerel P, Van Gool S. Paediatric neuroradiological aspects of Langerhans cell histiocytosis. Neuroradiology 2008;50(1):85–92.

35. Kilborn TN, The J, Goodman TR. Paediatric manifestations of Langerhans cell histiocytosis: a review of the clinical and radiological findings. Clin Radiol 2003;58(4):269–78.

36. Prayer D, Grois N, Prosch H, et al. MR imaging presentation of intracranial disease associated with Langerhans cell histiocytosis. AJNR Am J Neuroradiol 2004;25(5):880–91.

37. Carpinteri R, Patelli I, Casanueva FF, et al. Pituitary tumours: inflammatory and granulomatous expansive lesions of the pituitary. Best Pract Res Clin Endocrinol Metab 2009;23(5):639–50.

38. Gellner V, Kurschel S, Scarpatetti M, et al. Lymphocytic hypophysitis in the pediatric population. Childs Nerv Syst 2008;24(7):785–92.

39. Molitch ME, Gillam MP. Lymphocytic hypophysitis. Horm Res 2007;68(Suppl 5):145–50.

40. Rivera JA. Lymphocytic hypophysitis: disease spectrum and approach to diagnosis and therapy. Pituitary 2006;9(1):35–45.

41. Zumla A, George A, Sharma V, et al. The WHO 2014 global tuberculosis report—further to go. Lancet Glob Health 2015;3(1):e10–2.

42. Gunes A, Uluca U, Aktar F, et al. Clinical, radiological and laboratory findings in 185 children with tuberculous meningitis at a single centre and relationship with the stage of the disease. Ital J Pediatr 2015;41(1):75.

43. Springer P, Swanevelder S, van Toorn R, et al. Cerebral infarction and neurodevelopmental outcome in childhood tuberculous meningitis. Eur J Paediatr Neurol 2009;13(4):343–9.

44. Baumann RJ, Robertson WC Jr. Neurosarcoid presents differently in children than in adults. Pediatrics 2003;112(6 Pt 1):e480–6.

45. Smith JK, Matheus MG, Castillo M. Imaging manifestations of neurosarcoidosis. AJR Am J Roentgenol 2004;182(2):289–95.

46. Derman A, Shields M, Davis A, et al. Diseases of the sella and parasellar region: an overview. Semin Roentgenol 2013;48(1):35–51.

47. Shields R, Mangla R, Almast J, et al. Magnetic resonance imaging of sellar and juxtasellar abnormalities in the paediatric population: an imaging review. Insights Imaging 2015;6(2):241–60.

48. Osborn AG, Salzman KL, Thurnher MM, et al. The new World Health Organization Classification of Central Nervous System Tumors: what can the neuroradiologist really say? AJNR Am J Neuroradiol 2012;33(5):795–802.

49. Saleem SN, Said AH, Lee DH. Lesions of the hypothalamus: MR imaging diagnostic features. Radiographics 2007;27(4):1087–108.

50. Connor SE, Penney CC. MRI in the differential diagnosis of a sellar mass. Clin Radiol 2003;58(1): 20–31.

51. Ramesh S, Raju S. Suprasellar arachnoid cyst presenting with bobble-head doll syndrome: report of three cases. J Pediatr Neurosci 2015;10(1):18–21.

52. Takhtani D, Melhem ER, Carson BS. A heterotopic cerebellum presenting as a suprasellar mass with associated nasopharyngeal teratoma. AJNR Am J Neuroradiol 2000;21(6):1119–21.

53. Glastonbury CM, Osborn AG, Salzman KL. Masses and malformations of the third ventricle: normal anatomic relationships and differential diagnoses. Radiographics 2011;31(7):1889–905.

54. Razek AA, Castillo M. Imaging lesions of the cavernous sinus. AJNR Am J Neuroradiol 2009; 30(3):444–52.

55. Mitchell LA, Thomas PQ, Zacharin MR, et al. Ectopic posterior pituitary lobe and periventricular heterotopia: cerebral malformations with the same underlying mechanism? AJNR Am J Neuroradiol 2002;23(9):1475–81.

56. Brooks BS, el Gammal T, Allison JD, et al. Frequency and variation of the posterior pituitary bright signal on MR images. AJNR Am J Neuroradiol 1989; 10(5):943–8.

57. Choudhury K, Sharma S, Kothari R, et al. Primary extraosseous intracranial Ewing's sarcoma: Case report and literature review. Indian J Med Paediatr Oncol 2011;32(2):118–21.

# Extraparenchymal Lesions in Pediatric Patients

Mary Tenenbaum, MD

## KEYWORDS

• Extraparenchymal brain lesions • Dermoid • Epidermoid • Tumor • Choroid plexus

## KEY POINTS

• The differential diagnosis for extraparenchymal lesions in the pediatric age group differs from that in adults.
• Etiology can be either neoplastic or nonneoplastic.
• Be aware of concerning clinical symptoms necessitating imaging.

## INTRODUCTION

Extraparenchymal lesions are those arising from intracranial structures other than the brain parenchyma. When a mass is diagnosed, it is key to identify features suggesting whether the lesion arises from the brain parenchyma or from the extraparenchymal structures, because the origin and location of the tumor can guide treatment, including determination of the resectability of the lesion, surgical approach, and prognosis. However, the differentiation of intraparenchymal lesions from extraparenchymal lesions can be challenging, and close attention to the imaging features of the mass lesions is required.

The etiology of extraparenchymal lesions is variable. They include both true neoplasms as well as congenital lesions. Neoplasms may be either benign or malignant, and either primary or metastatic, although metastatic disease is less common in children than adults. On this note, the common lesions affecting the extraparenchymal structures in the pediatric population differ from the common entities encountered in the adult population. As such, age plays an important role in the differential diagnosis and evaluation of these lesions.[1]

In children, dominant symptoms depend on the age and location of the tumor. Infants may present with increasing head circumference, lethargy, and vomiting. Older children may also report headaches, worsening school performance, and focal neurologic deficits, including cranial nerve palsies (Box 1).[1,2]

Symptoms may progress rapidly, especially in the context of an aggressive, rapidly growing tumor, or may progress slowly over time when tumors are slow growing and less aggressive. Because some of the associated symptoms are common and nonspecific, in particular headaches, determining when it is appropriate to consider imaging to evaluate for an underlying lesion can be a clinical challenge. Some guidelines for imaging have been suggested in the literature, with concerning predictors for central nervous system lesions summarized in Box 2. The greater the number of predictors present, the greater the risk of an underlying surgical lesion.

## NORMAL ANATOMY AND IMAGING TECHNIQUE

Key anatomic locations to examine for extraparenchymal lesions are the ventricles, subarachnoid spaces, and meninges. If a lesion is extraparenchymal, there should be a margin between the lesion and the underlying brain. Typically, the

Disclosures: Nothing to disclose.
Department of Radiology, Baystate Medical Center, 759 Chestnut Street, Springfield, MA 01199, USA
E-mail address: Mary.Tenenbaum@baystatehealth.org

Neuroimag Clin N Am 27 (2017) 123–134
http://dx.doi.org/10.1016/j.nic.2016.08.005
1052-5149/17/© 2016 Elsevier Inc. All rights reserved.

underlying brain parenchyma will be displaced by an extraparenchymal lesion, rather than infiltrated or replaced by it, as with intraparenchymal lesions.[1] Extraparenchymal lesions usually result in less parenchymal edema than lesions arising from the brain parenchyma itself. In addition, an extraparenchymal lesion may result in less mass effect relative to its size than an intraparenchymal lesion. Other features suggestive of an extraparenchymal rather than intraparenchymal lesion include involvement of bone, crossing the midline

without involvement of cerebral commissures, and less severe presenting symptoms.[1]

When considering imaging technique, MR imaging is preferable to computed tomography (CT) scanning for the evaluation of intracranial masses. MR imaging has greater sensitivity, especially in the subarachnoid spaces and posterior fossa, greater ability to differentiate tumor from normal structures, better ability to characterize tissues, and superior capability to determining tumor extent compared with SCT scanning.

If CT scanning is performed, noncontrast imaging is highly valuable for assessment of the presence of hemorrhage and calcifications. Noncontrast imaging also allows for assessment of tumor density, which is a surrogate for tumor cellularity. Highly cellular tumors should be hyperdense on CT scanning, whereas less cellular tumors are less dense. CT scans can also suggest the presence of fat.

MR imaging protocols should include at least T1-weighted, T2-weighted, diffusion-weighted, gradient echo or susceptibility weighted imaging, and fluid-attenuated inversion recovery imaging, as well as postcontrast T1-weighted imaging in multiple planes. Other potentially useful sequences include high-resolution T2-weighted sequences and volumetric T1-weighted sequences, because these studies can allow greater anatomic definition of tumor involvement regarding size, extent, and more direct visualization of the tissues involved (**Table 1**).

## IMAGING FINDINGS AND PATHOLOGY

Extraparenchymal Lesions in Childhood
- Choroid plexus tumors
- Dermoid/epidermoid

**Table 1**
**Imaging protocols for CT and MR imaging**

| CT | MR imaging |
| --- | --- |
| Noncontrast | Multiplanar imaging should include T1, T2, FLAIR, diffusion, GRE or SWI, and postcontrast T1 |
| Postcontrast can be considered, but usually is not needed because MR imaging provides more information and is usually performed. | Additional sequences such as high resolution T2-weighted and volumetric T1-weighted images may be helpful. |

*Abbreviations:* CT, computed tomography; FLAIR, fluid-attenuated inversion recovery; GRE, gradient echo; SWI, susceptibility weighted imaging.

- Arachnoid cysts
- Meningiomas (rare in childhood)
- Schwannomas (rare in childhood)
- Lymphoma/leukemia
- Miscellaneous

## Choroid Plexus Tumors

Choroid plexus tumors arise from the epithelium of the choroid plexus. This category includes choroid plexus papillomas (World Health Organization grade I), atypical choroid plexus papillomas (World Health Organization grade II), and choroid plexus carcinomas (World Health Organization grade III). Radiologically, these entities cannot be distinguished accurately, and diagnosis must be made on histology. However, papillomas outnumber carcinomas by approximately 5:1. Choroid plexus tumors are rare, accounting for only 2% to 6% of pediatric brain tumors. Choroid plexus tumors in

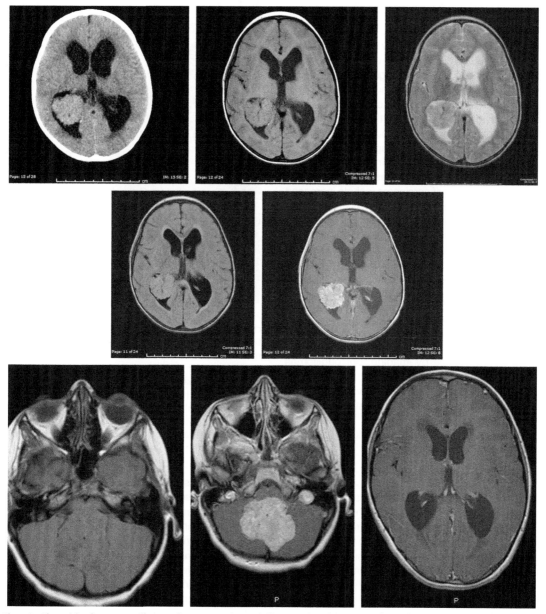

**Fig. 1.** Choroid plexus papilloma. (*Top row from left*) Axial computed tomography (CT), T1-weighted and T2-weighted images. (*Bottom row*) Axial fluid-attenuated inversion recovery (FLAIR) and postcontrast T1-weighted images. There is a hyperdense mass in the atrium of the right lateral ventricle on CT. The MR imaging images show a mass with avid frond like enhancement and central T2-weighted hypointense branching. There is associated hydrocephalus with transependymal cerebrospinal fluid flow demonstrated by periventricular FLAIR hyperintensity.

children most commonly arise in the lateral ventricles. Although they can occur at any age, choroid plexus papillomas usually present by 5 years of age in the pediatric population, and the most common reason for their discovery is severe hydrocephalus.[1,3,4] Hydrocephalus can occur in up to 80% of cases, and likely results from both overproduction of cerebrospinal fluid (CSF) by the tumor and impaired resorption, as well as obstruction.[5]

Choroid plexus papillomas have variable CT appearance, and can be isodense or hyperdense. Calcifications can be present. They are lobulated, and enhance homogeneously. On MR imaging (Fig. 1), they have a papillary appearance with branching pattern and may have cysts, septatations and/or, calcification. Hemorrhage may be demonstrated, especially in atypical choroid plexus papillomas and choroid plexus carcinomas. They enhance avidly. When arising in the fourth ventricle, they can extend through the outlet foramina and present as a cerebellopontine angle mass. Although there is considerable overlap in appearance between choroid plexus papillomas and carcinomas, features suggestive of carcinoma include increased heterogeneity, ill-defined margins, loss of branching pattern, restricted diffusion, and very high choline in the spectroscopy, owing to high cell density (Fig. 2).[6] Because choroid plexus carcinomas can metastasize, imaging of the spine should be performed to evaluate for leptomeningeal spread.[1,3,4]

Choroid Plexus Tumors
- Hydrocephalus is a key feature.
- Choroid plexus papilloma, atypical choroid plexus papilloma and carcinoma may be indistinguishable by imaging, but papillomas are much more common.
- Histology is needed for definitive diagnosis.
- Avidly enhancing masses, most commonly in the lateral ventricles.
- Consider spine imaging to evaluate for metastatic disease.

### Dermoid/Epidermoid

Both dermoids and epidermoids arise from congenital rests of tissue in the intracranial compartment. Epidermoids arise from the ectoderm only, whereas dermoids arise from both the ectoderm and mesoderm. Both lesions are more common in the posterior fossa than in the supratentorial compartment, with dermoids more often located in the midline; epidermoids can have a more variable location and greater off midline occurrence, especially in the cerebellopontine angle cistern. Given variability of location, the presentation is variable, including cranial neuropathies, and hydrocephalus, with these symptoms largely

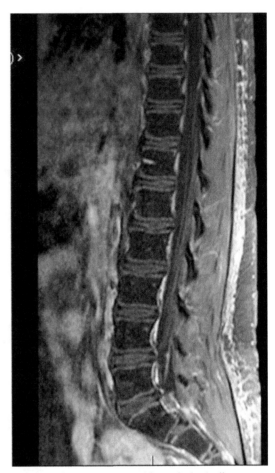

Fig. 2. Pediatric patient with pathologically proven choroid plexus carcinoma. Precontrast and postcontrast axial T1-weighted images show avidly enhancing mass centered in the fourth ventricle. This lesion has more irregular margins than the previous case of papilloma. Small nonenhancing cystic components are present. There is associated obstructive hydrocephalus. In this case, sagittal T1-weighted fat-saturated postcontrast imaging of the lumbar spine shows smooth and nodular leptomeningeal enhancement along the cauda equina indicating metastasis.

owing to a mass effect on adjacent structures. Dermoids may also present as chemical meningitis in the setting of rupture.[1,7–9]

On CT scanning, epidermoids may present with the same attenuation as CSF, making their detection challenging. On MR imaging (Figs. 3 and 4), however, epidermoids have a highly characteristic appearance with very high signal intensity on the diffusion-weighted image of an otherwise mildly heterogeneous cystic mass without enhancement. High-resolution T2-weighted imaging may be useful in assessing the boundaries and lobulated contour of these lesions, as well as the relationship to adjacent vessels and nerves.

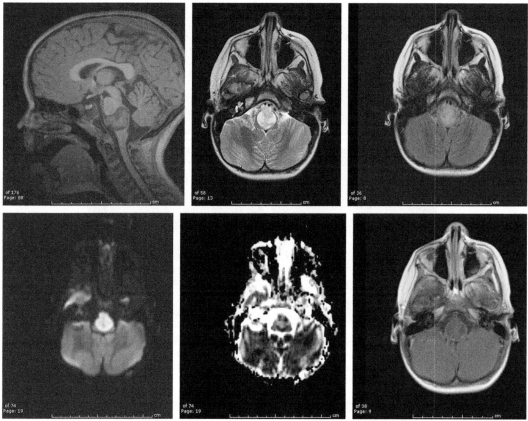

Fig. 3. A 33-month-old infant with progressive gait dysfunction. Sagittal T1-weighted, axial T2, axial T2-weighted fluid-attenuated inversion recovery, axial diffusion, apparent diffusion coefficient map (ADC map) and axial T1-weighted postcontrast images (*top to bottom, left to right*) show midline heterogeneous non enhancing cystic mass with very high signal intensity on DWI consistent with epidermoid tumor. The lesion compresses the brainstem.

On CT, dermoids typically appear as nonenhancing midline fat attenuation masses. On MR imaging (Fig. 5), they appear very similar to lipomas with intrinsic T1-weighted hyperintensity, which suppresses on fat-saturated imaging, and T2-weighted hypointensity. There may be variable signal cystic components. Close attention should be paid for evidence of T1-weighted hyperintense foci in the subarachnoid space, which would be indicative of a ruptured dermoid with chemical meningitis. When midline dermoid or epidermoid tumors are present, close examination for the presence of concurrent dermal sinus tracts is required, because they can present a source of recurrent infections[1,7–9] (Box 3).

## Arachnoid Cysts

Arachnoid cysts include congenital lesions of the arachnoid. Congenital arachnoid cysts expand by secretion and accumulation of CSF. Arachnoid cysts may also be acquired, and in this setting may result from previous trauma or inflammation with the development of loculation of CSF in regions of resultant scarring.[1]

Congenital arachnoid cysts most commonly occur sporadically, although there are some important syndromic associations, for example, polycystic kidney disease and Aicardi syndrome, where other congenital anomalies are typically demonstrated.[1]

Most arachnoid cysts are discovered incidentally and are asymptomatic. Although the true relationship between arachnoid cysts and clinical symptoms is unclear, large cysts can occasionally be associated with headaches, seizures, or neurologic deficits. Large cysts can also result in obstructive hydrocephalus. In addition, arachnoid cysts can rupture, resulting in subdural collections and midline shift. There can be associated hemorrhage.[10,11]

On both CT scans and MR imaging (Figs. 6–8), arachnoid cysts are well-marginated

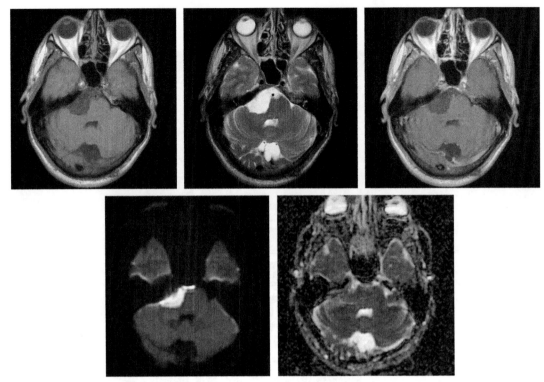

Fig. 4. (*Top*) Axial T1-weighted, T2-weighted, and T1-weighted postcontrast images. (*Bottom*) Diffusion trace and apparent diffusion coeficient images. A nonenhancing cystic mass with very high signal intensity on diffusion-weighted imaging in the right cerebellopontine angle cistern is consistent with an epidermoid. There is mass effect on the adjacent cerebellum and pons.

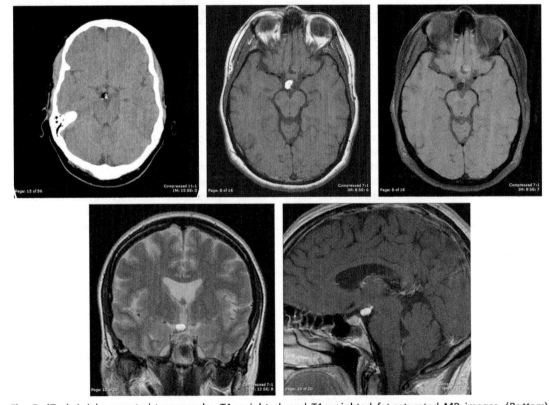

Fig. 5. (*Top*) Axial computed tomography, T1-weighted, and T1-weighted fat-saturated MR images. (*Bottom*) Coronal T2-weighted and sagittal T1-weighted postcontrast MR images. There is a right suprasellar fat containing mass with calcification consistent with a dermoid. Fat content is shown with suppression of signal on the T1-weighted fat-saturated sequence.

Box 3
Epidermoids and dermoids

*Epidermoids*

- May be indistinguishable from CSF on CT and T2

- High signal intensity on DWI is key to diagnosis, with similar appearance to CSF on other sequences (although some internal heterogeneity is usually present, especially on FLAIR)

- This is a common cerebellopontine angle cistern lesion, and a tendency to be off midline more than dermoids

*Dermoids*

- Fat attenuation midline mass on CT

- Fat signal similar to lipoma on MR imaging, but with some internal heterogeneity

- Be aware of chemical meningitis and look closely for evidence of rupture on MR imaging

- Look out for associated dermal sinus and infection

*Abbreviations:* CSF, cerebrospinal fluid; CT, computed tomography; DWI, diffusion-weighted imaging; FLAIR, fluid-attenuated inversion recovery.

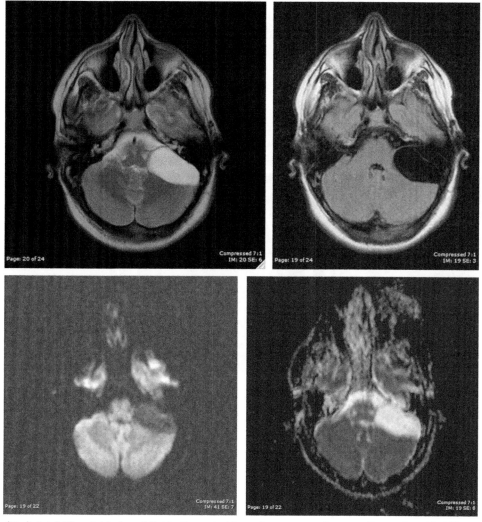

Fig. 6. (*Top*) Axial T2-weighted and fluid-attenuated inversion recovery images. (*Bottom*) Axial diffusion trace and apparent diffusion coefficient images. There is a well-circumscribed cystic structure in the left cerebellopontine angle cistern following cerebrospinal fluid signal on all sequences consistent with an arachnoid cyst. Note the lack of restricted diffusion, in contrast with the previous case of cerebellopontine angle cistern epidermoid.

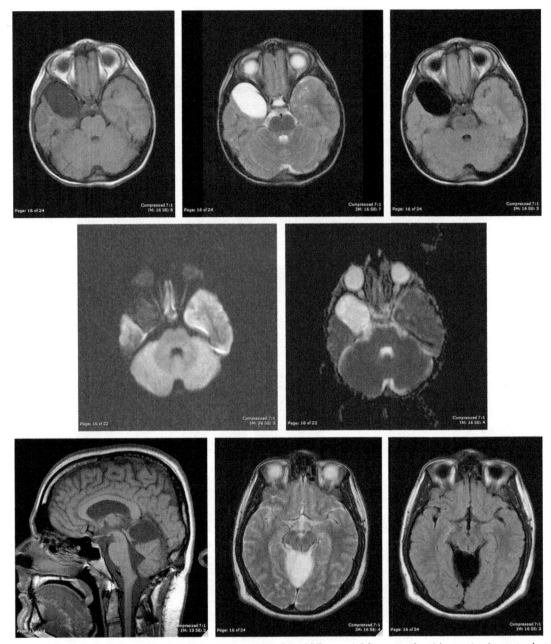

Fig. 7. A 4-year-old child with incidentally discovered right middle cranial fossa arachnoid cyst. Again, note that the lesion follows cerebrospinal fluid signal on all sequences. This is a very common location for arachnoid cysts.

homogeneous structures with attenuation and signal characteristics identical to CSF. If the cyst is of sufficient size, it can displace the adjacent brain parenchyma. They can occur in any region where an arachnoid is present, but are most commonly demonstrated in the sylvian fissures, followed by the cerebellopontine angle cisterns, cerebral convexity, suprasellar cistern, and retrocerebellar region. In the retrocerebellar region, the differential diagnosis also includes mega cisterna magna or Blake's pouch cyst.[1] Arachnoid cysts may also be intraventricular in location.

Arachnoid cysts
- Congenital or acquired
- Well-defined
- Identical to CSF
- Rarely symptomatic

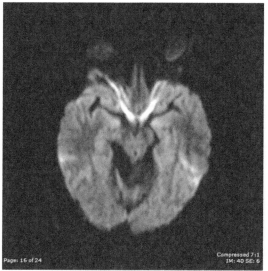
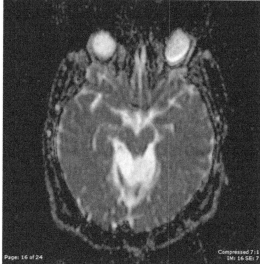

Fig. 8. Quadrigeminal plate cistern arachnoid cyst with mass effect on the tectum and cerebellum.

## Meningiomas

Meningiomas are tumors arising from meningocytes or the arachnoid cap cells of the meninges. These tumors are so rare in childhood that other dural based entities or calvarial lesions invading the dura, such as dural Langerhans cell histiocytosis, melanoma, Ewing sarcoma, plasma cell granulomas, and infantile myofibromatosis should be considered in the differential diagnosis.[1] However, if there is a history of type II neurofibromatosis, meningiomas can occur and, if they do, there is a far higher rate of malignant degeneration than in adults. Hence, when associated with neurofibromatosis, prognosis tends to be worse. Meningiomas can also occur as a complication of radiation therapy.[12–14]

Meningiomas appear as relatively isodense extra axial masses on CT scanning, with homogeneously enhancement. In children, a dural tail may be absent, possibly indicating an origin from ectopic rest tissue.[12–14]

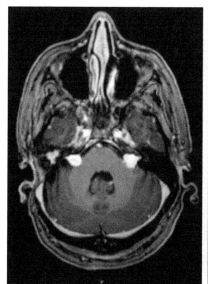
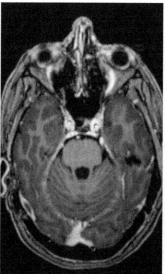
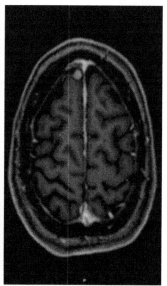

Fig. 9. Pediatric patient with history of type II neurofibromatosis. Postcontrast axial T1-weighted images show enhancing masses in both cerebellopontine angles consistent with bilateral vestibular schwannomas (*left*). There is also a schwannoma involving the left trigeminal nerve (*center*) and a small right frontal parasagittal presumed meningioma near the vertex without a dural tail (*right*).

## Schwannomas

Schwannomas arise from Schwann cells, which are the cells forming the myelin sheaths of nerves. In the intracranial compartment, they most commonly arise from the vestibular division of cranial nerve VII. As with meningiomas, these are far more frequently encountered in the adult than the pediatric population, and if found in a pediatric patient, type II neurofibromatosis should be considered. Bilateral vestibular

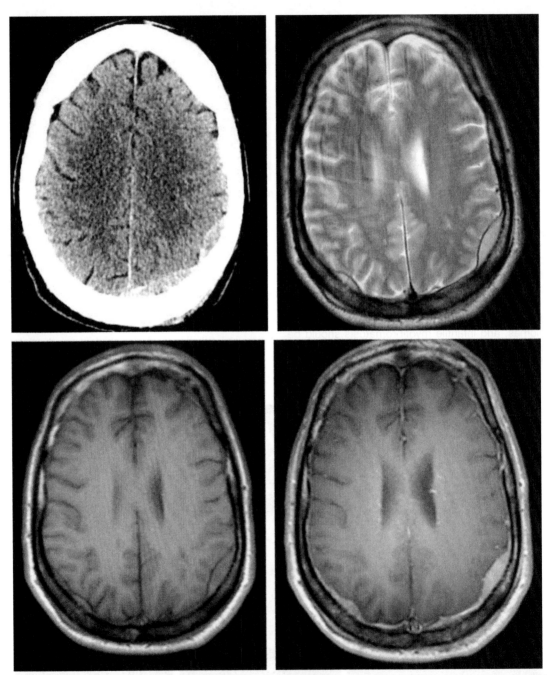

**Fig. 10.** (*Top*) Axial CT and axial T2-weighted MR imaging images. (*Bottom*) Precontrast and postcontrast axial T1-weighted images. Hyperdense extraaxial mass on computed tomography overlying the left parietal lobe with involvement of the adjacent extracalvarial soft tissues. On MR imaging, there is dural thickening, mass effect on the brain, and avid enhancement both of the left parietal lesion and of an additional right sided lesion. Biopsy showed lymphoma.

schwannomas are considered pathognomonic of type II neurofibromatosis (Fig. 9). Sporadic unilateral vestibular schwannomas have also been reported in childhood without syndromic association.[15,16]

These lesions appear as heterogeneous enhancing masses associated with the cranial nerves. The lesions can be largely solid and homogeneous, but can also have variable degree of central necrosis and cystic components, especially when they achieve large size. Schwannomas can contain hemorrhage. There may associated erosion of adjacent osseous structures, and if a vestibular schwannoma is encountered on CT scanning, evaluation of the caliber of the internal auditory canal is important, because expansion may be a clue to the presence of the underlying lesion. Enhancement is variable, depending in part on the degree of cystic change and necrosis.

## Lymphoma/Leukemia

Systemic malignancies rarely affect the intracranial compartment in childhood, but because leukemia and lymphoma are common childhood malignancies, intracranial involvement should be investigated. When the tumor involves the extraparenchymal spaces, presentations include hydrocephalus, enhancement of cranial nerves, and masses involving the meninges or calvarium.[1]

As hypercellular tumors, these entities are an important differential consideration for hyperdense extraaxial masses on CT scanning, and can affect both the dura and the calvarium, mimicking extraaxial hemorrhage. Careful attention should be payed to the source of extraaxial hyperdensity. However, on MR imaging evaluation (Fig. 10), the diagnosis of a mass rather than hematoma should be clear, because leukemia/lymphoma should show avid enhancement and lack intrinsic T1-weighted hyperintensity or susceptibility to suggest hemorrhage. Given the hypercellularity, restricted diffusion is also characteristic.

## Miscellaneous

Lesions primarily involving the calvarium can extend into the extraparenchymal spaces, in particular metastatic neuroblastoma. Langerhans cell histiocystosis can involve not only the calvarium and brain parenchyma, but can also involve the meninges and choroid plexus. Extramedullary hematopoiesis may also rarely involve the epidural space in the setting of chronic anemia, hemoglobinopathies, and myeloproliferative syndromes.[1]

## SUMMARY

Extraparenchymal lesions of childhood include neoplastic and nonneoplastic entities. Lesions affecting children are different from the most common entities affecting adults. Although there are imaging features that are highly suggestive of extraparenchymal origin, it can be difficult to distinguish extraparenchymal from intraparenchymal lesions. MR imaging is the examination of choice for evaluation of extraparenchymal lesions given higher sensitivity and anatomic detail. Syndromic associations should be considered, especially for unusual lesions in the pediatric age group such as meningioma and schwannoma.

## REFERENCES

1. Barkovich AJ, Raybaud C. Pediatric neuroimaging. 5th edition. Philadelphia: Lippincott, Williams, and Wilkins; 2012.
2. Medina LS, Pinter JD, Zurakowski D, et al. Children with headache: clinical predictors of surgical space occupying lesions and the role of neuroimaging. Radiology 1997;202:819–24.
3. Coates TL, Hinshaw DB Jr, Peckman N, et al. Pediatric choroid plexus neoplasms: MR, CT, and pathologic correlation. Radiology 1989;173(1):81–8.
4. Meyers SP, Khademian ZP, Chuang SH, et al. Choroid plexus carcinomas in children: MRI features and patient outcomes. Neuroradiology 2004;46: 770–80.
5. Jaiswal AK, Jaiswal S, Sahu RN, et al. Choroid plexus papilloma in children: diagnostic and surgical considerations. J Pediatr Neurosci 2009; 4(1):10–6.
6. Brandão LA, Poussaint TY. Pediatric brain tumors. Neuroimaging Clin N Am 2013;23:499–525.
7. Tsuruda JS, Chew WM, Moseley ME, et al. Diffusion-weighted MR imaging of the brain: value of differentiating between extraaxial cysts and epidermoid tumors. AJR Am J Roentgenol 1990;155(5): 1059–65.
8. Martinez-Lage J, Ramos J, Puche A, et al. Extradural dermoid tumours of the posterior fossa. Arch Dis Child 1997;77(5):427–30.
9. Higashi S, Takinami K, Yamashita J. Occipital dermal sinus associated with dermoid cyst in the fourth ventricle. AJNR Am J Neuroradiol 1995;16(4 Suppl):945–8.
10. Eidlitz-Markus T, Zeharia A, Cohen YH, et al. Characteristics and management of arachnoid cyst in the pediatric headache clinic setting. Headache 2014;54(10):1583–90.
11. Parsch CS, Krauss J, Hofmann E, et al. Arachnoid cysts associated with subdural hematomas and

hygromas: analysis of 16 cases, long-term follow-up, and review of the literature. Neurosurgery 1997; 40(3):483–90.

12. Greene S, Nair N, Ojemann JG, et al. Meningiomas in children. Pediatr Neurosurg 2008;44(1):9–13.

13. Darling CF, Byrd SE, Reyes-Mugica M, et al. MR of pediatric intracranial meningiomas. AJNR Am J Neuroradiol 1994;15(3):435–44.

14. Erdinçler P, Lena G, Sarioğlu AC, et al. Intracranial meningiomas in children: review of 29 cases. Surg Neurol 1998;49(2):136–40.

15. Hernanz-Schulman M, Welch K, Strand R, et al. Acoustic neuromas in children. AJNR Am J Neuroradiol 1986;7:519–21.

16. Pothula VB, Lesser T, Mallucci C, et al. Vestibular Schwannomas in Children. Otol Neurotol 2001;22: 903–7.

# Tumor and Tumorlike Masses in Pediatric Patients that Involve Multiple Spaces

Thangamadhan Bosemani, MD*, Andrea Poretti, MD

## KEYWORDS

- Tumor • Tumorlike • Multiple spaces • Intracranial • Children • MR imaging

## KEY POINTS

- The pediatric central nervous system is affected by tumors and tumorlike masses that involve multiple spaces.
- Neuroimaging plays an important role in distinguishing tumors from tumorlike masses.
- MR imaging may represent the best predictor of neurodevelopmental abnormalities, seizures, and requirement of neurosurgery in neurocutaneous melanosis.
- Histiocytic disorders, infectious or inflammatory processes, and neurocutaneous syndromes should be considered potential tumor mimics.

## INTRODUCTION

Brain tumors are the most common solid tumor of childhood, the second most common malignancy overall after leukemia and the leading cause of mortality among all childhood cancers.[1] Primary brain tumors have been categorized by the World Health Organization classification to include tumors of the neuroepithelium, cranial nerves, meninges, and sella and those of hematopoietic and germ cell origin.[2] Brain tumors typically form masses, which infiltrate or compress brain parenchyma. The tentorium cerebelli divides the brain parenchyma into supratentorial and infratentorial compartments. The meningeal layers covering the brain create potential anatomic spaces such as epidural, subdural, and subarachnoid. Masses may be confined to a single compartment/space or may extend across multiple compartments/spaces. Not every brain mass, however, represents a tumor or neoplasm. Tumorlike masses of the pediatric brain include histiocytic disorders, inflammatory lesions, vasculitis, ischemia, hemorrhage, vascular malformations, and malformations of brain development.[3]

The recognition of a brain mass on imaging is the first step in the workup. This recognition is followed by verifying its location, identifying it as a tumor and distinguishing it from tumorlike mimics, characterizing the tumor grade and type, and describing its characteristics (including vascularity, vascular permeability, and metabolic spectrum). Hence, imaging plays a vital role in establishing the correct diagnosis, establishing a therapeutic strategy, and influencing prognosis.

Disclosure: The authors report no conflicts of interest.
Section of Pediatric Neuroradiology, Division of Pediatric Radiology, The Russell H. Morgan Department of Radiology and Radiological Science, Charlotte R. Bloomberg Children's Center, The Johns Hopkins School of Medicine, Sheikh Zayed Tower, Room 4174, 1800 Orleans Street, Baltimore, MD 21287-0842, USA
* Corresponding author.
E-mail address: tbosema1@jhmi.edu

Neuroimag Clin N Am 27 (2017) 135–153
http://dx.doi.org/10.1016/j.nic.2016.08.006
1052-5149/17/© 2016 Elsevier Inc. All rights reserved.

MR imaging, including conventional (anatomic) and advanced (functional) sequences, is the study of choice.

This article reviews pediatric brain tumors that involve multiple spaces, including lymphoproliferative disorders, melanocytic lesions, metastasis, tumors of meningothelial cells, and tumors in children with neurofibromatosis type 1 (NF-1), neurofibromatosis type 2 (NF-2), and von Hippel-Lindau (VHL) disease. In addition, tumor-like masses, which include histiocytic disorders, inflammatory processes, infectious etiologies, and neurocutaneous syndromes, are reviewed. For each entity, epidemiology, pathophysiology, and neuroimaging findings are discussed. For tumorlike masses, features and findings that allow the correct differentiation from neoplastic masses are discussed.

## TUMORS ACROSS MULTIPLE SPACES
### Lymphoproliferative Disorders

Lymphoproliferative disorders in childhood include central nervous system (CNS) involvement in childhood leukemia and non-Hodgkin lymphoma (NHL), primary central nervous system lymphoma (PCNSL), and posttransplant lymphoproliferative disorder with CNS involvement (CNS PTLD). Lymphoproliferative disorders may extend across multiple spaces, such as the brain parenchyma, meninges, bone marrow, or calvarium.

### Central nervous system involvement in childhood leukemia
Acute lymphoblastic leukemia (ALL) is a common hematologic malignancy of the bone marrow in which precursor lymphoblasts, blocked at an early stage of differentiation, proliferate rapidly and replace normal hematopoietic cells of the bone marrow.[4] ALL is the most common childhood malignancy, accounting for approximately 25% of cancers and 80% of all leukemias in children.[4]

CNS involvement is typically clinically occult and discovered at the time of lumbar puncture. Children may present with cranial nerve deficits, seizure, altered mental status, headache, or other neurologic deficits.[5]

Primary neuroimaging manifestations of ALL include enlargement of the lateral ventricles (present before therapy, hence, representing hydrocephalus rather than atrophy), leukemic infiltration of CNS structures (meninges, parenchyma, bone marrow, orbit, and spine; Fig. 1A–D), and cerebrovascular complications (hemorrhage, cerebral infarction).[6]

Leukemic infiltration may involve the leptomeninges, subarachnoid space, or epidural space.

Meningeal thickening and enhancement can be either focal or diffuse on postcontrast T1-weighted images. Leptomeningeal enhancement of the brain may result from CNS leukemia/relapse, infection, or, rarely, both. Parenchymal leukemic infiltration is very uncommon, it is often hyperdense on CT, it is contiguous with a meningeal surface, and it enhances after contrast material administration.[6] On MR imaging, parenchymal leukemic CNS infiltration tends to be slightly hypointense on T1-weighted images and isointense to mildly hyperintense on T2-weighted and fluid-attenuated inversion recovery (FLAIR) images compared with gray matter.

Chloroma, also known as *granulocytic sarcoma*, is a focal extramedullary mass of immature myeloid cells of granulocytic lineage that infiltrate bone and soft tissue, most frequently occurring in myelogenous leukemia.[7] Chloromas most commonly arise in the skull, orbits, and sinuses (Fig. 2).

Spinal involvement is frequent in leukemia and lymphoma, either as initial manifestation or in relapse, with bone marrow or meningeal infiltration (Fig. 1E, F). MR imaging of the bone marrow shows low-signal-intensity leukemic infiltrates on T1-weighted images.[6] Subarachnoid nodules, enhancement, and sugar coating of the nerve roots and cauda equina consistent with leptomeningeal seeding are seen on contrast-enhanced T1-weighted images.

Primary cerebrovascular complications are related to leukocytosis, thrombocytopenia, sepsis, or coagulopathy. Hemorrhage is the most common cerebrovascular complication. Hemorrhage can be identified on conventional MR imaging sequences such as T1 and T2 and on advanced sequences such as susceptibility-weighted imaging. Hemorrhage may show mass effect, midline shift, and perifocal edema.

More common than primary leukemic infiltration and primary cerebrovascular complications are treatment-related changes of the CNS including infection, acute neurotoxicity, demyelination, and hemorrhage.[6]

### Central nervous system involvement in childhood non-Hodgkin lymphoma
CNS involvement in NHL is identified by either malignant cells in the cerebrospinal fluid or by cranial nerve palsy on physical examination, which guides further management.[8] About 6% of childhood/adolescent NHL patients are CNS positive during the course of the disease.[9] On MR imaging, leptomeningeal disease with meningeal thickening and enhancement may be seen. MR imaging is highly sensitive for the presence

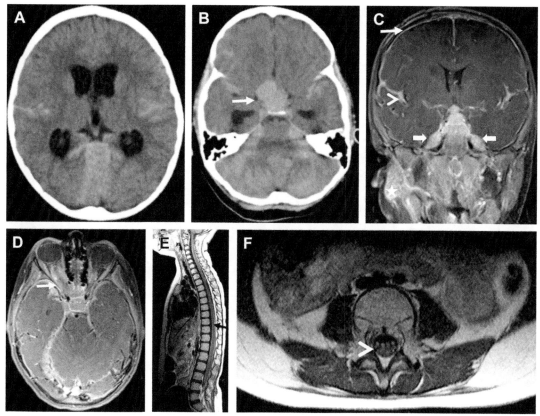

Fig. 1. A 4-year-old girl with ALL presents with altered mental status. (*A, B*) Axial noncontrast CT images of the brain show ventriculomegaly, diffuse hyperdense material in the sulci, and a contiguous hyperdense lobulated mass in the suprasellar cistern (*arrow*), consistent with leukemic infiltration. (*C*) Coronal T1 postcontrast image shows pachymeningeal (*arrow*) and leptomeningeal (*arrow head*) enhancement. Lobulated masslike enhancement in the suprasellar cistern extends to bilateral cavernous sinuses (*block arrows*). Enhancement in the superficial lobe of the right parotid gland (*star*) is shown. (*D*) Axial T1 postcontrast image shows lobulated masslike enhancement extending from the suprasellar cistern in to both orbits, right greater than left, which surrounds the intraorbital portion of the right optic nerve (*arrow*). (*E*) Sagittal and (*F*) axial T1 postcontrast images of the spine show diffuse leptomeningeal enhancement (*arrow*) and thickening with enhancement of the cauda equina nerve roots (*arrow head*). The constellation of findings is consistent with leukemic infiltration extending across multiple spaces.

of meningeal pathologic conditions, but nonspecific for the disease entity. For example, benign meningeal enhancement may be observed after diagnostic or therapeutic lumbar puncture. Soft tissue masses arising from the maxillofacial or pharynx may have trans-spatial extension to the skull base or intracranial compartment (Fig. 3). In addition, parenchymal mass lesions similar to PCNSL may be seen.

*Primary central nervous system lymphoma*
PCNSL represents a rare subtype of NHL restricted to the CNS.[10] Children with immune deficiency syndromes are at increased risk for PCNSL development; however, most reported cases occur in immunocompetent patients.[11] In PCNSL, lesions are typically multiple and located

within the brain parenchyma. Deep brain structures such as basal ganglia, thalami, cerebellum, and brainstem are most commonly involved, whereas infiltration of the cerebral hemispheres and isolated meningeal involvement are less frequent. Lesions are typically isointense to hyperintense on T2-weighted images and hypointense or isointense on unenhanced T1-weighted MR images.[12] Enhancement is shown after administration of contrast. Because of tumor hypercellularity, water diffusion is often restricted, making them appear hyperintense on trace of diffusion maps (diffusion-weighted imaging [DWI]) with matching low apparent diffusion coefficient values. Microhemorrhages and calcifications are rare in PCNSL, thus, differentiating them from high-grade gliomas.

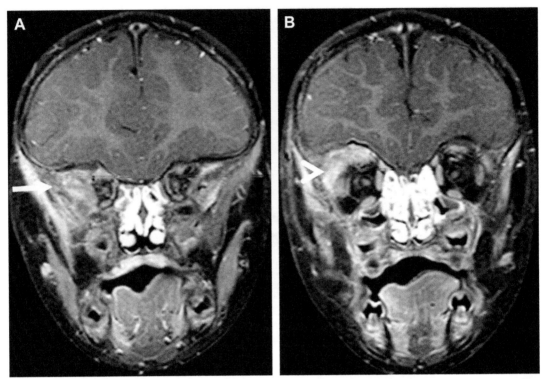

**Fig. 2.** A 22-month-old boy with acute myelogenous leukemia and chloroma. (*A*, *B*) Coronal T1 postcontrast images show an enhancing mass arising from the right sphenoid wing (*arrow*) with intraorbital extension and infiltration of the lacrimal gland (*arrow head*).

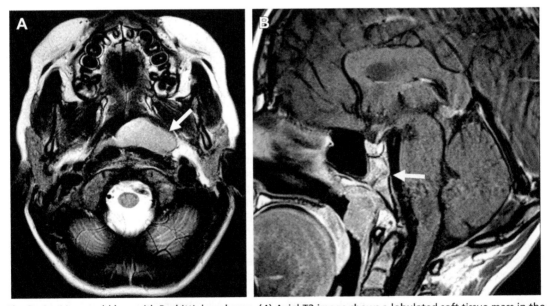

**Fig. 3.** An 11-year-old boy with Burkitt's lymphoma. (*A*) Axial T2 image shows a lobulated soft tissue mass in the left adenoidal tonsillar pillar extending to the nasopharynx (*arrow*). (*B*) Sagittal T1 postcontrast image shows the enhancing soft tissue mass in the nasopharyngeal region with infiltration of the clivus (*arrow*) and basisphenoid.

### Posttransplant lymphoproliferative disorder with central nervous system involvement

CNS PTLD in children is uncommon and can prove diagnostically challenging. Lung, liver, heart, and intestinal transplant patients have a higher risk of CNS PTLD development compared with kidney and bone marrow allograft recipients.[13] Multifocal parenchymal lesions are typically seen in CNS PTLD with MR imaging characteristics similar to those of PCNSL. However, intraparenchymal hemorrhage is an uncommon feature of PCNSL and hence a potential distinguishing feature.[13]

### Primary Melanocytic Lesions

Congenital melanocytic nevi (CMN) can be single or multiple and are present at birth or arise within the first few weeks of life. Multiple CMN can be associated with neurologic abnormalities of the CNS, traditionally termed *neurocutaneous melanosis* (NCM).[14] NCM (OMIM 249400) is caused by somatic mutation in the *NRAS* gene on chromosome 1p13 and is defined by the presence of multiple (>3) or giant CMN and infiltration of brain or leptomeninges by abnormal melanin deposits.

In children with 2 or more CMN at birth, MR Imaging of the neural axis is the modality of choice to search for CNS involvement and should be performed in the first year of life (ideally within the first 6 months because of myelination obscuring the signal from melanin).[14] Myelination may obscure melanin deposits beyond the age of 6 months, as both myelin and melanin appear bright on T1-weighted MR images and hypointense on T2-weighted MR images. MR imaging is the best predictor of neurodevelopmental abnormalities, seizures, and requirement for neurosurgery in childhood.[15] MR imaging neither rules out nor predicts those who will ultimately have symptoms.[16] A total of 60% to 70% of patients with NCM are symptomatic.[17]

Melanin, methemoglobin, lipid, protein, calcium, iron, copper, and manganese are a few substances that appear hyperintense on T1-weighted images. In NCM, the typical location for melanin deposition is in the anterior regions of the temporal lobes (amygdala), cerebellum, pons, and leptomeninges (Fig. 4A).[15,17] When melanosis is present around the cerebellum and pons, hypoplasia of the cerebellum (primarily of the vermis) and pons is typically seen, and the condition may be misdiagnosed as pontocerebellar hypoplasia. The fourth ventricle may be enlarged mimicking a Dandy-Walker malformation. In addition to

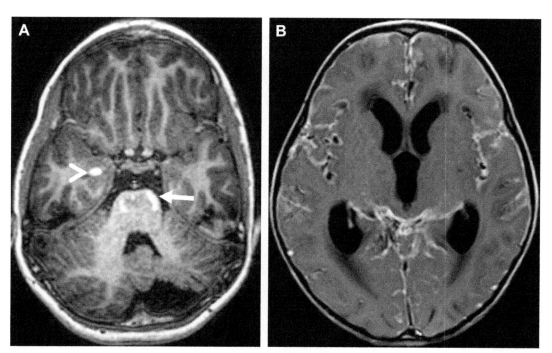

Fig. 4. Neurocutaneous melanosis. (*A*) Axial T1-weighted image shows hyperintense signal in the anterior aspect of the pons (*arrow*) and right mesial temporal lobe (*arrow head*) consistent with neurocutaneous melanosis. In addition, mild asymmetry in size of the cerebellar hemisphere is noted. (*B*) Postcontrast T1-weighted image shows diffuse nodular leptomeningeal enhancement and communicating hydrocephalus. Findings are consistent with progressive leptomeningeal melanocytosis.

T1 hyperintensity on the precontrast images, diffuse nodular enhancement may be present postcontrast with progressive leptomeningeal melanocytosis (Fig. 4B). Progressive leptomeningeal melanocytosis or melanoma (defined by progressive growth of the lesion, presence of surrounding edema or mass effect, or presence of central necrosis) of the brain and spine is associated with a poor prognosis. Proliferating leptomeningeal deposits are associated with uncontrolled communicating hydrocephalus and or increasing intracranial pressure (see Fig. 4B). Spinal arachnoid cysts are a common finding in children with NCM.

## Metastasis

The CNS is a rare site of metastasis from a solid extracranial primary tumor in children. The most common solid primary tumors reported in children are sarcomas, neuroblastomas, nephroblastomas, and germ cell tumors.[18] Metastasis may be in an intradural or extradural location. Intradural lesions may involve the leptomeninges, brain, or spinal cord, and are typically of hematogenous spread. Extradural lesions typically arise from contiguous structures such as bone, skin, or soft tissues. Extradural lesions may also be reached by venous plexus or lymph channels. MR imaging is the study of choice to search for metastasis. Metastasis may be multiple and extend across multiple compartments (Fig. 5). Neuroimaging features of brain metastasis include perifocal edema, mass effect, and avid contrast enhancement. Metastases are subcortical- or cortical-based lesions, which are T1 isointense and T2 hyperintense.[19]

## Meningothelial Cell Lesions

Meningiomas in children account for less than 3% of all primary CNS tumors with a slight male predominance.[20] Although meningiomas represent the most common dura-based neoplasm in the pediatric population, they have a predilection for occurring in unusual sites such as intraventricular and infratentorial regions. Meningiomas can be characterized into 3 clinical groups: (1) spontaneously arising meningiomas, (2) NF-2-associated meningiomas, and (3) radiation-induced meningiomas.[21] Multiplicity of meningiomas is associated with NF-2 (Fig. 6) and postradiation. Cystic components in meningiomas are more commonly found in children than in adults. In addition, pediatric meningiomas are often large, grow rapidly, and are more frequently malignant compared with meningiomas in adults.

Typical MR signal characteristics of meningiomas are (1) isointense to gray matter on

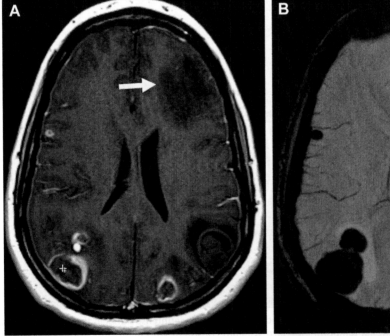
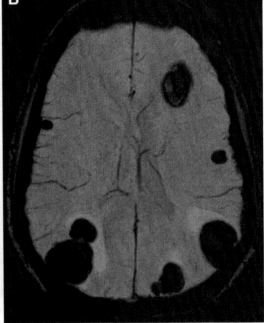

Fig. 5. An 18-year-old woman with metastatic malignant peripheral nerve sheath tumor. (A) Axial T1 postcontrast image shows numerous enhancing masses with perifocal edema (arrow). (B) Axial susceptibility-weighted imaging shows susceptibility within the masses consistent with hemorrhage.

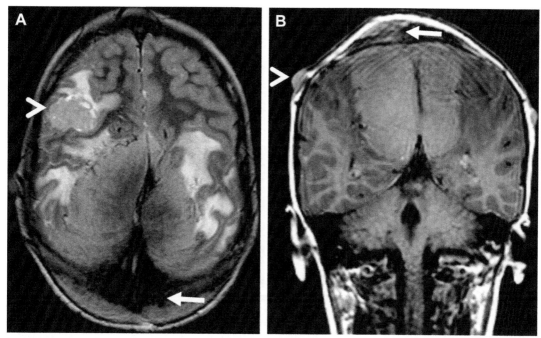

Fig. 6. A 10-year-old boy with NF-2 and multiple meningiomas. (*A*) Axial T2-weighted image shows a posterior interhemispheric falx meningioma with perifocal edema in bilateral frontal lobes and adjacent calvarial hyperostosis (*arrow*). Additional right frontal meningioma with surrounding edema (*arrow head*) is shown. (*B*) Coronal T1 postcontrast image shows enhancement of the posterior interhemispheric falx meningioma with calvarial hyperostosis and intradiploic extension (*arrow*). Scalp lesions consistent with neurofibromas are shown (*arrow head*).

T1-weighted images, (2) isointense to hyperintense to gray matter on T2-weighted and FLAIR images, (3) heterogeneous postcontrast enhancement, (4) calcification, (5) peritumoral edema, (5) bone erosion, and (6) hyperostosis.[21] Dural tail is typically seen in radiation induced tumors and NF-2. Perfusion-weighted imaging may be helpful in differentiating meningeal tumors from neuroepithelial tumors because the last ones show persistence of abnormal relaxivity after the bolus of contrast because of the absence of the blood–brain barrier.

## Neurofibromatosis Type 1

NF-1 (OMIM 162200) is the most common neurocutaneous syndrome with a prevalence of 1 in 2500 to 3000 individuals.[22] It is an autosomal dominant disorder caused by heterozygous mutation in the neurofibromin gene on chromosome 17q11.2. Neurofibromin is widely expressed with high levels in the nervous system and acts as a tumor suppressor. Neurofibromin reduces cell growth and proliferation by negative regulation of the cellular proto-oncogene p21RAS and by control of the serine threonine kinase mTOR (mammalian target of rapamycin).[23] Impaired neurofibromin function predisposes to benign and malignant tumor formation.

The main clinical manifestations of NF-1 involve the skin and the nervous system, but the complications are variable and may involve most of the body systems.[24]

Neuroimaging abnormalities in NF-1 include intracranial neoplasms, parenchymal T2- hyperintense lesions, cerebral vasculopathy, and sphenoid wing dysplasia. Intracranial neoplasms include glioma and plexiform neurofibroma.[25] Gliomas generally develop in different spaces/compartments including the optic pathways, brainstem, and, rarely, cerebellum. Optic pathway gliomas are the most frequent neoplasms seen in about 15% of children with NF-1 and are typically low-grade pilocytic astrocytomas. Optic pathway gliomas appear as concentrically enlarged irregular optic nerves or an enlarged optic chiasm, with T2-hyperintense signal (Fig. 7). The tumor may extend from the intraorbital compartment to the chiasm and the optic pathways. The degree of gadolinium contrast enhancement does not correlate with tumor grade.

## Neurofibromatosis Type 2

NF-2 (OMIM 101000) is an autosomal dominant neurocutaneous syndrome characterized by schwannomas, meningiomas, ependymomas,

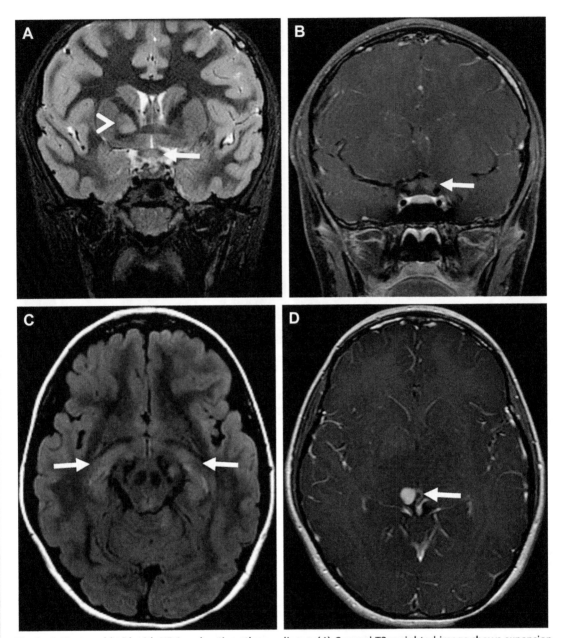

**Fig. 7.** A 12-year-old girl with NF-1 and optic pathway glioma. (*A*) Coronal T2-weighted image shows expansion of the optic chiasm with hyperintense signal (*arrow*) and unidentified bright object in the right globus pallidum (*arrow head*). (*B*) Coronal T1 postcontrast image shows expansion and enhancement of the prechiasmatic segments of the optic nerves, left greater than right (*arrow*), consistent with gliomas. (*C*) Axial FLAIR image shows hyperintense signal in bilateral optic pathways (*arrows*). (*D*) Axial T1 postcontrast image shows a glioma in the right dorsal thalamus (*arrow*).

and ocular abnormalities. It results from a defect in neurofibromin 2, a tumor suppressor gene situated on chromosome 22q11 that encodes the protein Merlin (moesin-ezrin-radixin–like protein), also called *Schwannomin*.[26]

The presence of bilateral vestibular schwannomas is a characteristic feature of NF-2 (Fig. 8).

Schwannomas arising from the cochlear nerve or facial nerve are relatively less common. Schwannomas are typically mildly hypointense on T2-weighted images, isointense on T1-weighted images, and enhance avidly with gadolinium contrast.[25] Schwannomas are eccentrically located with respect to the nerve.

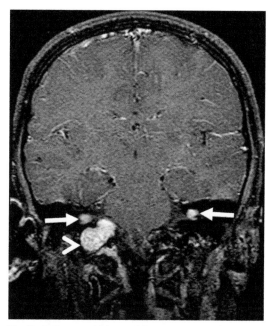

Fig. 8. A 6-year-old boy with NF-2. Coronal T1 post-contrast image shows bilateral avidly enhancing vestibular schwannomas in the internal auditory canals (*arrows*). In addition, a bilobed enhancing mass involving the right hypoglossal nerve is shown (*arrow head*).

Intracranial meningiomas are the second most common tumor in NF-2. Meningiomas typically occur over the convexities and may be multiple (see Fig. 6). Meningiomas are T2 hypointense and T1 isointense and have variable degrees of calcification. Gadolinium contrast enhancement has an inverse relationship to the degree of calcification.

## von Hippel-Lindau Disease

VHL (OMIM 193300) is an autosomal dominant neurocutaneous syndrome characterized by various benign and malignant tumors of the CNS, kidneys, adrenal glands, inner ear, reproductive adnexal organs, retinal, cerebellar, and spinal hemangioblastomas and endolymphatic sac tumors. VHL results from a germline mutation in the *VHL* tumor suppressor gene on chromosome 3p25.3, which inactivates one of the *VHL* alleles, with the carriers of this mutation being subject to a second inactivating event (2-hit hypothesis).[27] CNS hemangioblastoma is observed in 65% of patients with VHL and is a defining feature in VHL.[28]

The cerebellum is the most common location (about 65%) for CNS hemangioblastomas. They are highly vascular benign World Health

Organization grade 1 tumors that show solid enhancement and appear to be pial based, therefore, are peripherally located in the cerebellum (Fig. 9). Hemangioblastomas are T1 isointense and T2 hyperintense. Heterogeneous T2 signal may be seen in the presence of intralesional hemorrhage. Mural nodules are well demarcated and show homogenous enhancement. Flow voids if present appear T2 hypointense with superficial heterogeneous enhancement. Peritumoral vasogenic edema is typically mild. In VHL, multiple lesions may occur simultaneously. Additional lesions may be present along the spinal cord. Imaging of the entire neural axis is consequently advised.

## TUMORLIKE MASSES ACROSS MULTIPLE SPACES
### Histiocytic Disorders

Histiocytic disorders affecting the CNS in children include (1) Langerhans cell histiocytosis (LCH), (2) juvenile xanthogranuloma (JXG), (3) Erdheim-Chester disease, (4) Rosai-Dorfman disease (RDD), and (5) hemophagocytic lymphohistiocytosis (HLH).

### Langerhans cell histiocytosis
LCH is a rare group of disorders of the monocyte-macrophage system and includes the subtypes

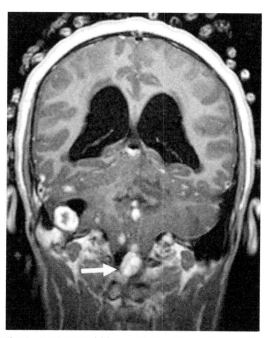

Fig. 9. A 16-year-old boy with Von Hippel-Lindau disease. Coronal T1 postcontrast image shows numerous hemangioblastomas within the cerebellum and in the cervicomedullary junction (*arrow*).

histiocytosis X, eosinophilic granuloma, Hand-Schuller-Christian disease, and Letterer-Siwe disease.[29] In CNS-LCH, cranial and intracranial changes on MR imaging include (1) lesions of the craniofacial bone, skull base, and sinus (**Fig. 10**); (2) intracranial, extra-axial changes (hypothalamic-pituitary region, meninges, circumventricular organs); (3) intracranial, intra-axial changes

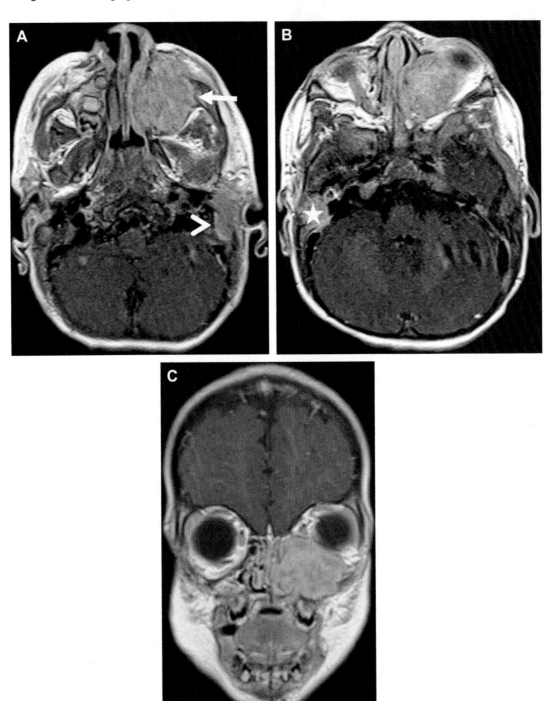

**Fig. 10.** A 16-month-old boy with LCH and multiple craniofacial region masses. (*A, B*) Axial T1 postcontrast images show a soft tissue mass centered in the left maxillary region with extension to the left nasal region (*arrow*) and mass in the left temporal (*arrow head*) and right temporal bones (*star*). (*C*) Coronal T1 postcontrast image shows trans-spatial extension of the left maxillary sinus mass to the orbit and nasal ethmoidal region on the left.

(white matter and gray matter); and (4) cerebral or cerebellar atrophy.[29] Hypothalamic pituitary axis involvement is the most common in CNS-LCH and is characterized by absence of normal bright signal in the posterior pituitary gland on T1-weighted image, often associated with thickening (3 mm) and enhancement (gradual enhancement without washout) of the pituitary stalk. Neurodegeneration is the next most common form of CNS-LCH, characterized by gray-matter changes mainly involving dentate nuclei and basal ganglia.[30]

Masslike lesions may be dural-based or space-occupying parenchymal lesions (rare). Dural-based masses may be single or multiple, subdural or epidural in location, and typically hypointense to isointense on T1-weighted images and hypointense on T2-weighted images with inconstant contrast enhancement. Space-occupying parenchymal lesions may be randomly distributed or take a vascular distribution. They may be of variable size, exert mass effect, and show contrast enhancement. Contrast enhancement pattern may be nodular, ringlike, or homogenous mass–like.[30]

### Juvenile xanthogranuloma

JXG is primarily a benign cutaneous disorder of non-Langerhans histiocytic proliferation, usually confined to childhood.[31] CNS involvement in isolation is rare. Lesions may be dural based in the frontoparietal region or located in the Meckel's cave. The lesions are typically isointense on T1-weighted images and show enhancement. Their location and MR signal characteristics mimic other primary intracranial tumors, such as meningioma, schwannoma, nerve sheath tumor, ependymoma, glioma, and RDD as well as granulomatous lesions such as neurosarcoidosis and tuberculosis.[31]

### Erdheim-Chester disease

Erdheim-Chester disease is an extremely rare disease that is histologically indistinguishable from JXG but arises in characteristic clinical patterns in adults.[32]

### Rosai-Dorfman disease

RDD is a rare, benign idiopathic histioproliferative disorder typically characterized by massive but painless cervical lymphadenopathy. CNS involvement occurs only in 5% of patients, and isolated CNS involvement is extremely rare.[33] The typical imaging appearance of intracranial RDD is a dural-based enhancing mass mimicking meningioma. Typical location of the lesion is parasphenoidal. Lesion may arise from the cerebral parenchyma or brain stem. Lesions may be extracalvarial in location (**Fig. 11**). Intra-axial lesions are typically isointense to brain on T1- and T2-weighted images with peripheral enhancement.[34]

### Hemophagocytic lymphohistiocytosis

HLH is a rare multisystem disorder characterized by the proliferation and infiltration of lymphocytes and histiocytes in the liver, spleen,

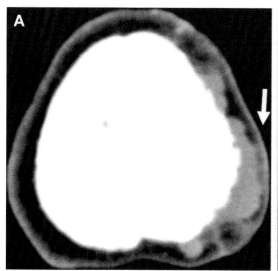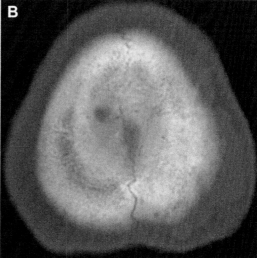

Fig. 11. A 16-year-old girl with RDD. (*A*) Axial noncontrast CT image at the left parietal vertex scalp shows lobulated soft tissue masses (*arrow*). (*B*) Axial CT in bone kernel shows adjacent left parietal bone hyperostosis.

lymph nodes, bones, and CNS.[35] CNS involvement has been reported in up to 73% of patients.[36] Patients with more aggressive disease and adverse outcome frequently have CNS involvement. Neurologic symptoms may be the initial or sole presentation of the disease and may include seizures, impaired consciousness, meningismus, hypotonia, and microcephaly. These symptoms are not specific and may mimic other more common inflammatory diseases of the brain, such as acute disseminated encephalomyelitis and vasculitis. Laboratory findings including cytopenias, elevated liver enzymes and hyperbilirubinemia, coagulopathy, hypertriglyceridemia, hyperferritinemia, and hypofibrinogenemia support the diagnosis of HLH. Neuroimaging findings may also facilitate an early diagnosis of HLH and include (1) multilobal, bilateral, mostly symmetric, scattered T2-hyperintense and FLAIR-hyperintense lesions involving the gray or white matter in the supratentorial and infratentorial regions, mostly periventricular (**Fig. 12**), juxtacortical, or cerebellar, while thalamus, basal ganglia, and brain stem are rarely involved; (2) nodular or ring enhancement of aforementioned parenchymal lesions; (3) diffuse leptomeningeal enhancement; (4) mild ventriculomegaly with prominent extraaxial cerebrospinal fluid spaces; and (5) reduced diffusion restriction with low apparent diffusion coefficient values in enhancing lesions, thalamus, basal ganglia, and cortical mantle.[35,36] The presence of symmetric lesions typically sparing the basal ganglia and thalami favors HLH compared with acute disseminated encephalomyelitis on neuroimaging.[37]

## Inflammatory Processes

### Inflammatory pseudotumor

Inflammatory pseudotumor is a pathologic term used to describe a reactive, inflammatory nonneoplastic phenomenon. Inflammatory pseudotumors are histopathologically characterized by a collagenous stroma of different vascularization, spindle cells, and a polyclonal mononuclear infiltrate, which may affect any organ system. Inflammatory pseudotumors affecting primarily the CNS are rare.[38] Lesions may be located in 5 anatomic regions: (1) intraparenchymal, (2) meningeal, (3) mixed intraparenchymal and meningeal lesions, (4) intraventricular, and (5) contiguous intracranial extension between the sphenoidal sinus, pterygopalatine fossa, or right nasal cavity.[38] Intraparenchymal lesions show avid postcontrast enhancement and perifocal edema. The presence of necrosis, hemorrhage, or calcification may further impart a tumoral appearance.

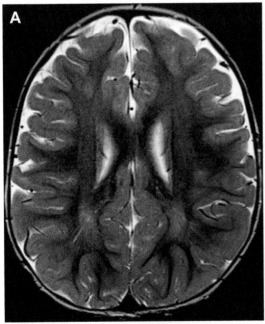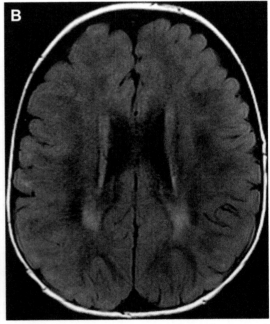

**Fig. 12.** A 19-month-old boy with HLH. (*A*) Axial T2- and (*B*) FLAIR-weighted images show symmetric hyperintense signal in the periventricular and periatrial white matter.

## Primary angiitis of the central nervous system

CNS vasculitis encompasses a broad spectrum of disorders that result in inflammation and destruction of the blood vessels of the brain, spinal cord, and meninges. Primary angiitis of the CNS (PACNS) is an idiopathic vasculitis confined to the CNS. CNS vasculitis is considered secondary when it occurs in the setting of a multisystem inflammatory disease, such as a systemic vasculitis or lupus, or an infection, such as varicella zoster virus.[39] PACNS may cause ischemic stroke and optic neuritis, and its clinical presentation encompasses acquired neurologic deficits such as seizures, movement disorders, progressive cognitive decline, and reduced visual function.[40] Early recognition with rapid initiation of immunosuppressive treatment can lead to significant improvement or even complete resolution of neurologic deficits.[40]

Two distinct subtypes of PACNS are recognized in children: (1) angiography-positive PACNS affecting large and medium-sized vessels and (2) angiography-negative PACNS involving small-sized vessels.[41]

In angiography-positive PACNS, children typically present with strokelike symptoms, and MR imaging findings are consistent with focal acute ischemia in a vascular distribution. The diagnosis of angiography-positive PACNS is confirmed by conventional digital subtraction angiography or magnetic resonance angiography, which may show stenosis, tortuosity, beading, and occlusion of the proximal large-sized and medium-sized vessels.[41] Gadolinium-enhanced magnetic resonance angiography adds important information by showing vessel wall enhancement and thickening in more than 85% of patients.

In angiography-negative PACNS, children may present with systemic features, including fever, malaise, and flulike symptoms. MR imaging findings are typically multifocal, bilateral or unilateral, or symmetric or asymmetric and can involve both gray and white matter. Digital subtraction angiography findings are normal. Lesions are not restricted to a vascular territory. Absence of diffusion restriction and leptomeningeal and parenchymal enhancement are suggestive of an inflammatory process rather than ischemia and helps distinguish it from demyelinating diseases.[41] Elective brain biopsy is required to confirm the diagnosis.

## Tumefactive demyelination

Acute demyelination is an acquired inflammatory illness characterized by neuroimaging features of single or multiple lesions in the brain, optic nerve, or spinal cord.[42] Tumefactive demyelination is uncommon in children. Tumefactive demyelination needs to be distinguished from tumor because of surgical complications of brain biopsy, including death, and the potential for worsening of demyelinating plaques by radiotherapy. In addition, a proportion of children with tumefactive demyelination are at risk for a future diagnosis of multiple sclerosis, which requires specific therapy.[42]

Lesions are typically multiple and are most commonly located in the frontoparietal regions. Enhancement of lesions is seen in approximately 50% of patients. Rim enhancement may occur but is often circumferential without orientation toward the ventricle (**Fig. 13**).[43] Tumefactive demyelination can be distinguished from tumor by the presence of multiple lesions, absence of cortical involvement, and decrease in lesion size or detection of new lesions on serial imaging.[42]

## Pseudotumoral hemicerebellitis

Hemicerebellitis is a rare inflammatory disorder involving one cerebellar hemisphere that affects children.[44] Pseudotumoral hemicerebellitis is a diagnosis primarily based on neuroimaging findings, in which mass effect and edema may mimic tumor in the unilateral cerebellar hemisphere. Neuroimaging features include T2-hyperintense signal of the cortex and subcortical white matter, contrast enhancement along the folia, and effacement of the fourth ventricle (**Fig. 14**). The signal changes, ill-defined expansion of the hemisphere, and fourth ventricular effacement represent the tumorlike appearance. Supratentorial hydrocephalus may be seen secondary to mass effect on the fourth ventricle. Advanced MR imaging techniques such as DWI and magnetic resonance spectroscopy have a limited role in characterizing pseudotumoral hemicerebellitis.

## Infectious Processes

### Brain abscess

Intracranial infections in children are rare and can progress rapidly leading to devastating and permanent neurologic sequelae. Intracranial infections are grouped into 3 main categories based on their location: epidural abscess, subdural empyema, and brain abscess. They arise most frequently from direct extension of infections in surrounding structures (sinusitis, otitis media) but also from hematogenous spread, skull trauma, or surgery.[45]

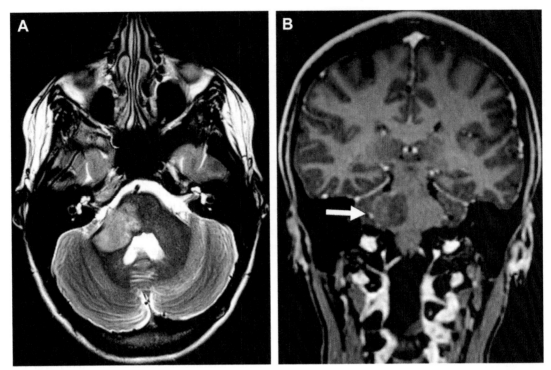

**Fig. 13.** A 17-year-old girl with multiple sclerosis. (*A*) Axial T2-weighted image shows a mass in the right pons with extension to the right middle cerebellar peduncle. (*B*) Coronal T1 postcontrast image shows subtle enhancement along the lateral aspect of the mass (*arrow*). Findings were consistent with tumefactive demyelination.

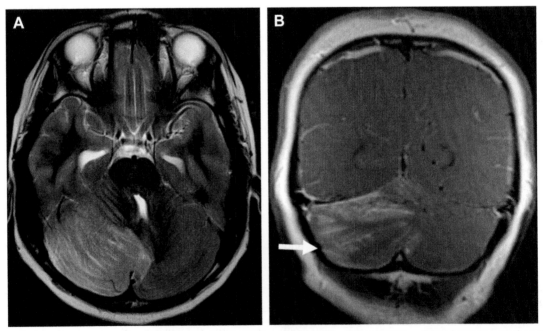

**Fig. 14.** A 7-year-old girl with right pseudotumoral hemicerebellitis. (*A*) Axial T2-weighted MR image shows ill-defined expansion of the right cerebellar hemisphere with hyperintense signal of the cortex and white matter and mass effect on the fourth ventricle. (*B*) Coronal T1 postcontrast image shows marked enhancement of the cerebellar foliae (*arrow*).

Brain abscesses begin as focal regions of brain suppuration or cerebritis and evolve into discrete purulent fluid collections with an enhancing capsule. Brain abscesses develop secondary to sinusitis, otitis, or dental infections in more than half of cases.[45] Hematogenous spreads of abscesses are generally multifocal in the distribution of the middle cerebral artery. Large brain abscesses typically have mass effect and perifocal edema.

Imaging findings during the early cerebritis phase are T2-hyperintense and T1-hypointense signal with patchy enhancement. In the later phase, the T1-hypointense signal becomes better demarcated, with T2-hyperintense signal both in the cavity and surrounding parenchyma.[46] Postcontrast images show a ring of enhancement (Fig. 15). Abscesses grow toward the white matter, away from the better-vascularized gray matter, with thinning of the medial wall. DWI shows diffusion restriction within the lesion confirming the presence of purulent fluid and distinguishing it from necrotic tumors.

### Acute necrotizing encephalopathy

Acute necrotizing encephalopathy of childhood is a novel type of parainfectious, noninflammatory encephalopathy originally described in East Asia.[47] The disease manifests a few days after a nonspecific viral illness such as influenza A and B, parainfluenza, varicella, and human herpes virus type 6. The initial presentation is followed by a progressive and rapid deterioration culminating in coma. Imaging establishes the diagnosis. Bilateral thalamic involvement continuous with lesions in the lateral putamina and external/extreme capsules is a prerequisite. Lesions are also common in the internal capsule, upper brainstem tegmentum, pons, cerebral periventricular white matter, and cerebellar deep nuclei and white matter, sparing other CNS regions.[47] The lesions are typically T2 hyperintense and FLAIR hyperintense and show restricted diffusion (Fig. 16) but may often cavitate and become T2 hypointense and T1 hyperintense, reflecting the hemorrhagic component. Involvement of the pons is a poor prognostic factor. Neuropathology finds edema, perivascular hemorrhage, and necrosis without astrogliosis or inflammatory cell infiltration. Early recognition of acute necrotizing encephalopathy is important because early treatment with steroids is essential. A familial genetic predisposition (point mutations in the *RANBP2* gene) has been found and allows identification of additional, at-risk individuals in an affected family.

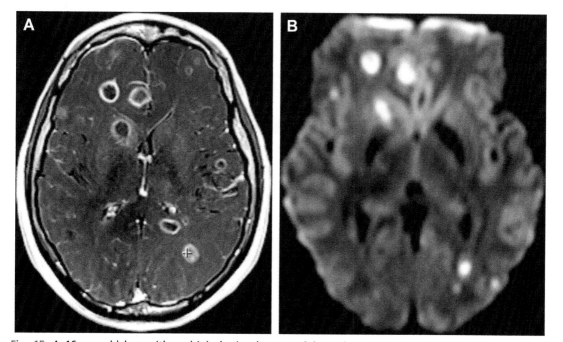

Fig. 15. A 16-year-old boy with multiple brain abscesses. (A) Axial T1 postcontrast image shows numerous enhancing parenchymal lesions with perifocal edema. (B) Axial trace diffusion image shows diffusion restriction consistent with the presence of purulent material.

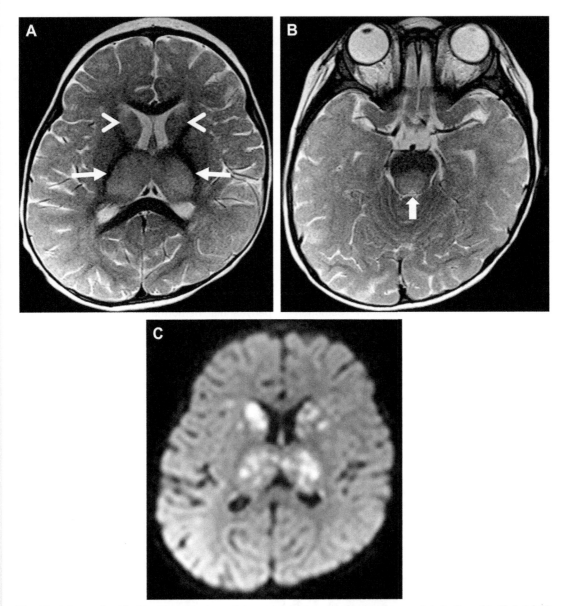

**Fig. 16.** A 9-month-old girl with acute necrotizing encephalopathy after influenza A infection. (*A, B*) Axial T2-weighted images show hyperintense signal in the bilateral thalami (*arrows*), caudate nuclei (*arrow heads*), and dorsal pons (*arrow*). (*C*) Axial trace diffusion image shows multiple foci of diffusion restriction in the thalami and deep gray nuclei.

## Neurocutaneous Syndromes

Neurocutaneous diseases include a group of developmental disorders with involvement of skin and central or peripheral nervous systems. Encephalocraniocutaneous lipomatosis is a sporadically occurring neurocutaneous disease characterized by the presence of skin lesions (eg, the nevus psiloliparus) and ocular (eg, choristomas) and CNS anomalies.[48] The most common neuroimaging finding is the presence of intracranial lipomas, frequently of cerebello-pontine location, or intradural or extradural spinal lipomatosis (**Fig. 17**).[49] Lipomas can be large and extend across multiple spaces. Arachnoid cyst is a frequent presentation caused by congenital abnormalities of the meninges. In addition, asymmetric intracranial changes include complete or partial atrophy of a hemisphere, porencephalic cysts, ventriculomegaly or hydrocephalus, and calcifications.[48]

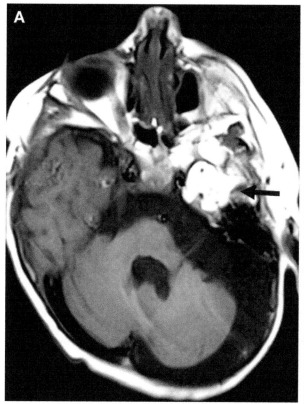
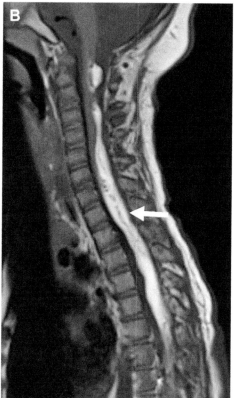

Fig. 17. Encephalocraniocutaneous lipomatosis. (A) Axial T1-weighted image shows left cerebellar hypoplasia and T1 bright lipoma infiltrating the left petrous temporal bone (arrow). (B) Sagittal T1-weighted image of the cervical spine shows epidural location of intraspinal lipoma (arrow). (From Michael GA, Poretti A, Huisman TA. Neuroimaging findings in Encephalocraniocutaneous Lipomatosis. Pediatr Neurol 2015;53(5):462–3; with permission.)

## SUMMARY

Brain masses are common findings in pediatric neuroradiology. Neuroimaging plays a key role in the workup of brain masses and allows (1) the identification of a brain mass, (2) determination of location if confined to a single versus multiple spaces, and (3) differentiation of tumor from tumorlike masses.

Clinical history and neurologic examination are key components in assisting the neuroimaging evaluation. Neuroimaging facilitates an accurate diagnosis, prompts early therapy, and influences prognosis and overall survival.

## REFERENCES

1. Ostrom QT, Gittleman H, Liao P, et al. CBTRUS statistical report: primary brain and central nervous system tumors diagnosed in the United States in 2007-2011. Neuro Oncol 2014;16(Suppl 4):iv1–63.
2. Louis DN, Ohgaki H, Wiestler OD, et al. The 2007 WHO classification of tumours of the central nervous system. Acta Neuropathol 2007;114:97–109.
3. Huisman TA. Tumor-like lesions of the brain. Cancer Imaging 2009;9(Spec No A):S10–3.
4. Katz AJ, Chia VM, Schoonen WM, et al. Acute lymphoblastic leukemia: an assessment of international incidence, survival, and disease burden. Cancer Causes Control 2015;26:1627–42.
5. Pui CH, Howard SC. Current management and challenges of malignant disease in the CNS in paediatric leukaemia. Lancet Oncol 2008;9:257–68.
6. Vazquez E, Lucaya J, Castellote A, et al. Neuroimaging in pediatric leukemia and lymphoma: differential diagnosis. Radiographics 2002;22:1411–28.
7. Porto L, Kieslich M, Schwabe D, et al. Central nervous system imaging in childhood leukaemia. Eur J Cancer 2004;40:2082–90.
8. Sandlund JT, Murphy SB, Santana VM, et al. CNS involvement in children with newly diagnosed non-Hodgkin's lymphoma. J Clin Oncol 2000;18:3018–24.
9. Salzburg J, Burkhardt B, Zimmermann M, et al. Prevalence, clinical pattern, and outcome of CNS involvement in childhood and adolescent non-Hodgkin's lymphoma differ by non-Hodgkin's lymphoma

subtype: a Berlin-Frankfurt-Munster Group Report. J Clin Oncol 2007;25:3915–22.

10. Thorer H, Zimmermann M, Makarova O, et al. Primary central nervous system lymphoma in children and adolescents: low relapse rate after treatment according to Non-Hodgkin-Lymphoma Berlin-Frankfurt-Munster protocols for systemic lymphoma. Haematologica 2014;99:e238–41.

11. Abla O, Weitzman S, Blay JY, et al. Primary CNS lymphoma in children and adolescents: a descriptive analysis from the International Primary CNS Lymphoma Collaborative Group (IPCG). Clin Cancer Res 2011;17:346–52.

12. Haldorsen IS, Espeland A, Larsson EM. Central nervous system lymphoma: characteristic findings on traditional and advanced imaging. AJNR Am J Neuroradiol 2011;32:984–92.

13. Gheorghe G, Radu O, Milanovich S, et al. Pathology of central nervous system posttransplant lymphoproliferative disorders: lessons from pediatric autopsies. Pediatr Dev Pathol 2013;16:67–73.

14. Waelchli R, Aylett SE, Atherton D, et al. Classification of neurological abnormalities in children with congenital melanocytic naevus syndrome identifies MRI as the best predictor of clinical outcome. Br J Dermatol 2015;173(3):739–50.

15. Bekiesinska-Figatowska M, Szczygielski O, Boczar M, et al. Neurocutaneous melanosis in children with giant congenital melanocytic nevi. Clin Imaging 2014;38:79–84.

16. Alikhan A, Ibrahimi OA, Eisen DB. Congenital melanocytic nevi: where are we now? Part I. Clinical presentation, epidemiology, pathogenesis, histology, malignant transformation, and neurocutaneous melanosis. J Am Acad Dermatol 2012;67:495.e1-17 [quiz: 512–4].

17. Ramaswamy V, Delaney H, Haque S, et al. Spectrum of central nervous system abnormalities in neurocutaneous melanocytosis. Dev Med Child Neurol 2012; 54:563–8.

18. Suki D, Khoury Abdulla R, Ding M, et al. Brain metastases in patients diagnosed with a solid primary cancer during childhood: experience from a single referral cancer center. J Neurosurg Pediatr 2014; 14:372–85.

19. Porto L, Jarisch A, Zanella F, et al. The role of magnetic resonance imaging in children with hematogenous brain metastases from primary solid tumors. Pediatr Hematol Oncol 2010;27:103–11.

20. Rushing EJ, Olsen C, Mena H, et al. Central nervous system meningiomas in the first two decades of life: a clinicopathological analysis of 87 patients. J Neurosurg 2005;103:489–95.

21. Pinto PS, Huisman TA, Ahn E, et al. Magnetic resonance imaging features of meningiomas in children and young adults: a retrospective analysis. J Neuroradiol 2012;39:218–26.

22. Williams VC, Lucas J, Babcock MA, et al. Neurofibromatosis type 1 revisited. Pediatrics 2009;123: 124–33.

23. Ferner RE. The neurofibromatoses. Pract Neurol 2010;10:82–93.

24. Ferner RE, Gutmann DH. Neurofibromatosis type 1 (NF1): diagnosis and management. Handb Clin Neurol 2013;115:939–55.

25. Nandigam K, Mechtler LL, Smirniotopoulos JG. Neuroimaging of neurocutaneous diseases. Neurol Clin 2014;32:159–92.

26. Lloyd SK, Evans DG. Neurofibromatosis type 2 (NF2): diagnosis and management. Handb Clin Neurol 2013;115:957–67.

27. Monsalve J, Kapur J, Malkin D, et al. Imaging of cancer predisposition syndromes in children. Radiographics 2011;31:263–80.

28. Kanno H, Kuratsu J, Nishikawa R, et al. Clinical features of patients bearing central nervous system hemangioblastoma in von Hippel-Lindau disease. Acta Neurochir (Wien) 2013;155:1–7.

29. Prayer D, Grois N, Prosch H, et al. MR imaging presentation of intracranial disease associated with Langerhans cell histiocytosis. AJNR Am J Neuroradiol 2004;25:880–91.

30. Chaudhary V, Bano S, Aggarwal R, et al. Neuroimaging of Langerhans cell histiocytosis: a radiological review. Jpn J Radiol 2013;31:786–96.

31. Tamir I, Davir R, Fellig Y, et al. Solitary juvenile xanthogranuloma mimicking intracranial tumor in children. J Clin Neurosci 2013;20:183–8.

32. Allen CE, Kelly KM, Bollard CM. Pediatric lymphomas and histiocytic disorders of childhood. Pediatr Clin North Am 2015;62:139–65.

33. Varan A, Sen H, Akalan N, et al. Pontine Rosai-Dorfman disease in a child. Childs Nerv Syst 2015; 31:971–5.

34. Di Rocco F, Garnett MR, Puget S, et al. Cerebral localization of Rosai-Dorfman disease in a child. Case report. J Neurosurg 2007;107:147–51.

35. Guandalini M, Butler A, Mandelstam S. Spectrum of imaging appearances in Australian children with central nervous system hemophagocytic lymphohistiocytosis. J Clin Neurosci 2014;21: 305–10.

36. Goo HW, Weon YC. A spectrum of neuroradiological findings in children with haemophagocytic lymphohistiocytosis. Pediatr Radiol 2007;37: 1110–7.

37. Deiva K, Mahlaoui N, Beaudonnet F, et al. CNS involvement at the onset of primary hemophagocytic lymphohistiocytosis. Neurology 2012;78: 1150–6.

38. Hausler M, Schaade L, Ramaekers VT, et al. Inflammatory pseudotumors of the central nervous system: report of 3 cases and a literature review. Hum Pathol 2003;34:253–62.

39. Rodriguez-Pla A, Monach PA. Primary angiitis of the central nervous system in adults and children. Rheum Dis Clin North Am 2015;41:47–62, viii.

40. Benseler S, Pohl D. Childhood central nervous system vasculitis. Handb Clin Neurol 2013;112: 1065–78.

41. Cellucci T, Benseler SM. Central nervous system vasculitis in children. Curr Opin Rheumatol 2010; 22:590–7.

42. Yiu EM, Laughlin S, Verhey LH, et al. Clinical and magnetic resonance imaging (MRI) distinctions between tumefactive demyelination and brain tumors in children. J Child Neurol 2014; 29:654–65.

43. Morin MP, Patenaude Y, Sinsky AB, et al. Solitary tumefactive demyelinating lesions in children. J Child Neurol 2011;26:995–9.

44. Jabbour P, Samaha E, Abi Lahoud G, et al. Hemicerebellitis mimicking a tumour on MRI. Childs Nerv Syst 2003;19:122–5.

45. Bonfield CM, Sharma J, Dobson S. Pediatric intracranial abscesses. J Infect 2015;71(Suppl 1):S42–6.

46. Foerster BR, Thurnher MM, Malani PN, et al. Intracranial infections: clinical and imaging characteristics. Acta Radiol 2007;48:875–93.

47. Mastroyianni SD, Gionnis D, Voudris K, et al. Acute necrotizing encephalopathy of childhood in non-Asian patients: report of three cases and literature review. J Child Neurol 2006;21:872–9.

48. Moog U. Encephalocraniocutaneous lipomatosis. J Med Genet 2009;46:721–9.

49. Moog U, Jones MC, Viskochil DH, et al. Brain anomalies in encephalocraniocutaneous lipomatosis. Am J Med Genet A 2007;143A:2963–72.

# Neuroimaging of Peptide-based Vaccine Therapy in Pediatric Brain Tumors: Initial Experience

Andre D. Furtado, MD[a], Rafael Ceschin, BS[a,b],
Stefan Blüml, PhD[c], Gary Mason, MD[d],
Regina I. Jakacki, MD[d], Hideho Okada, MD[e],
Ian F. Pollack, MD[f,g], Ashok Panigrahy, MD[a],*

## KEYWORDS

- Pseudoprogression • Vaccine therapy • Pediatric brain tumors • MR spectroscopy

## KEY POINTS

- Peptide-based immunotherapy for pediatric brain tumors is associated with the presence of treatment-related heterogeneity, including that of pseudoprogression.
- Conventional MR imaging has limitations in the assessment of treatment-related heterogeneity, particularly regarding distinguishing true tumor progression from efficacious treatment responses.
- Advanced neuroimaging techniques, including diffusion magnetic resonance (MR), perfusion MR, and MR spectroscopy (MRS), may add value in the assessment of treatment-related heterogeneity.
- Recent delineation of specific response criteria for immunotherapy of adult brain tumors (Immunotherapy Response Assessment in Neuro-Oncology [iRANO]) is likely to be relevant to the pediatric population.

## INTRODUCTION

There has been significant progress in the field of immunotherapy, within oncology, with recent Food and Drug Administration approval of immunotherapeutics for metastatic melanoma and non–small cell lung cancer and the advent of multiple immunotherapy clinical trials for primary and metastatic adult brain tumors.[1–4] These adult immunotherapy studies have identified unique responses in regard to treatment response heterogeneity (as characterized by pseudoprogression, delayed responses, therapy-induced inflammation, and so forth) and resulting radiographic challenges. As such, new guidelines have been recently published by the iRANO group to allow for refinement of response assessment criteria for neuro-oncology patients

Disclosure: See last page of the article.
[a] Department of Radiology, University of Pittsburgh, 3600 Forbes Avenue, Pittsburgh, PA 15213, USA;
[b] Department of Bioinformatics, University of Pittsburgh, 5607 Baum Boulevard, Suite 500, Pittsburgh, PA 15206, USA; [c] Department of Radiology, Children's Hospital of Los Angeles, Keck School of Medicine, University of Southern California, Los Angeles, CA 90007, USA; [d] Department of Pediatrics, University of Pittsburgh, 4401 Penn Avenue, Pittsburgh, PA 15224, USA; [e] Department of Neurosurgery, University of California, San Francisco, 505 Parnassus Avenue, M-779, San Francisco, CA 94143, USA; [f] Department of Neurosurgery, University of Pittsburgh, 200 Lothrop Street, Pittsburgh, PA 15213, USA; [g] Children's Hospital of Pittsburgh, University of Pittsburgh Cancer Institute, University of Pittsburgh School of Medicine, University of Pittsburgh, 4401 Penn Avenue, Pittsburgh, PA 15224, USA
* Corresponding author. Department of Pediatric Radiology, Children's Hospital of Pittsburgh of UPMC, 4401 Penn Avenue, Pittsburgh, PA 15224.
E-mail address: panigrahya@upmc.edu

Neuroimag Clin N Am 27 (2017) 155–166
http://dx.doi.org/10.1016/j.nic.2016.09.002
1052-5149/17/© 2016 Elsevier Inc. All rights reserved.

receiving immunotherapy.[4] These iRANO criteria suggest that among adult patients who demonstrate imaging findings meeting RANO (response assessment in neuro-oncology) criteria for progressive disease within 6 months of initiating immunotherapy, including the development of new lesions, confirmation of radiographic progression on follow-up imaging is recommended provided that the adult patient is not significantly worse clinically.[4]

The authors' institutions is currently engaged in multiple peptide-based vaccine trials for children with diffuse intrinsic pontine glioma (DIPG), recurrent high-grade glioma, recurrent low grade-glioma, and recurrent ependymoma.[5–7] The authors have recently described the occurrence of heterogeneous treatment response (including pseudoprogression), which has remarkable similarity with what has been seen in some adult immunotherapy studies. The purpose of this review article is to highlight the authors' initial experience with regard to the emerging radiographic challenges related to heterogeneous treatment response, including that of pseudoprogression, with the use of peptide-based vaccine therapy in pediatric brain tumors.

The authors' initial experience with some of the advanced neuroimaging techniques, including diffusion MR and MRS, is also described to help address some of these radiographic challenges.

## CONVENTIONAL MR IMAGING

The authors have noted multiple forms of treatment-related heterogeneity in different pilot studies of peptide-based vaccine therapy for pediatric brain tumors, particularly in DIPG, recurrent supratentorial high-grade tumors, and recurrent low-grade gliomas. Conventional MR imaging supplemented with MRS, diffusion MR, and perfusion MR was typically performed serially at regular intervals depending on the specific protocol while on the peptide-based vaccine therapy (Fig. 1) (ie, every 6 weeks for newly diagnosed patients receiving radiation). The different forms of treatment-related heterogeneity that have resulted in radiographic challenges include (1) pseudoprogression, characterized by transient enlargement of the tumor with associated clinical symptoms, recently published for the authors' DIPG cohort (Fig. 2A) and recurrent low-grade

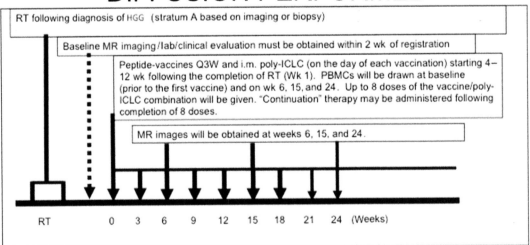

Fig. 1. Example of timing of MR imaging scans for new diagnosis of high-grade pediatric glioma treated with radiation and serial peptide-based vaccine therapy. The time of conventional MR imaging during the course of peptide-vaccine therapy for this particular stratum (A) of the vaccine study was approximately every 6 weeks after initiation of therapy. Straum A of included new diagnosis of high-grade gliomas based on imaging (DIPG) or biopsy and included initial radiotherapy followed by peptide-based vaccine. Note, additional time points of imaging were obtained during clinical pseudoprogression. The timing of serial MR imaging was different for different strata. Diffusion imaging was integrated with all conventional MR imaging scans. MRS and perfusion MR were performed in conjunction with only certain conventional MR imaging scan for logistic reasons. HGG, high grade glioma; i.m., intramuscular; PBMC, peripheral blood mononuclear cell; Q3W, every 3 weeks; RT, radiotherapy.

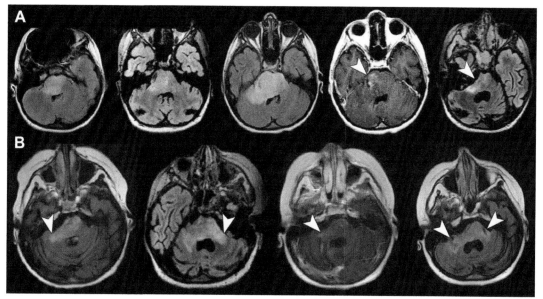

Fig. 2. (*A*) (*Top*) Tumor pseudoprogression. (*Left*) MR baseline before and after radiation immediately before vaccine therapy. Tumor is unchanged from diagnosis. (*Middle*) After 15 weeks' post–first vaccine dose, the patient had tumor enlargement (nonenhancing fluid-attenuated invasion recovery [FLAIR] hyperintensity) and worsened neurologic symptoms. (*Right*) Steroids were started and the MR findings (*arrowheads*) and symptoms improved. (*B*) (*Bottom*) Development of additional lesions: same patient as Fig. 2A, but after first pseudoprogression later in the course of the peptide vaccine therapy. Note the development of small lesions (*left, arrowhead*) (hyperintense FLAIR signal abnormality in the middle cerebellar peduncle (first in the right middle cerebellar peduncle and then left middle cerebellar peduncle, *arrowheads*) that undergo subsequent cystic necrosis and shrinkage on follow-up scans (*right, arrowheads*).

glioma cohort[5,6]; (2) development of different types of noncystic and cystic focal signal abnormalities within the DIPG cohort and recurrent supratentorial high-grade glioma cohort (discussed later; Fig. 3); (3) development of both contiguous (Fig. 2B) and remote smaller lesions that eventually regress and/or undergo necrosis; and (4) one portion of the tumor responding to treatment while another portion of the tumor appears to be growing (see Fig. 7).

In a series of 21 children with DIPG treated with peptide-based vaccines at the authors' institution, 4 children (19%) had documented pseudoprogression based on imaging and clinical criteria: 1 child had transient tumor enlargement in association with acute neurologic deterioration 4 months after beginning vaccination that later regressed and culminated in a sustained partial response (see Fig. 2A) and 3 other children had symptomatic pseudoprogression, with transient neurologic deterioration and tumor enlargement followed by stabilization on decreasing steroid doses. After the episode of pseudoprogression, the patient with the subsequent partial response developed contiguous lesions in the bilateral middle cerebellar peduncle later in the course of peptide-based vaccine therapy. These lesions eventually

underwent shrinkage and necrosis (see Fig. 2B). Cases of pseudoprogression were also noted in other types of pediatric brain tumors treated with the peptide vaccine, including a cervicomedullary biopsy-proved anaplastic astrocytoma lesion (see Fig. 3), recurrent supratentorial high-grade gliomas, and recurrent low-grade gliomas.[5,6]

The authors also observed an unusually high incidence of focal cystic and noncystic signal intensity changes (likely representing evolving necrosis) in a pediatric DIPG population treated with the peptide-based vaccine. When these changes were classified into 4 categories based on T2 signal characteristics and postcontrast enhancement characteristics (Fig. 4), 81% of these children developed focal areas of noncystic changes during immunotherapy, with an average time between starting vaccine to development of noncystic changes of 4.8 months (from 38 days to 10.8 months), and 57% developed focal cystic changes, with an average time of 6.5 months (from 1.2 months to 10.6 months) after the initiation of therapy. Of all the patients who developed cystic necrosis, 82% had noticeable enhancement in the region prior to the development of the necrosis. A small subset of patients had areas of enhancement that were stable or decreased in

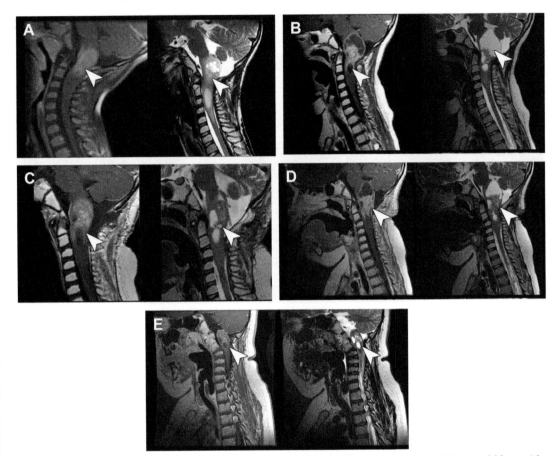

Fig. 3. Biopsy-proved pseudoprogression of a cervical medullary anaplastic astrocytoma: 4.5-year-old boy with a biopsy-proved cervicomedullary anaplastic glioma ([A] baseline, *arrowheads*) who developed worsening neck pain after his fourth vaccine, which became increasingly severe immediately after his fifth vaccine, 6.5 months after diagnosis, 4 months after completion of irradiation, and 3 months after beginning vaccination. He exhibited neurologic worsening and MR imaging showed formation of a necrotic cyst superior to the tumor in the medullary region (B, *arrowhead*). Vaccines were withheld, and the cyst continued to increase in size; his neck pain became debilitating and he underwent laminectomy and cyst decompression 2.5 months later (C, *arrowheads*). He had rapid clinical improvement and resolution of the cyst on subsequent MR imaging scan. Biopsies showed no mitotically active tumor, and he resumed vaccine therapy. Six weeks later, he developed clinical and radiographic worsening with recurrence of neck pain. An MR imaging showed re-accumulation of the cyst and increased enhancement and size of the solid component, which prompted discontinuation of the vaccine regimen (D, *arrowheads*). He was started on palliative oral chemotherapy and has shown a dramatic clinical improvement over the next 3 months and is back at school and almost completely off steroids. Five years later, the patient is still alive with small stable residual lesion (E, *arrowheads*).

size on subsequent examinations. Studies are ongoing at the authors' institution to correlate these patterns of focal signal abnormality with survival and pseudoprogression. These findings underscore the concept that conventional MR imaging has limitations in the ability to assess different forms of treatment-related imaging heterogeneity. The authors' initial experience with the use of advanced neuroimaging modalities (ie, MRS, diffusion MR, and perfusion MR) to evaluate treatment response is described.

## MAGNETIC RESONANCE SPECTROSCOPY

MRS provides a metabolic evaluation of the sampled tissue. In vivo intracellular metabolites with concentrations of 0.1 μmol/g to 0.5 μmol/g or higher can be assessed. Abnormal choline (Cho) metabolism is a common endpoint for many forms of cancer. Cho-containing metabolites are involved in the synthesis and breakdown of cell membranes. Because growing tumors require the net synthesis of cell membranes to

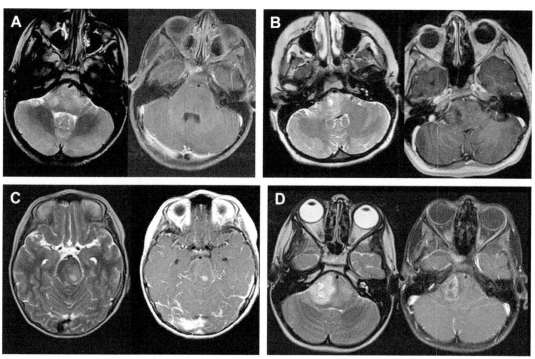

Fig. 4. Focal changes in pediatric DIBG during immunotherapy (Right T2WI, Left post contrast T1WI). Areas of noncystic changes without enhancement (*A*), areas of noncystic changes with enhancement (*B*), areas of cystic changes without enhancement (*C*), and areas of cystic changes with peripheral enhancement (*D*).

support cell proliferation, the in vivo measurement of Cho provides surrogate information on tumor growth rates. Brain tumors generally have elevated levels of Cho, with higher Cho levels observed in more aggressive tumors.[8–10] Another metabolic feature of aggressive tumors is a prominent signal from mobile lipids,[11,12] although the time course is less predictable. Lipids (and lactate) can accumulate in cystic/necrotic areas but may also be recycled by tumor cells and/or surrounding cells for de novo cell membrane synthesis and for oxidation in the tricarboxylic acid cycle. Lipids may increase as tumors progress, for example, from grade III astrocytoma to glioblastoma.[12] Myo-inositol is well regarded as a marker of gliosis[13] as well as an important osmolyte whose regulation across the plasma membrane is a key cellular mechanism for mediating osmotic stress in astrocytes.[14,15] In in vivo human studies, myo-inositol is consistently elevated in the setting of chronic inflammation, such as in multiple sclerosis and other neuroinflammatory central nervous system conditions,[16–18] likely reflecting ongoing astrogliosis. Myo-inositol is generally elevated in ependymoma and gliomas, which are typically characterized by a high fraction of glial cells.[19–21] Histopathologic studies have suggested there is increased reactive gliosis in individual tumors

marked by an elevated myo-inositol concentration,[22,23] and in a recent study, elevated myo-inositol distinguished tissue inflammation from tumor proliferation in adult glioblastoma patients treated with radiation therapy and adjuvant therapy.[24] The authors are currently exploring the hypothesis that alterations in myo-inositol may be a predictor of outcome in certain forms of pediatric tumors treated with the peptide-based vaccines [in particular the DIPG cohort (Fig. 5)]. A key observation was the stability of serial MRS spectra in the setting of clinical and radiographic pseudoprogression (see Fig. 5). Specifically, the MRS spectra were stable comparing 3 time points of imaging: baseline, at the time of pseudoprogression, and after pseudoprogression. When the cases of pseudoprogression (eg, case shown in Fig. 2) were specifically looked at, there was serial stability in the Cho-to-creatine ratio, myo-inositol, and lipids/lactate (see Fig. 5). From these preliminary observations, the authors hypothesize that the stability of certain metabolite ratios (including Cho-to-creatine ratio) may distinguish treatment response and pseudoprogression from true progression in the setting of peptide-based treatment of high-grade gliomas (including DIPG). Likewise, stability in lipids/lactate and myo-inositol also may have the potential to distinguish

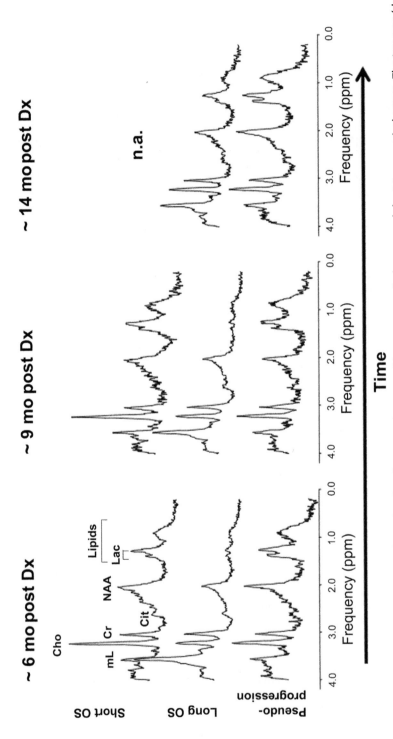

**Fig. 5.** Comparison of pseudoprogression case (from Fig. 2) with averaged spectra of long-term survival group and short-term survival group. The top row (short-term survival) shows that there is increase in the Cho-to-creatine ratio between the first 2 time points. The middle row shows that in the long-term survival group there is relative stability in the Cho-to-creatine ratio over time. The bottom row shows the MRS for the pseudoprogression case from Fig. 2, in which there is preservation of Cho-to-creatine ratio across time points. Metabolite levels, including myo-inositol and lipids/lactate, remain stable across all 3 time points in the patient with pseudoprogression (*bottom row*). Cit, citrate; Cr, creatine; Dx, diagnosis; Lac, lactate; n.a., not available; NAA, N-acetylaspartate; OS, overall survival; ppm, parts per million.

pseudoprogression from true progression. These findings underscore the importance in obtaining serial MRS data at baseline and different points of therapy, including at the time of pseudoprogression. These preliminary observations need to be confirmed in large-scale multicenter studies.

## DIFFUSION-WEIGHTED MR IMAGING

Diffusion refers to random (brownian) motion of molecules due to heat. In clinical imaging, the authors evaluate the mean diffusivity of water molecules assuming isotropy in each voxel. In vivo, the limitation of diffusion-weighted imaging is that the diffusion of water molecules is due not only to heat but also to active transport, flow along pressure gradients, and changes in membrane permeability. The apparent diffusion coefficient (ADC) is a quantitative diffusion constant calculated from different b values (different gradient amplitudes) to reflect the diffusion of water molecules through different tissues, expressed in units of $mm^2/s$.[25] Higher ADC values mean increased water motion and lower ADC values mean decreased (restricted) water motion. Although untreated brain tumors demonstrate increased ADC values compared with the normal brain as a result of disruption of normal cellular integrity, densely cellular tumors demonstrate relative lower ADC values. Baseline low minimum ADC values have

been associated with worse clinical outcome as determined by the authors and other investigators.[26,27] The effect of radiation therapy can be divided in acute, early-delayed, and late-delayed radiation changes. A transient increase in ADC has been reported between 3 months and 5 months after radiation,[28] likely the result from tissue damage, vasodilation, and edema.[29] With time, the ADC values decrease, which is particularly noticeable in children with DIPG (Fig. 6). Using serial functional diffusion maps (sfDM), the authors' group demonstrated that children with DIPG status postradiation, who had tumor pseudoprogression during immunotherapy, had higher fitted average log-transformed parametric response mapping ratios and fractional decreased ADC compared with those without pseudoprogression.[30] Moreover, focal increase in ADC signal preceded the appearance of cystic necrosis (see Fig. 6). Serial parametric response mapping of ADC seems a promising method to assess treatment response in children with DIPG treated with peptide-based vaccinations.

## PERFUSION MR IMAGING

The 3 major types of perfusion MR in the authors' studies of pediatric brain tumors treated with peptide-based vaccine therapy include dynamic susceptibility contrast (DSC), dynamic contrast

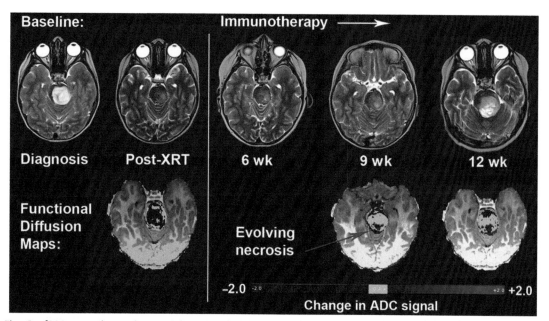

Fig. 6. sfDM to evaluate the spatial-temporal changes in ADC measurements in pediatric DIPG treated with peptide-based vaccination. sfDM demonstrates decrease in ADC signal after radiation (*blue voxels, left bottom*). During immunotherapy, focal increase in ADC signal (*red voxels, right bottom*) preceded the appearance of necrosis. The stability of the ADC signal (*green voxels, right bottom*) is consistent with treatment-related necrosis rather than tumor progression. XRT, radiation therapy.

enhancement, and arterial spin labeling (ASL). DSC MR imaging, also known as bolus-tracking MR imaging, is based on serial measurements of MR imaging signal change within a region of interest during the first pass of exogenous, paramagnetic, nondiffusible contrast agent, typically a gadolinium-based contrast agent (GBCA). Under normal conditions, the local susceptibility effect induced by intravascular compartmentalization of GBCA translates into a signal drop on T2 spin-echo or T2 gradient-echo (T2* GRE) echo-planar imaging. Higher-grade brain tumors tend to have increased microvascular circulation related to tumoral angiogenesis and, as a result, larger blood volume on DSC signal intensity time curves.[31] This technique is valuable for guidance of stereotactic biopsy. One of the limitations of DSC is when there is severe disruption of the brain-blood barrier causing inaccurate estimation of intravascular blood volume due to extravasation of GBCA (T1-dominant contrast leakage).[32,33] In contrast to DSC imaging, dynamic contrast-enhanced imaging measures an increase in MR imaging signal proportional to the concentration of GBCA in the region of interest using T1-weighted imaging, providing an evaluation of the wash-in and wash-out contrast kinetics within tumors as a result of tumor perfusion, vessel permeability, and volume of the extravascular-extracellular space.[34] One alternative without the administration of intravenous contrast is the ASL, which consists of labeling protons in the blood in supplying vessels outside the imaging plane. Subtraction of the images obtained with and without labeling allows calculation of tissue perfusion, which is proportional to the cerebral blood flow.[35] ASL may be a reliable alternative to DSC with several advantages in children because it does not require intravenous administration of contrast, can be repeated multiple times, and has the potential to provide quantitative cerebral blood flow.[36] In a recent article by the Pediatric Brain Tumor Consortium, there was no association between progression-free survival and relative cerebral blood volume assess by DSC at baseline, or when perfusion values were used as time-dependent variables, in children with brain tumor treated with radiation and molecularly targeted agents (gefitinib and tipifarnib).[27]

The potential role of DSC, dynamic contrast-enhanced, and ASL imaging in assessing pediatric brain tumor treated with immunotherapy is currently being investigated at the authors' institution. As a pilot study, the authors examined diffusion and perfusion correlates of heterogeneous treatment response in peptide-based therapy for pediatric DIPG. The hypothesis that correlations between ADC (cellularity) and ASL (vascularity) would differ between brainstem glioma (DIPG) groups treated with and without vaccine therapy was tested. ADC and ASL images of 19 pediatric DIPG patients (n = 11 on vaccine therapy and n = 8 not on vaccine therapy) were acquired at 1.5T. After registration, tumor regions were manually segmented. A correlation analysis between mean ADC and ASL in the tumor and unaffected gray matter was conducted using linear regression. Statistically significant correlation between mean ADC and ASL was seen in DIPG regions of patients on vaccine (R = −0.358, P = .0256). No statistically significant association was seen in the mean ADC and ASL of the DIPG in patients treated with standard radiation and radiochemotherapy (nonvaccine) (R = 0.006, P = .9770). As such, a unique inverse correlation of perfusion and diffusion (with increased perfusion associated with decreased ADC or increased cellularity) was noted in the vaccine therapy DIPG group compared with the nonvaccine therapy group. This may reflect identification of a unique treatment response within the vaccine group. Validation in a larger dataset and correlation with outcome is currently being pursued.

## 23NA–MAGNETIC RESONANCE AND 3'-[18F] FLUORO-3'-DEOXYTHYMIDINE IMAGING

23Na-MR is a useful noninvasive technique to assess proliferation. In neoplastic tissue, sustained depolarization of the cell membrane precedes the high rate of mitotic activity that characterizes abnormal tumor growth, leading to concomitant increase in intracellular 23Na concentration (ISC) as demonstrated in several human neoplasms. Further characterization of this rise in ISC in several types of human carcinoma/glial cell lines has established a positive correlation between proliferative activity and increased intracellular $Na^+/K^+$ ratio. The increase in ISC leads to a concomitant increase in the total tissue 23Na concentration over the tumor volume.[37–43] 23Na concentration was altered in several of the authors' pediatric patients with brain tumors treated with immunotherapy. The highest concentrations were observed in high-grade supratentorial astrocytomas (Fig. 7). Preliminary observations were that a decrease in 23Na signal portends a good treatment response, possibly earlier than other imaging methods. The authors are currently evaluating the utility of 23Na-MR to help characterize heterogeneous treatment response in different types of pediatric brain tumors undergoing peptide-based vaccine therapy.

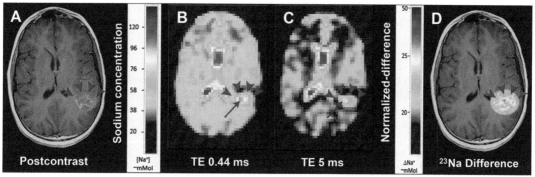

**Fig. 7.** <sup>23</sup>Na-MR of a necrotic lesion in pediatric subject. (*A*) Shows a ring-enhancing necrotic lesion (*red arrowheads*); this lesion was a new recurrent lesion, separate from a lesion in the frontal lobe (not shown) that has initially responded to peptide-based vaccine therapy. (*B*) Short-echo <sup>23</sup>Na-MR and (*C*) longer-echo <sup>23</sup>Na-MR showing total/extracellular sodium and increased foci in the periphery of lesion (*red arrows*). (*D*) Coregistered targeted subtracted overlap image show that the periphery of the necrosis (*red arrowheads*) had increased ICS (*red and yellow voxels*) and decreased central ICS (*bluish voxels*) representing tumor-related cavitation/necrosis confirmed to be a recurrent tumor by follow-up. TE, echo time.

All the MR biomarkers being studied (conventional MR imaging, MRS, ADC, ASL, and sodium) have limitations in the assessment of new large necrotic lesions, which have been observed in a significant percentage of malignant gliomas treated with immunotherapy in the authors' current clinical trials. 3'-[18F] fluoro-3'-deoxythymidine ([18F]-FLT) PET may be particularly valuable for these patients. [18F]-FLT is a pyrimidine analog and a biomarker for thymidine kinase 1 activity during the S phase of DNA synthesis. Previous investigations have demonstrated a high correlation between [18F]-FLT uptake and proliferation rate.[44–56] The potential advantages of [18F]-FLT over fludeoxyglucose F 18 in high-grade gliomas include improved signal-to-noise ratio and significantly greater specificity for proliferation over treatment-related necrosis.[57,58] In addition, there is research to support that [18F]-FLT may distinguish between tumor proliferation and inflammation, which may be useful in the assessment of pseudoprogression.[59–62] The authors use [18F]-FLT to label solid tumor around areas of necrosis, thereby potentially providing an indicator of tumor proliferation. The authors are currently in the process of developing an MR-PET protocol to perform [18F]-FLT imaging in pediatric brain tumor patients treated with peptide-based vaccine therapy.

## SUMMARY

Potential benefits of peptide-based immunotherapy for pediatric brain tumors have been identified with pilot studies performed at the authors' institution. Different forms of treatment-related heterogeneity are described, which has resulted in radiographic challenges, including the determination of pseudoprogression versus true tumor progression by conventional MR imaging. Initial results suggest that advanced neuroimaging techniques, including diffusion MR, perfusion MR, and MRS, may add value to the assessment of treatment-related heterogeneity. Future work may help identify which imaging approach is superior. Initial observations suggest that recent delineation of specific response criteria for immunotherapy of adult brain tumors (iRANO) is likely to be relevant to the pediatric brain tumor population, and further validation in multicenter pediatric brain tumor peptide-based vaccine studies are warranted.

## DISCLOSURES

UPCI (University of Pittsburgh Cancer Institute) Clinical Research Services for regulatory management; Andres Salazar and Oncovir, Inc. for provision of poly-ICLC; physicians who referred their patients; and the patients and families who participated in this trial. This study was supported by National Institutes of Health grants R21CA149872 and P01NS40923 and the UPCI Immunological Monitoring Core and Biostatistics Shared Resource Facility, supported in part by National Institute of Health (NIH) award P30CA47904; grants from the Pediatric Low-Grade Glioma Initiative via the National Brain Tumor Society, the Ian's (Ian Yagoda) Friends Foundation Grant, Society of Pediatric Radiology Pilot Award, and the Ellie Kavalieros Fund of the Children's Hospital of Pittsburgh Foundation; and the Pediatric Clinical and Translational Research Center, supported by the NIH through grant numbers UL1 RR024153 and

UL1TR000005. R. Ceschin was supported by an NLM grant 5T15LM00705927.

## CONFLICTS OF INTEREST

H. Okada is an inventor in the US Patent Application No. 60,611, 797 (Utility Patent Application) "Identification of An IL-13 Receptor Alpha2 Peptide Analogue Capable of Enhancing Stimulation of Glioma-Specific CTL Response." An exclusive licensing agreement has been completed on this application between the University of Pittsburgh and Stemline, Inc. Due to the potential conflicts of interest, H. Okada did not solely interpret any data in the current study. Dr R.I. Jakacki is currently employed by AstraZeneca.

## ACKNOWLEDGMENTS

We thank Vince Lee for technical assistance and Fern Wasco for research coordination. Also, the authors would like to acknowledge the important contribution of Jack Schnur to the content of this article.

## REFERENCES

1. Kantoff PW, Higano CS, Shore ND, et al. Sipuleucel-T immunotherapy for castration-resistant prostate cancer. N Engl J Med 2010;363(5):411–22.
2. Hodi FS, O'Day SJ, McDermott DF, et al. Improved survival with ipilimumab in patients with metastatic melanoma. N Engl J Med 2010;363(8):711–23.
3. Robert C, Long GV, Brady B, et al. Nivolumab in previously untreated melanoma without BRAF mutation. N Engl J Med 2015;372(4):320–30.
4. Okada H, Weller M, Huang R, et al. Immunotherapy response assessment in neuro-oncology: a report of the RANO working group. Lancet Oncol 2015;16:534–42.
5. Pollack IF, Jakacki RI, Butterfield LH, et al. Immune responses and outcome after vaccination with glioma-associated antigen peptides and poly-ICLC in a pilot study for pediatric recurrent low-grade gliomasdagger. Neuro Oncol 2016;18(8):1157–68.
6. Pollack IF, Jakacki RI, Butterfield LH, et al. Antigen-specific immune responses and clinical outcome after vaccination with glioma-associated antigen peptides and polyinosinic-polycytidylic acid stabilized by lysine and carboxymethylcellulose in children with newly diagnosed malignant brainstem and nonbrainstem gliomas. J Clin Oncol 2014;32(19):2050–8.
7. Yeung JT, Hamilton RL, Okada H, et al. Increased expression of tumor-associated antigens in pediatric and adult ependymomas: implication for vaccine therapy. J Neurooncol 2013;111(2):103–11.
8. Astrakas LG, Zurakowski D, Tzika AA, et al. Noninvasive magnetic resonance spectroscopic imaging biomarkers to predict the clinical grade of pediatric brain tumors. Clin Cancer Res 2004;10(24):8220–8.
9. Shimizu H, Kumabe T, Shirane R, et al. Correlation between choline level measured by proton MR spectroscopy and Ki-67 labeling index in gliomas. AJNR Am J Neuroradiol 2000;21(4):659–65.
10. Tamiya T, Kinoshita K, Ono Y, et al. Proton magnetic resonance spectroscopy reflects cellular proliferative activity in astrocytomas. Neuroradiology 2000;42(5):333–8.
11. Negendank W, Sauter R. Intratumoral lipids in 1H MRS in vivo in brain tumors: experience of the Siemens cooperative clinical trial. Anticancer Res 1996;16(3B):1533–8.
12. Murphy PS, Rowland IJ, Viviers L, et al. Could assessment of glioma methylene lipid resonance by in vivo (1)H-MRS be of clinical value? Br J Radiol 2003;76(907):459–63.
13. Brand A, Richter-Landsberg C, Leibfritz D. Multinuclear NMR studies on the energy metabolism of glial and neuronal cells. Dev Neurosci 1993;15(3–5):289–98.
14. Wiese TJ, Dunlap JA, Conner CE, et al. Osmotic regulation of Na-myo-inositol cotransporter mRNA level and activity in endothelial and neural cells. Am J Physiol 1996;270(4 Pt 1):C990–7.
15. Paredes A, McManus M, Kwon HM, et al. Osmoregulation of Na(+)-inositol cotransporter activity and mRNA levels in brain glial cells. Am J Physiol 1992;263(6 Pt 1):C1282–8.
16. Kapeller P, Ropele S, Enzinger C, et al. Discrimination of white matter lesions and multiple sclerosis plaques by short echo quantitative 1H-magnetic resonance spectroscopy. J Neurol 2005;252(10):1229–34.
17. Bruhn H, Frahm J, Merboldt KD, et al. Multiple sclerosis in children: cerebral metabolic alterations monitored by localized proton magnetic resonance spectroscopy in vivo. Ann Neurol 1992;32(2):140–50.
18. Chang L, Lee PL, Yiannoutsos CT, et al. A multicenter in vivo proton-MRS study of HIV-associated dementia and its relationship to age. Neuroimage 2004;23(4):1336–47.
19. Davies NP, Wilson M, Harris LM, et al. Identification and characterisation of childhood cerebellar tumours by in vivo proton MRS. NMR Biomed 2008;21(8):908–18.
20. Panigrahy A, Krieger MD, Gonzalez-Gomez I, et al. Quantitative short echo time 1H-MR spectroscopy of untreated pediatric brain tumors: preoperative diagnosis and characterization. AJNR Am J Neuroradiol 2006;27(3):560–72.
21. Panigrahy A, Bluml S. Neuroimaging of pediatric brain tumors: from basic to advanced magnetic

resonance imaging (MRI). J Child Neurol 2009; 24(11):1343–65.

22. Hattingen E, Raab P, Franz K, et al. Myo-inositol: a marker of reactive astrogliosis in glial tumors? NMR Biomed 2008;21(3):233–41.

23. Amstutz DR, Coons SW, Kerrigan JF, et al. Hypothalamic hamartomas: correlation of MR imaging and spectroscopic findings with tumor glial content. AJNR Am J Neuroradiol 2006; 27(4):794–8.

24. Srinivasan R, Phillips JJ, Vandenberg SR, et al. Ex vivo MR spectroscopic measure differentiates tumor from treatment effects in GBM. Neuro Oncol 2010;12(11):1152–61.

25. Mukherjee P, Berman JI, Chung SW, et al. Diffusion tensor MR imaging and fiber tractography: theoretic underpinnings. AJNR Am J Neuroradiol 2008;29(4): 632–41.

26. Okada H, Lieberman FS, Walter KA, et al. Autologous glioma cell vaccine admixed with interleukin-4 gene transfected fibroblasts in the treatment of patients with malignant gliomas. J Transl Med 2007;5:67.

27. Poussaint TY, Kocak M, Vajapeyam S, et al. MRI as a central component of clinical trials analysis in brainstem glioma: a report from the Pediatric Brain Tumor Consortium (PBTC). Neuro Oncol 2011; 13(4):417–27.

28. Kitahara S, Nakasu S, Murata K, et al. Evaluation of treatment-induced cerebral white matter injury by using diffusion-tensor MR imaging: initial experience. AJNR Am J Neuroradiol 2005;26(9):2200–6.

29. Wong CS, Van der Kogel AJ. Mechanisms of radiation injury to the central nervous system: implications for neuroprotection. Mol Interv 2004;4(5): 273–84.

30. Ceschin R, Kurland BF, Abberbock SR, et al. Parametric response mapping of apparent diffusion coefficient as an imaging biomarker to distinguish pseudoprogression from true tumor progression in peptide-based vaccine therapy for pediatric diffuse intrinsic pontine glioma. AJNR Am J Neuroradiol 2015;36(11):2170–6.

31. Law M, Yang S, Babb JS, et al. Comparison of cerebral blood volume and vascular permeability from dynamic susceptibility contrast-enhanced perfusion MR imaging with glioma grade. AJNR Am J Neuroradiol 2004;25(5):746–55.

32. Cha S. Dynamic susceptibility-weighted contrast-enhanced perfusion MR imaging in pediatric patients. Neuroimaging Clin N Am 2006;16(1): 137–47, ix.

33. Calamante F. Perfusion MRI using dynamic-susceptibility contrast MRI: quantification issues in patient studies. Top Magn Reson Imaging 2010; 21(2):75–85.

34. Choyke PL, Dwyer AJ, Knopp MV. Functional tumor imaging with dynamic contrast-enhanced magnetic resonance imaging. J Magn Reson Imaging 2003; 17(5):509–20.

35. Pollock JM, Tan H, Kraft RA, et al. Arterial spin-labeled MR perfusion imaging: clinical applications. Magn Reson Imaging Clin N Am 2009; 17(2):315–38.

36. Yang Y, Frank JA, Hou L, et al. Multislice imaging of quantitative cerebral perfusion with pulsed arterial spin labeling. Magn Reson Med 1998;39(5):825–32.

37. Bartha R, Megyesi JF, Watling CJ. Low-grade glioma: correlation of short echo time 1H-MR spectroscopy with 23Na MR imaging. AJNR Am J Neuroradiol 2008;29(3):464–70.

38. Cameron IL, Smith NK, Pool TB, et al. Intracellular concentration of sodium and other elements as related to mitogenesis and oncogenesis in vivo. Cancer Res 1980;40(5):1493–500.

39. Ouwerkerk R, Bleich KB, Gillen JS, et al. Tissue sodium concentration in human brain tumors as measured with 23Na MR imaging. Radiology 2003; 227(2):529–37.

40. Thulborn KR, Davis D, Adams H, et al. Quantitative tissue sodium concentration mapping of the growth of focal cerebral tumors with sodium magnetic resonance imaging. Magn Reson Med 1999;41(2): 351–9.

41. Turski PA, Houston LW, Perman WH, et al. Experimental and human brain neoplasms: detection with in vivo sodium MR imaging. Radiology 1987; 163(1):245–9.

42. Boada FE, Tanase C, Davis D, et al. Non-invasive assessment of tumor proliferation using triple quantum filtered 23/Na MRI: technical challenges and solutions. Conf Proc IEEE Eng Med Biol Soc 2004;7: 5238–41.

43. Schepkin VD, Lee KC, Kuszpit K, et al. Proton and sodium MRI assessment of emerging tumor chemotherapeutic resistance. NMR Biomed 2006;19(8): 1035–42.

44. Chen W, Cloughesy T, Kamdar N, et al. Imaging proliferation in brain tumors with 18F-FLT PET: comparison with 18F-FDG. J Nucl Med 2005;46(6):945–52.

45. Shields AF, Grierson JR, Dohmen BM, et al. Imaging proliferation in vivo with [F-18]FLT and positron emission tomography. Nat Med 1998;4(11):1334–6.

46. Backes H, Ullrich R, Neumaier B, et al. Noninvasive quantification of 18F-FLT human brain PET for the assessment of tumour proliferation in patients with high-grade glioma. Eur J Nucl Med Mol Imaging 2009;36(12):1960–7.

47. Hatakeyama T, Kawai N, Nishiyama Y, et al. 11C-methionine (MET) and 18F-fluorothymidine (FLT) PET in patients with newly diagnosed glioma. Eur J Nucl Med Mol Imaging 2008;35(11):2009–17.

48. Saga T, Kawashima H, Araki N, et al. Evaluation of primary brain tumors with FLT-PET: usefulness and limitations. Clin Nucl Med 2006;31(12):774–80.

49. Ullrich R, Backes H, Li H, et al. Glioma proliferation as assessed by 3'-fluoro-3'-deoxy-L-thymidine positron emission tomography in patients with newly diagnosed high-grade glioma. Clin Cancer Res 2008;14(7):2049–55.

50. Chen W, Delaloye S, Silverman DH, et al. Predicting treatment response of malignant gliomas to bevacizumab and irinotecan by imaging proliferation with [18F] fluorothymidine positron emission tomography: a pilot study. J Clin Oncol 2007; 25(30):4714–21.

51. Choi SJ, Kim JS, Kim JH, et al. [18F]3'-deoxy-3'-fluorothymidine PET for the diagnosis and grading of brain tumors. Eur J Nucl Med Mol Imaging 2005; 32(6):653–9.

52. Yamamoto Y, Ono Y, Aga F, et al. Correlation of 18F-FLT uptake with tumor grade and Ki-67 immunohistochemistry in patients with newly diagnosed and recurrent gliomas. J Nucl Med 2012;53(12): 1911–5.

53. Wardak M, Schiepers C, Dahlbom M, et al. Discriminant analysis of (1)(8)F-fluorothymidine kinetic parameters to predict survival in patients with recurrent high-grade glioma. Clin Cancer Res 2011;17(20):6553–62.

54. Spence AM, Muzi M, Link JM, et al. NCI-sponsored trial for the evaluation of safety and preliminary efficacy of 3'-deoxy-3'-[18F]fluorothymidine (FLT) as a marker of proliferation in patients with recurrent gliomas: preliminary efficacy studies. Mol Imaging Biol 2009;11(5):343–55.

55. Corroyer-Dulmont A, Pérès EA, Petit E, et al. Detection of glioblastoma response to temozolomide combined with bevacizumab based on muMRI and muPET imaging reveals [18F]-fluoro-L-thymidine as an early and robust predictive marker for treatment efficacy. Neuro Oncol 2013;15(1):41–56.

56. Schwarzenberg J, Czernin J, Cloughesy TF, et al. 3'-deoxy-3'-18F-fluorothymidine PET and MRI for early survival predictions in patients with recurrent malignant glioma treated with bevacizumab. J Nucl Med 2012;53(1):29–36.

57. Enslow MS, Zollinger LV, Morton KA, et al. Comparison of 18F-fluorodeoxyglucose and 18F-fluorothymidine PET in differentiating radiation necrosis from recurrent glioma. Clin Nucl Med 2012;37(9):854–61.

58. Jain R, Narang J, Sundgren PM, et al. Treatment induced necrosis versus recurrent/progressing brain tumor: going beyond the boundaries of conventional morphologic imaging. J Neurooncol 2010;100(1):17–29.

59. van Waarde A, Jager PL, Ishiwata K, et al. Comparison of sigma-ligands and metabolic PET tracers for differentiating tumor from inflammation. J Nucl Med 2006;47(1):150–4.

60. van Waarde A, Cobben DC, Suurmeijer AJ, et al. Selectivity of 18F-FLT and 18F-FDG for differentiating tumor from inflammation in a rodent model. J Nucl Med 2004;45(4):695–700.

61. Grivennikov SI, Karin M. Inflammation and oncogenesis: a vicious connection. Curr Opin Genet Dev 2010;20(1):65–71.

62. van Waarde A, Elsinga PH. Proliferation markers for the differential diagnosis of tumor and inflammation. Curr Pharm Des 2008;14(31):3326–39.

# Advanced MR Imaging in Pediatric Brain Tumors, Clinical Applications

Maarten Lequin, MD, PhD*, Jeroen Hendrikse, MD, PhD

## KEYWORDS

• MR • Advanced imaging • Pediatric • Brain tumor

## KEY POINTS

- A combination of conventional and advanced MR imaging sequences is recommended to make the correct diagnosis in pediatric patients suspected to have a brain tumor.
- In the work-up of brain tumors at least diffusion-weighted imaging/diffusion tensor imaging, MR spectroscopy (MRS), and a perfusion MR technique should be included in the imaging protocol.
- MRS data may play an important role in assessing therapeutic response and therefore should be interpreted by experienced neuroradiologists.
- Arterial spin labeling is a promising noninvasive perfusion sequence that may become an important biomarker for tumor diagnosis and tumor grading.
- Future advances in molecular biology will alter neuroradiologic concepts and thinking and add information to that obtained from conventional and advanced MR imaging techniques, which will benefit pediatric patients with brain tumors.

## INTRODUCTION

Imaging of brain tumors has significantly improved with the use of advanced magnetic resonance (MR) techniques, such as MR spectroscopy (MRS), perfusion-weighted imaging, diffusion-weighted imaging (DWI), diffusion tensor imaging (DTI), susceptibility-weighted imaging (SWI), and functional MR (fMR) imaging.[1–10] Conventional MR imaging techniques provide anatomic/structural information about the brain. Unlike conventional imaging, advanced MR techniques also provide physiologic and functional information concerning metabolism; hemodynamics; and, with diffusion-weighted technique, information on brain tumor cellularity. Recently, the introduction of DNA methylation profiling for molecular classification has been proposed, which outperforms the current histopathologic classification and thus might serve as a basis for the next World Health Organization classification scheme for central nervous system (CNS) tumors. In the future, this may have a great impact on the correlation between advanced imaging assessment and the newly proposed molecular classification. This overview is based on the literature between the currently used histopathologic classifications of pediatric brain tumors and their characteristics on advanced MR imaging techniques. In the near future it will be mandatory to scan with advanced imaging protocols in all pediatric brain tumors, classified by their molecular phenotype to reevaluate their diagnostic value.

Neuroradiology, Department of Radiology and Nuclear Medicine, University Medical Center Utrecht, Heidelberglaan 100, 3584 CX Utrecht, Netherlands
* Corresponding author.
*E-mail address:* m.h.lequin@umcutrecht.nl

Neuroimag Clin N Am 27 (2017) 167–190
http://dx.doi.org/10.1016/j.nic.2016.08.007
1052-5149/17/© 2016 Elsevier Inc. All rights reserved.

The most useful clinical applications of these advanced MR techniques in pediatric brain tumors, stratified by the current classification, are discussed here.

1. DWI approaches (DWI, DTI, diffusion kurtosis imaging [DKI])
2. MRS (single-voxel [SV] imaging, and chemical shift imaging [CSI])
3. Perfusion-weighted techniques (dynamic susceptibility contrast [DSC] technique; dynamic contrast-enhanced [DCE]; and arterial spin labeling [ASL], a noncontrast technique)
4. Other advanced MR imaging sequences, useful for diagnosis and presurgical planning in children suspected to have a brain tumor (SWI and fMR imaging)

## Diffusion-Weighted Imaging Technique (Diffusion-Weighted Imaging, Diffusion Tensor Imaging, Diffusion Kurtosis Imaging)

DWI is commonly used by (pediatric) neuroradiologists in everyday clinical practice. Although it is no longer a novel imaging technique, it provides information that is not obtainable using conventional MR sequences and is therefore discussed in this article.

The additional information is obtained by measuring the mobility of water molecules, assuming a process of random, unrestricted, but potentially hindered diffusion. The diffusion probability distribution function, the chance of a particular proton diffusing from one location to another in a given time, is thus considered a gaussian distribution, with the standard deviation relating to the apparent diffusion coefficient (ADC). The ADC value depends on the complexity of the cytoarchitecture, determined by, for example, cell membranes, intracellular organelles, and the rapid exchange of protons between different compartments (Fig. 1). The cytoarchitecture of the tumor can inhibit random brownian motion and thus causes water diffusion to deviate from strict gaussian behavior. This restricted diffusion appears hyperintense on the diffusion trace map and dark on the ADC map (Fig. 2). In clinical practice and research, ADC maps and ADC values have been used to assess tumor cellularity and tumor grade (Fig. 3). Recently, Poretti and colleagues[4] showed that tumor grade as estimated by ADC values could be better assessed only from the solid, contrast-enhancing part of the tumor rather than the entire tumor. Further, ADC values can also be used to assay treatment response and detect tumor recurrence and even to differentiate tumor recurrence from pseudoprogression.[5]

Although mainly used in the treatment scheme of high-grade gliomas in adults, antiangiogenic drugs may also be a treatment option in pediatric patients with brain tumors. DWI based on ADC analyses is less affected by vascular permeability changes caused by antiangiogenic treatment than contrast-enhanced T1-weighted imaging and is therefore a good imaging marker of treatment outcomes. However, clinicians should beware of areas of restricted diffusion that may appear after antiangiogenic treatment, which were stable on follow-up MR imaging studies, and therefore are more consistent with necrosis than tumor recurrence/progression.[6]

There are studies focusing on treatment-induced changes in ADC values by comparing pretreatment and early posttreatment measures.[7] Some reports even advocate the use of functional diffusion map methods by voxel-wise subtraction of the pretreatment and posttreatment ADC maps for accurate assessment of changes in ADC values at all tumor locations.[8] Also ADC value changes over time, suggesting that serial MR (DWI) imaging may be useful to investigate possible changes in volume of low-ADC regions within the tumor.

Although the results from DWI and quantitative ADC look promising and DWI imaging is easy and quick to perform, clinicians should keep in mind that variations in equipment (even from the same brand) and acquisition parameters can result in significant differences in calculated ADC values. Even using ratios by comparing with normal-appearing brain tissue as a reference may produce inconsistent results. This possibility is especially important in follow-up scanning, making it sometimes more difficult to differentiate between tumor growth and necrosis. Second, brain tumors may become more heterogeneous after treatment, which may influence ADC values and result in inaccurate diagnosis of tumor progression. Some investigators suggest histogram-based methods but this is a time-consuming approach.[9]

### Diffusion tensor imaging

The diffusion-weighted technique not only uses the magnitude of the diffusion but can also provide the direction of diffusion and is therefore sensitive to directional movements of water molecules using DTI. DTI has been used extensively for the identification of functional white matter tracts in vivo. In neuro-oncology, DTI has the potential to establish spatial relationships between normal-appearing white matter and tumor borders and provide clinically valuable information on

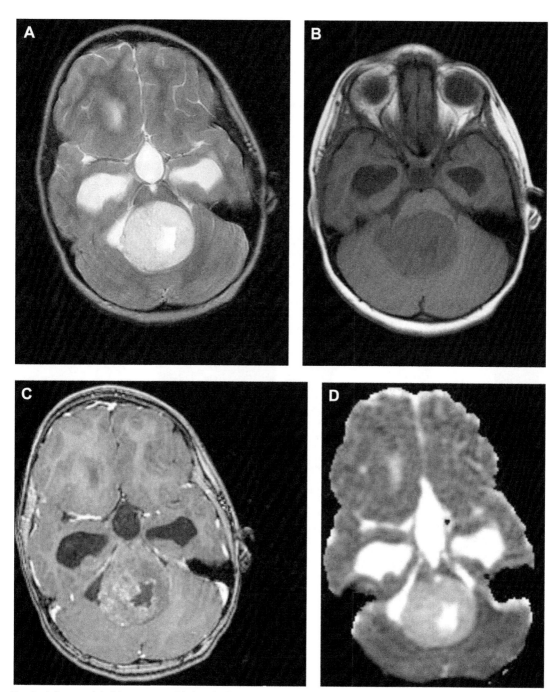

Fig. 1. A 5-year-old girl presents with headache and vomiting. There is a midline solid tumor, with cystic components compromising the cerebellar vermis. On the T2 (A) and T1 without (B) and with contrast (C) it is difficult to suggest the correct diagnosis. Looking at the ADC map (D) no restriction is seen, which is most consistent with a pilocytic astrocytoma.

possible progression of tumor into the surrounding white matter tracts and visualization of displacement or loss of white matter tracts as a result of tumor behavior and postoperative status.

In gray matter, it is usually sufficient to characterize diffusion properties with a single ADC, because measured water diffusivity is largely independent of the orientation of the tissue. However, in anisotropic areas, such as white matter, where diffusivity is known to depend on the orientation of the tissue, a single ADC is not able to describe the orientation-dependent water mobility in the

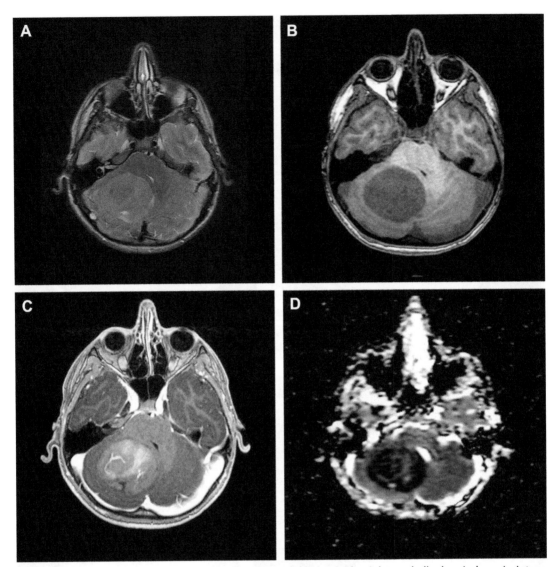

Fig. 2. A 14-year-old boy presents with ataxia. There is a solid lesion in the right cerebellar hemisphere, isointense to the cerebellar cortex on the T2 (*A*), suggesting a high cellular tumor. The lesion is hypointense on T1 (*B*) and presents with nonhomogeneous enhancement (*C*). ADC map (*D*) is most helpful to make the diagnosis of medulloblastoma, once there is restricted diffusion.

tissue. Brain tumors not only invade gray matter but also white matter and may severely displace white matter tracts (Fig. 4). To avoid accidental resection or transection of important white matter tracts, accurate localization of these tracts may be obtained using DTI.

If the decision is surgery, DTI can address issues such as the best surgical approach to avoid damage to major white matter tracts, minimizing adverse neurologic outcomes.

*Diffusion kurtosis imaging*

Recently, van Cauter and colleagues[10] showed that DKI is better at distinguishing between

low-grade and high-grade gliomas in adults than DTI or the most simple approach, DWI. The investigators stated that, using DKI, additional information on microstructure and microdynamics in gliomas could be obtained by exploring nongaussian diffusion properties. This ability is helpful in differentiating between low-grade and high-grade gliomas. DKI uses a similar pulse sequence to those used in DWI and DTI. However, the important difference is the use of higher and at least 2 nonzero b-values. The advantage of DKI is that, besides kurtosis parameters (axial, radial, and mean kurtosis), it also generates all conventional DTI parameters (fractional anisotropy, radial

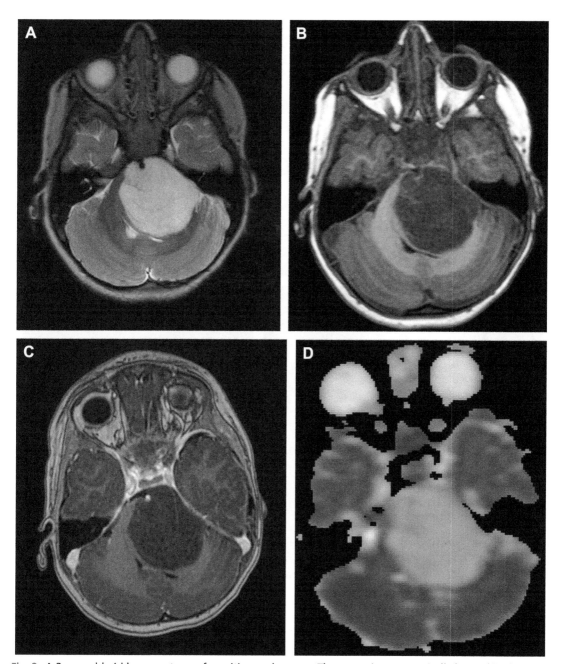

**Fig. 3.** A 3-year-old girl has symptoms of vomiting and nausea. The tumor is asymmetrically located in the pons, well demarcated. The tumor is hyperintense on T2 (*A*), hypointense on T1 (*B*), with nearly no enhancement (*C*; axial T1 with contrast). The ADC map (*D*) shows no diffusion restriction, but on histology it was a high-grade tumor, grade III astrocytoma.

diffusivity, axial diffusivity, and mean diffusivity) and therefore allows comparison with published DTI data on brain tumor grading. Another advantage of using higher b-values is that the diffusion signal decay is no longer monoexponential, and may result in greater imaging contrast between different tissue types, and may improve brain

tumor characterization.[11] A disadvantage is the longer scanning time. To date there is only evidence that DKI can help to differentiate between groups of patients with low-grade and high-grade gliomas but not on an individual level. Larger prospective studies need to be performed, not only in adults but also in children with brain

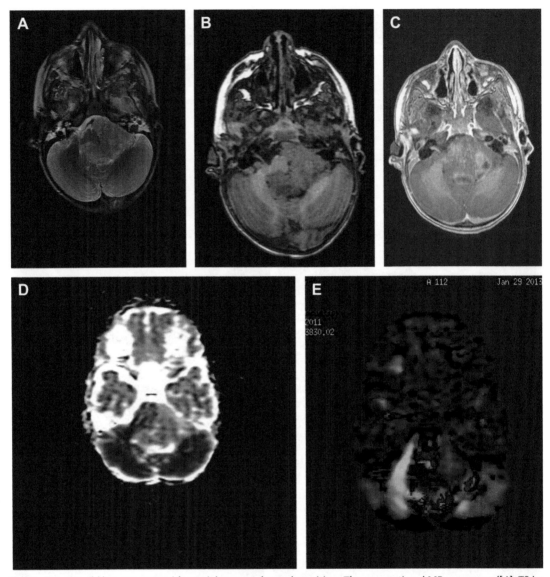

**Fig. 4.** A 1-year-old boy presents with cranial nerve palsy and vomiting. The conventional MR sequences ([A], T2 image, [B], T1 image, and [C], T1 image with contrast) show extension of the tumor to the left cerebellar-pontine angle, suggesting an ependymoma. Also the ADC map (D) shows no severe diffusion restriction. The structural map (colored direction map) (E) shows invasion of the left middle cerebellar peduncle, favoring the diagnosis of ependymoma.

tumors, to validate the power of DKI as a new noninvasive biomarker in grading gliomas or other types of brain tumors.

### Magnetic Resonance Spectroscopy (Magnetic Resonance Spectroscopy, Single-Voxel Imaging, and Chemical Shift Imaging)

MRS provides radiologists with the opportunity to gain information on biochemical and cellular metabolite analyses of brain tissue. Proton MRS is the most commonly used MRS technique.[3] There are multiple metabolite peak assessments possible, depending on the echo time (TE) used. Five predominant metabolite peaks can be identified:

1. Choline (Cho)-containing compounds, which reflect membrane turnover and cellularity.
2. Creatine (Cr), which represents energy synthesis and serves as an internal control for determining metabolite ratios given its relative stability, except in instances of energy failure (tumor necrosis).
3. N-acetyl aspartate (NAA), which is found mostly in neurons but may also be found in glial cells

and serves mostly as a marker of neuronal cells.

4. Lactate, which results from anaerobic metabolism and is seen not only in necrotic tumors but also in low-grade tumors, like pilocytic astrocytomas. A lactate peak can be seen in hypoxic or infarcted tissue and also in brains of children with metabolic diseases.

5. Lipids can appear when there are increased cellular and myelin breakdown products or nonviable necrotic tissue. Lipids may also be shown in cystic lesions such as pilocytic astrocytomas.

Many other metabolites can be detected, especially with short TE (35 milliseconds) and when using higher field strengths (3 T or higher). In the literature, multiple articles focus on MRS and its use in children with a suspected brain tumor. On a 1.5-T MR system, the most commonly used proton MRS technique in children suspected to have a brain tumor is short TE (<35 milliseconds). This short TE allows additional metabolite peaks such as myoinositol (mI, a glial cell marker), glycine, glutamine/glutamate (Glx), taurine (Tau), alanine (Ala), and citrate (Cit) to be identified. These metabolites can be useful in suggesting histology and its biological behavior or malignancy grade of a brain tumor. The observable MR metabolites provide powerful information, but many notable metabolites are not detectable in brain MR spectra; for example, DNA, RNA, most proteins, enzymes, and phospholipids are missing. Some key neurotransmitters, such as acetylcholine, dopamine, and serotonin, are also absent with either their concentrations being too low, or the molecules being invisible to MRS.

Proton MRS can be used for diagnosing and differentiating brain tumor types, as well as predicting tumor grade and pretherapy/biopsy planning. Also, posttherapy assessment, including differentiating radiation necrosis from tumor recurrence, is possible because normal brain metabolite levels after treatment favor edema and postsurgical changes. Tzika and colleagues[12] showed that the metabolic profile of a brain tumor obtained with MRS gives additional information that is not provided by other tumor imaging parameters, such as enhancement, diffusion, and relative cerebral blood volume. The MR spectroscopic hallmark of brain tumors relative to normal brain tissue is increased choline and decreased NAA levels.

In general, the grading of the tumor increases when NAA and creatine levels are decreased, and choline, lactate, and lipid levels are increased.

Very malignant tumors have high metabolic activity and deplete their energy storages, resulting in reduced creatine levels. Very high cellular tumors with rapid growth have high choline levels. Lipids are found in necrotic portions of tumors, and lactate appears when tumors outgrow their blood supply and start using anaerobic glycolysis.

However, pilocytic astrocytoma, a grade I low-grade tumor, usually shows very low levels of NAA and Cr, and high choline, lipid, and lactate levels in the spectra, mimicking aggressive lesions.

For an accurate assessment of the tumor biology, the spectroscopic voxel should preferably be placed over the enhancing part of the tumor, avoiding areas of necrosis, hemorrhage, calcification, cysts, or cerebrospinal fluid.

As mentioned earlier, MRS can also play an important role in assessing therapeutic response. For example, early detection of treatment failure is important because an ineffective treatment can be modified before a significant progression of disease.

MRS data can be obtained in SV or multivoxel mode.

### Single-voxel technique

In SV mode, the most commonly used methods for volume selection/excitation are stimulated echo acquisition mode (STEAM) and point-resolved spectroscopy sequence (PRESS). In general, shorter TEs are better achieved with STEAM; however, it is more sensitive to motion. In theory, for the same total TE, the signal of PRESS is twice as great as that of STEAM; PRESS is also less sensitive to motion. To date, PRESS seems to be the most commonly used method of volume selection in clinical neuro-oncology practice. The major advantage of SV 1H-MRS is its short acquisition time (approximately 3 minutes compared with about 7–9 minutes for multivoxel).

With a short TE of 35 milliseconds or less, metabolites with both short and long T2 relaxation times can be detected. With a long TE of 288 milliseconds, only metabolites with a long T2 are seen, producing a spectrum containing primarily NAA, creatine, and choline. One other helpful TE is 144 milliseconds because it inverts lactate below baseline at 1.3 ppm and therefore makes it easily distinguishable from lipids and macromolecules, which resonate at the same concentration (**Fig. 5**).

As a general rule, SV, short-TE MRS is used to make the initial diagnosis, because the signal/noise ratio is high and all metabolites, which can be used for further characterizing the brain tumor, are represented. Its major flaw is that it

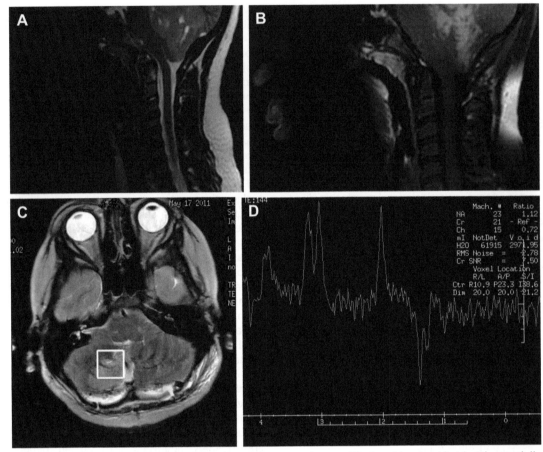

**Fig. 5.** The first row shows sagittal T2 (*A*) and T1 with contrast images (*B*) of an 11-year-old girl with a medulloblastoma. Postoperative (*C*) spectra with intermediate TE of 144 milliseconds (within 48 hours after resection of medulloblastoma) shows lactate peak below baseline (*D*) compatible with ischemia on the medial site of the right cerebellar hemisphere, probably caused by prolonged instrumental pressure.

lacks spatial resolution and cannot be used to better define the extent of a brain tumor, especially in brain tumors known to spread easily, like high-grade gliomas. Some brain tumors on imaging and histology are heterogeneous, and, therefore, SV spectroscopy cannot be used to map regional metabolic variations. Therefore, SV spectroscopy alone cannot reliably define the highest-grade components of the tumor. It may also involve significant averaging with low-grade parts of a tumor or even with adjacent normal brain tissue.

### Multivoxel technique

Multivoxel MRS, a chemical shift technique (CSI) using either a short or long TE, can be used to further characterize different regions of a tumor and to assess the brain parenchyma around or adjacent to the tumor. This method is best for detection of infiltrating malignant cells beyond the enhancing margins of tumors. Particularly in

the case of cerebral high-grade gliomas, increased choline levels are frequently detected in edematous regions of the brain outside the enhancing mass (**Fig. 6**).[3] CSI can also be used to assess the response to therapy and to search for tumor recurrence. It is possible to scan in a two-dimensional (2D) or three-dimensional (3D) mode. The 3D CSI method is especially sensitive for detecting small areas of recurrence. A major drawback is its long scanning time (in children it may result in a higher portion of MR scanning under general anesthesia) and its low signal/noise ratio caused by its smaller voxel size, resulting in less reliable MR spectra. Also, acquisitions from larger volumes increase the risk for inhomogeneity of the magnet field and inadequate water suppression. 2D CSI MRS has also been used to help biopsy planning by showing areas of highest choline levels.

Quantitative rather than qualitative, MRS has been recently suggested for the assessment of

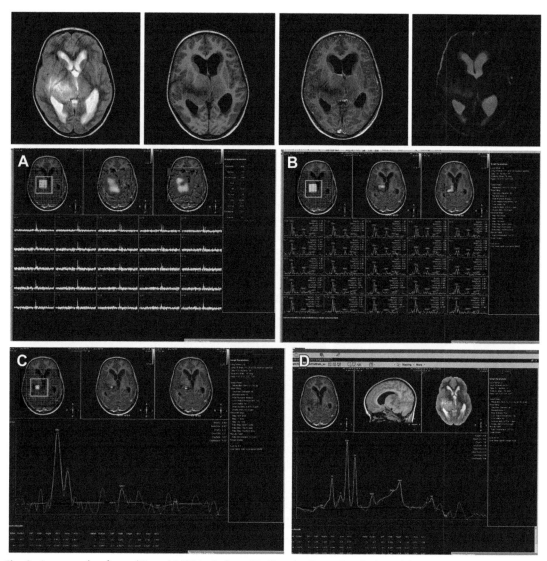

Fig. 6. An example of a multivoxel MRS technique (A–C) and a SV MRS technique (D) in a 6-year-old girl with an anaplastic astrocytoma. Note the high choline peak and low NAA, suggesting a high-grade tumor with prominent cell-membrane turnover. The top row images shows conventional sequences of T2W image, T1W image, T1W image with contrast and ADC image, respectively.

the metabolic profiles of pediatric brain tumors. Although absolute concentrations and concentration ratios of the prominent metabolites of the 1H-MR spectrum (NAA, Cr, tCho [total Choline], ml) provide important diagnostic information, less prominent spectral features, such as increased Tau in medulloblastomas or reduced guanidinoacetate in astrocytomas, also proved to be relevant for the discrimination of different tumors (Fig. 7).[13] This quantitative MRS may help improve preoperative diagnosis of specific tumors. However, in daily practice, MRS should be used with standardized acquisition and processing methods, and easy-to-follow rules for quality control. Also, the interpretation is complex and

requires expert knowledge to have an impact on clinical decision making (Fig. 8). Fully automated processing and quantitation can be helpful but in inexperienced hands it is cumbersome.

In summary, our suggested protocol in pediatric patients suspected to have a brain tumor is:

1. Initial diagnosis, SV MRS with short TE (35 milliseconds) in suspected brain tumor area and 2D CSI for defining the preferable area for biopsy. On both MRS sequences, the area with contrast enhancement should be included and areas with cerebrospinal fluid, hemorrhage, and calcifications should be avoided (Fig. 9).

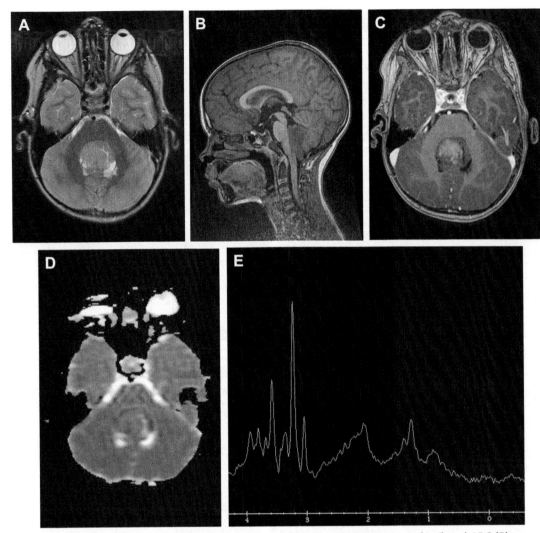

**Fig. 7.** A 5-year-old boy presents with a midline tumor. Conventional MR sequences (*A–C*) and ADC (*D*) suggest medulloblastoma. Single-voxel MRS (*E*) shows high choline and increased taurine, favoring the diagnosis of medulloblastoma and closely related to high risk of cerebrospinal fluid spread. This diagnosis was confirmed on the spinal MR.

2. Postoperative 24-hour to 72-hour MR scan. Depending on the amount of residual tumor seen on the conventional images and what the surgeon suspects to have left behind, SV, 2D CSI, or 3D CSI with short TE can be done. Because of landmark changes and other postoperative alterations, like bleeding, hemostasis material, and infarction of surrounding brain parenchyma, interpretation of the MRS spectra can be challenging. SV is less sensitive for postoperative changes and therefore, for routine postoperative scanning, the best choice. However, if the suspected residual tumor area is small, then 2D or 3D CSI may be better options.

3. Follow-up MRS can be included in the scanning protocol if treatment response seems to be inadequate. Some clinicians advocate using 3D CSI in every follow-up scan to detect small tumor recurrence. In brainstem gliomas, SV is the best method because of interpretation problems with CSI spectra caused by magnetic field inhomogeneity at the skull base.

All metabolites that are detectable with MRS and that could help in differentiating among pediatric brain tumors are summarized in **Tables 1** and **2**. Therapeutic response assessment, radiation necrosis, and differential diagnosis for focal brain tumor are discussed briefly. Extensive

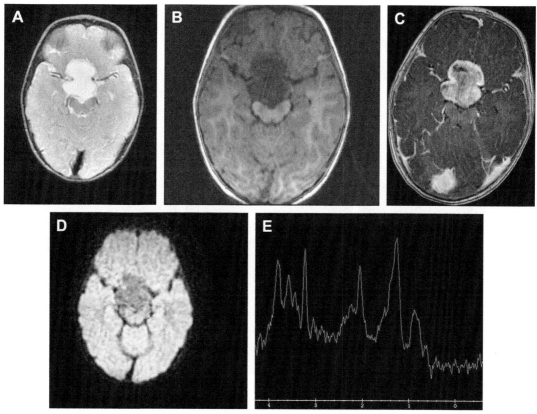

Fig. 8. A 1-year-old boy with a pilomyxoid astrocytoma, located at the suprasellar region, in the midline. The T2-weighted image (*A*), T1 (*B*), and T1 with contrast (*C*) and no diffusion restriction on DWI (*D*) suggest a low-grade tumor like a pilocytic astrocytoma. Note the higher choline peak compared to the creatine peak, elevated lipid peak, favoring the diagnosis of pilomyxoid astrocytoma (*E*).

description of possible brain tumor types in the posterior fossa and supratentorial are addressed in other articles.

### Therapeutic response assessment

As stated earlier, 2D or 3D CSI is the best technique to assess a small recurrence within the surgical bed, especially when MRS can detect an increase in the Cho peak. Second, clinicians must take into account whether radiation therapy has been given, because this may result in low NAA peaks in the surrounding gray and white matter, compared with normal NAA levels in healthy controls. In the case of medulloblastomas, a higher total choline and taurine level may suggest metastatic disease, which may have a different therapeutic response (see Fig. 7). In brainstem glioma, if the citrate peak is reduced compared with the pretreatment situation, this may indicate malignant transformation, or result from chronic steroid administration, radiotherapy, and/or chemotherapy.[14] Also, increased total choline and lipid levels can suggest malignant transformation. In grade II astrocytomas, a citrate

peak may indicate a more aggressive behavior and higher chance for recurrence and metastases, and therapeutic response assessment should be tailored for patients with this kind of tumor.

### Radiation necrosis

Radiation necrosis could be a diagnostic challenge for neuroradiologists. Most of the time conventional imaging is inconclusive and advanced MR imaging techniques are necessary (Figs. 10 and 11). Typically, radiation necrosis develops months to several years after radiation therapy.

Besides perfusion-weighted imaging, MRS can be helpful to differentiate between tumor progression and radiation necrosis. On MRS, a high lipid/lactate peak, low NAA peak, and a low choline peak compared with the spectra of normal-appearing brain parenchyma and with the spectra of the pretreatment brain tumor are suggestive of radiation necrosis.

High choline peaks may be shown after radiation therapy because of tumor cell death. In these cases, information obtained from other advanced MR imaging techniques, such as perfusion-weighted MR

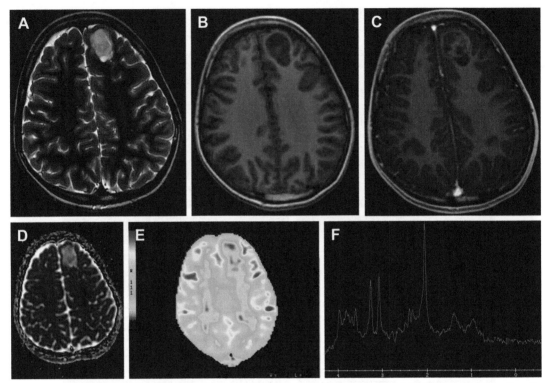

**Fig. 9.** A 12-year-old girl presents with focal seizures. The T2 (*A*), T1 (*B*), and T1 with contrast (*C*), as well as the ADC value (*D*), suggest a low-grade tumor. ASL shows the lesion has low perfusion (*E*). MRS (*F*) shows increased myoinositol peak compatible with a glial tumor. Low choline level also suggests a low-grade tumor. On histology it was a low-grade oligodendroglioma.

imaging, as well as follow-up with MRS, may be helpful in characterizing the lesion.

## Pseudoprogression

In the pediatric population, pseudoprogression is less an issue than in the adult population, because of a lower occurrence of high-grade brain tumors

**Table 1**
**Peaks of metabolites in infratentorial brain tumors**

| ml | Tau | Cho | Cr | Cit | Glx/Glu | NAA | Lac | Lip | Ala | Cho/Cr | Cho/NAA | ml/Cr | Tumor |
|----|-----|-----|----|-----|---------|-----|-----|-----|-----|--------|---------|-------|-------|
|    | ↑   | ↑   |    |     | ↑       | ↓   | ↑   | ↑   | ↑   | ↑      |         |       | MB |
| ↑  |     | ↑   | ↑  |     | ↑       |     |     |     |     |        |         |       | Ependymoma |
| ↑↑ |     |     | ↑  |     | ↓       |     |     |     |     |        |         |       | CPP |
|    |     |     |    |     | ↓       |     |     |     |     |        |         |       | CPC |
|    |     |     |    |     |         |     |     |     | ↑   |        |         |       | Meningioma |
| ↓  |     | ↑   |    |     |         |     | ↑   |     | ↑   |        |         |       | Glioblastoma |
|    |     | ↑   |    |     |         | ↓   |     | ↑   |     |        |         |       | ATRT |
|    |     | ↑   | ↓  |     |         | ↓   | ↑   |     |     | ↑      |         | ↑     | Pilocytic astrocytoma |
| ↓  |     |     | ↑  |     |         |     |     |     |     | ↑      | ↑       |       | BSG |
| ↑  |     | ↑   | ↓  | ↑   |         | ↓   | ↑   |     |     | ↑      | ↑       |       | Diffuse astrocytoma |
|    |     |     |    |     |         |     |     |     |     | ↑      |         | ↓     | Pilomyxoid |

*Abbreviations:* ATRT, atypical teratoid rhabdoid tumor; BSG, brainstem glioma; CPC, choroid plexus carcinoma; CPP, choroid plexus papilloma; Lac, lactate; Lip, lipids; MB, medulloblastoma.

**Table 2**
**Peaks of metabolites in supratentorial brain tumors**

| ml | Tau | Cho | Cr | Cit | Glx/Glu | NAA | Lac | Lip | Ala | Cho/Cr | Cho/NAA | ml/Cr | Tumor |
|----|-----|-----|----|-----|---------|-----|-----|-----|-----|--------|---------|-------|-------|
|    |     | ↑   |    |     |         | ↓   | ↑   | ↑   |     |        |         |       | PNET |
|    |     | ↑   |    |     |         | ↓   |     |     |     |        |         |       | ATRT |
| ↑  |     |     |    |     |         |     |     |     |     |        |         |       | Low grade oligodendroglioma |
|    |     | ↑   |    |     |         |     | ↑   |     | ↑   | ↑      |         |       | Oligo high grade |
| ↑  |     |     |    |     |         |     |     |     |     |        | ↑       |       | DNET |
| ↑  |     |     |    |     |         |     |     |     |     |        |         |       | DIG/DACI |
| ↑  |     |     |    |     |         | ↓   |     |     |     |        |         |       | Ganglioglioma/ gangliocytoma |
| ↑  | ↓   | ↓   |    |     |         |     |     |     |     |        |         |       | CPP |
| ↓  | ↑   | ↓   |    |     |         |     | ↑   |     |     |        |         |       | CPC |
| ↑  |     |     |    | ↑   |         |     |     |     |     |        |         |       | SEGA |
|    | ↑   |     |    |     | ↑       |     |     |     | ↑   | ↑      |         |       | Meningioma |
|    | ↑   | ↑   |    |     | ↑       |     |     |     |     |        |         |       | Germinoma |
| ↑  |     | ↑   |    |     |         | ↓   |     | ↑   |     |        |         |       | Pineoblastoma |

*Abbreviations:* DACI, desmoplastic astrocytoma of infancy; DIG, desmoplastic infantile ganglioglioma; DNET, dysembryoplastic neuroepithelial tumor; PNET, primitive neuroectodermal tumor; SEGA, subependymal giant cell astrocytoma.

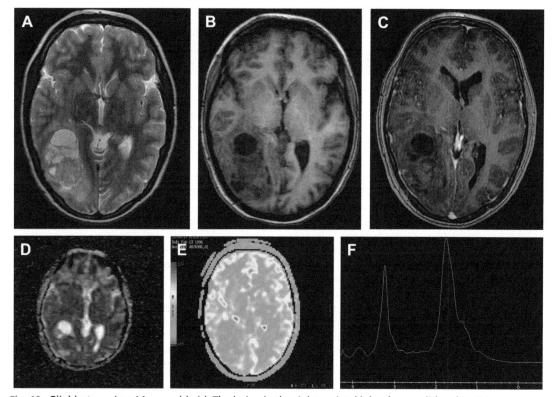

Fig. 10. Glioblastoma in a 14-year-old girl. The lesion in the right parietal lobe shows solid and cystic components on T2 (*A*) and T1 (*B*) and nearly no enhancement (*C*). Some areas in the tumor show low ADC values (*D*). On ASL there is moderate perfusion (*E*). Spectrum suggests high-grade tumor with increased choline and lipid peaks and reduced NAA and creatine peaks (*F*).

**A**    **B**    **C**

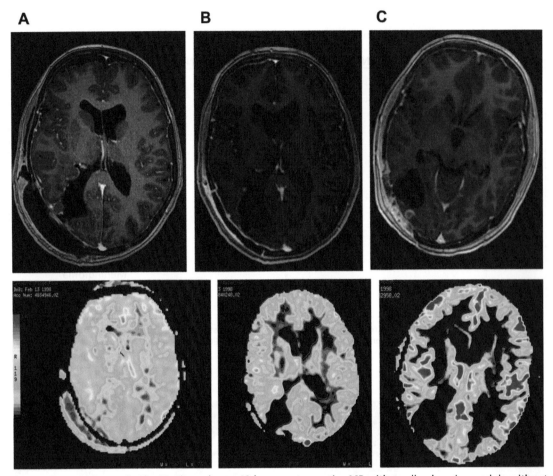

Fig. 11. Same patient as in Fig. 10. First column: 48-hour postoperative MR with small enhancing nodule without hyperperfusion on ASL (*A*). Two weeks later, another enhancing lesion more lateral-anterior to the postoperative cavity. Recurrence or pseudoprogression? (*B, second column*) Three months later, enhancing lesion caudomedial without hyperperfusion, probably fibrotic tissue. Previous hyperperfused area lateral-anterior no longer visible, so it was pseudoprogression (*C*).

(Fig. 12) treated with postoperative adjuvant radiation therapy and temozolomide chemotherapy. Pseudoprogression often appears several weeks to months after radiation therapy. The causative factor is a transient interruption of myelin synthesis secondary to damage to oligodendrocytes as a result of radiation injury.

Accurate distinction between tumor recurrence and treatment effects can also be difficult in children. DWI and PET scans (with 11C-methionine) may provide the answer in many cases, but sometimes MRS can give additional information. Because of new treatment strategies, radiologists can no longer rely on changes in enhancement within the old tumor region. Enlargement of an enhancing lesion may represent pseudoprogression.

Although perfusion and permeability may help distinguish pseudoprogression from true tumor progression, follow-up MR imaging with contrast is the only established technique to confidently distinguish these lesions.

*Pseudoresponse*
To date, MRS has not provided any additional value in the diagnosis of pseudoresponse. Pseudoresponse has been noticed since the introduction of antiangiogenic therapies targeting vascular endothelial factor (VEGF), such as bevacizumab, a recombinant humanized monoclonal antibody to VEGF-A, or the VEGF receptor, such as cediranib, a pan-VEGF receptor tyrosine kinase inhibitor normalization of leaky tumor blood vessels. These agents can cause reduction in enhancement within 1 to 2 days after administration, with a radiographic response observed in 25% to 60% of patients.[15] However, this impressive radiographic response does not translate into increased overall survival. It is thought that

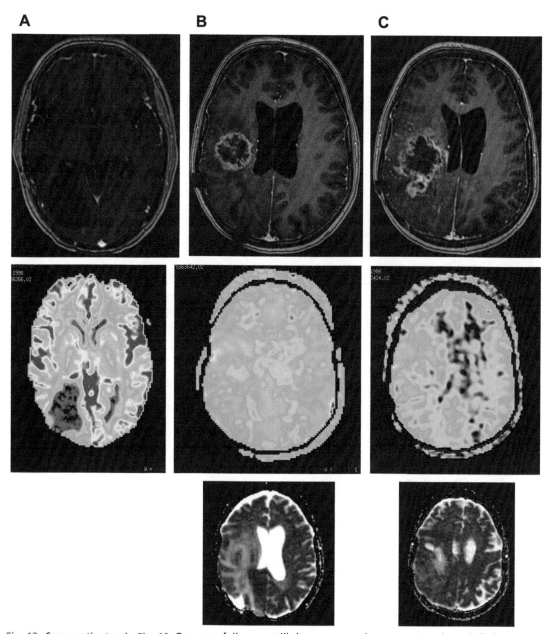

**Fig. 12.** Same patient as in **Fig. 10.** One-year follow-up still shows some enhancement caudomedially but no hyperperfused areas on ASL (*A, first column*). Second column (*B*) shows recurrent tumor anterior to the operative area, but in the radiation treatment field. Note the increased perfusion on the ASL and the low ADC value area of the enhancing tumor. Two months later, the recurrent tumor enlarges rapidly and shows an infiltrative growth pattern (*C, third column*).

the rapid radiographic response represents a direct action on blood vessel permeability rather than a true antitumor effect; a phenomenon termed pseudoresponse. A further confounder in radiographic assessment of therapy response is the tendency for antiangiogenic agents to promote progression of nonenhancing disease by selecting for an invasive tumor phenotype capable of co-opting existing blood vessels and no longer relying on angiogenesis.[16]

### Differential diagnosis

It may be difficult or even impossible to distinguish between a necrotic tumor and an abscess, even with contrast-enhanced MR imaging. Most of the time DWI can give the answer and in some cases MRS can be of additional help (**Figs. 13** and **14**). If in the cystic/necrotic part of the mass acetate, succinate, and amino acid (valine, alanine, leucine) peaks are visible, a pyogenic abscess is the most likely diagnosis.[17]

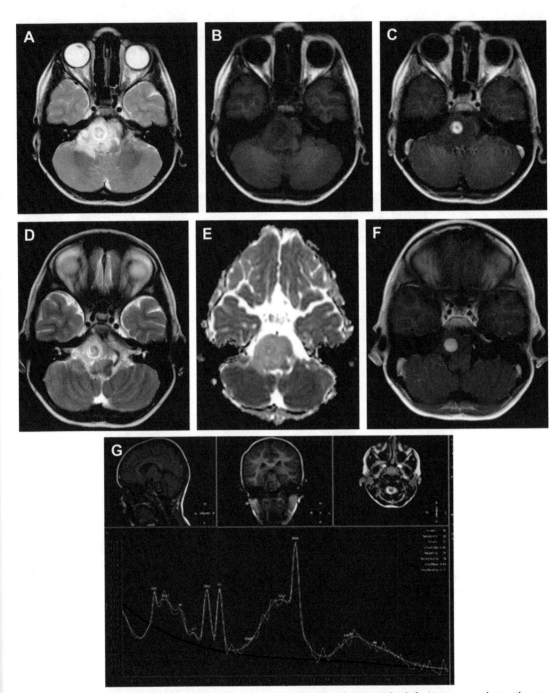

**Fig. 13.** An 8-year-old boy presents with a deviation of the head and eyes to the left. Upper row shows the conventional MR sequence characteristics on the initial MR scan (*A–C*). Differential diagnoses include brain abscess, tumor, or vascular malformation. Second row MR scan 3 days later with T2 (*D*) and with ADC (*E*) showing no restricted diffusion except for a rim in the enhancing lesion (*F*). SV MRS (35 milliseconds) shows a normal spectrum (*G*). No increased choline peak suggesting tumor. No clear lactate peak suggesting abscess. Cavernous hemangioma with some internal bleeding?

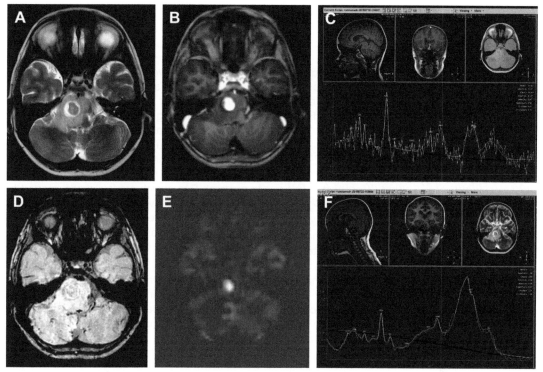

**Fig. 14.** MR 12 days later in the same patient as **Fig. 13** shows enlargement of the brainstem lesion (*A, B*). MRS shows a change in the spectra (*C*). Now there is a prominent choline peak favoring brain tumor. Susceptibility-weighted image (*D*) shows no bleeding in the tumor and no other bleeding ruling out a cavernous hemangioma. ASL shows high CBF (cerebral blood flow), suggesting high-grade tumor (*E*). On the MR 9 days later, MRS shows high choline peak, lower NAA, and a high lipid/lactate, characteristic of a high-grade brain tumor (*F*). On histology it was a primitive neuroectodermal tumor.

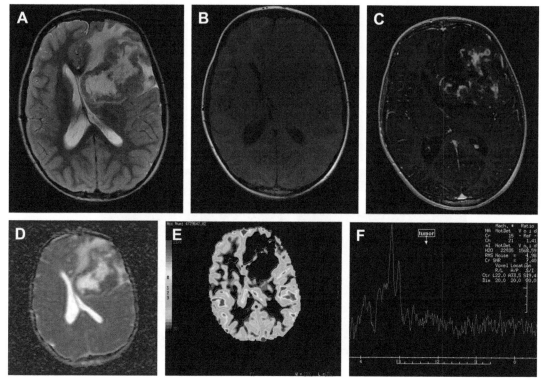

**Fig. 15.** Supratentorial anaplastic ependymoma: 6-year-old boy with irritability, and signs of high intracranial pressure. There is a large lesion with perifocal edema on T2 (*A*) in the left frontal lobe, with heterogeneous enhancement (*B, C*). The ADC map (*D*) shows restriction in the tumor wall. The DSC shows low perfusion (*E*). Spectra show increase of the Cho peak, presence of lipids, along with reduction of the NAA and Cr peaks (*F*).

In pseudotumoral demyelinating lesions, MRS may shows increased choline, lactate, and lipid levels, caused by inflammatory response, mimicking neoplasm. Increase of glutamate and glutamine levels shown with short-TE MRS favors demyelination rather than tumor.[18]

### Contrast Perfusion MR Imaging (Dynamic Susceptibility Contrast MR Imaging, Dynamic Contrast-Enhanced MR Imaging, and Arterial Spin Labeling; A Noncontrast Technique)

#### Dynamic susceptibility contrast MR imaging

Imaging the passage of an injected MR imaging contrast bolus can be used to investigate the perfusion characteristics of brain tumors. With DSC MR imaging the passage of the MR imaging contrast agent is used to investigate tumor characteristics based on the T2* effects, in which the (relative) cerebral blood volume (CBV) is the most important parameter used for the characterization of brain tumors. A higher (relative) CBV is correlated with a higher tumor grade both in adults and in children. In a recent DSC perfusion study of 63 pediatric patients with brain tumors, the relative CBV was a good method to exclude high-grade tumors in patients with low relative CBV values. However, the specificity in this study was low because a subgroup of low-grade tumors also showed higher relative CBV values.[19]

Interesting findings may be shown in pediatric brain tumors such as medulloblastomas and pilocytic astrocytomas (PAs). Despite being aggressive grade IV tumors, medulloblastomas may not present with high blood volumes in the perfusion study. In contrast, PAs, which are low grade (grade I tumors), often present with very high blood volumes.

Knowledge of these unexpected findings is helpful in order to consider the appropriate diagnosis.

#### Dynamic contrast-enhanced MR imaging

With DCE MR imaging, permeability characteristics of brain tumors can be assessed based on dynamic imaging of changes using T1 in the brain tumor regions. With DCE MR imaging, vascular permeability parameters such as the transfer coefficient (K-trans) can be determined. At present, most DSC perfusion MR imaging studies are reported for brain tumor evaluation in children (**Figs. 15** and **16**).

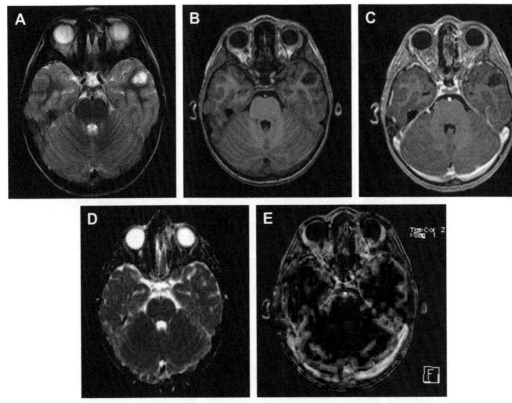

Fig. 16. A 7-year-old girl presents with temporal epileptic focus on the left. Conventional MR images show a high-signal-intensity lesion on T2 (*A*), hypointense on T1 (*B*), subcortical, in the left temporal lobe. No enhancement (*C*), no restricted diffusion (*D*), hypoperfused on the DSC study (*E*). Histology confirmed a dysembryoplastic neuroepithelial tumor.

## Arterial spin labeling MR imaging

ASL MR imaging is a noncontrast method to assess the perfusion in brain tumors and has been the focus of clinical research of many groups around the world. In general, ASL MR imaging is performed by magnetically labeling the arterial water in the feeding arteries to the brain. After labeling the arterial blood the MR sequence is built in such way that a delay (typically 1–2 seconds) allows the labeled water molecules to flow into the brain tissue and exchange with the brain tissue water. Consequently, a small change (a few percent) occurs in the magnetization of the brain tissue water. In itself this small percentage change is not visible but a control image is also acquired and a subtraction of labeled and control images is performed that results in a perfusion-weighted MR image. Because the signal/noise ratio of a single subtracted label control image is low, typically a series of 20 to 40 labeled and control pairs are acquired, which results in ASL MR imaging scan times of 3 to 5 minutes. Two main flavors of ASL perfusion methods are available on many MR imaging scanners. The first is pulsed ASL and the second is (pseudo) continuous ASL. These methods differ in the way the blood in the neck region is labeled. With pulsed ASL a thick excitation slab labels all the blood in the neck region at 1 point in time (spatial labeling of the blood in the arteries). With (pseudo) continuous ASL a thin excitation slab is used in which the blood in the neck region is labeled during 1.5 to 2.0 seconds (temporal labeling of the blood in the arteries). In a recent article the consensus was that pseudocontinuous ASL with certain labeling and delay parameters provides the best images for use in most clinical scenarios. More recently,[20] a study compared pseudocontinuous ASL with pulsed ASL in a series of 61 children. The result from this study was that pseudocontinuous ASL resulted in a better image quality compared with the pulsed ASL method.[21] Quantitatively both methods resulted in the same cerebral blood flow values. Also interesting from this study was that in 75% of the scans the image quality was good enough for this comparison, which shows that there is a high percentage of patients in whom ASL might result in noninterpretable results; for instance, because of motion artifacts.

Similar to its use in adults, ASL perfusion MR imaging may be a useful method to estimate tumor grade in children. In adults, tumor grade was correlated with higher ASL perfusion signal. In a recent study, Yeom and colleagues[22] showed that high-grade brain tumors (grades 3 and 4) have high ASL MR imaging perfusion signal intensity, whereas low-grade tumors (grades 1 and 2) have low ASL perfusion signal intensity. ASL perfusion MR imaging was performed in 54 children with a mean age of 7.5 years, before treatment. Using region of interest analysis, the maximum relative tumor blood flow was obtained. The largest portions of tumors were astrocytic tumors in this study. ASL perfusion MR imaging was not able to distinguish tumor histologic subtypes, except that there was a higher ASL perfusion signal in posterior fossa medulloblastomas compared with PAs.

However, more research is needed concerning the use of ASL perfusion MR imaging in patients with brain tumors. Areas of interest are the correlation between (pretreatment) ASL perfusion signal and patient prognosis. For instance, **Fig. 17** shows ASL perfusion signal in 2 patients with a medulloblastoma. In one patient, ASL perfusion images show low perfusion signal, whereas in the other patient the ASL perfusion signal is high. These differences in perfusion signal may have prognostic consequences. Furthermore, another unexplored area is the use of ASL perfusion signal in the postoperative evaluation of children treated for brain tumors. For instance, being able to discriminate between treatment effects (radiotherapy) and recurrent tumor growth, which may show contrast enhancement on postcontrast T1-weighted MR imaging images. Higher perfusion ASL signal can be expected in high-grade recurrent tumors compared with possibly low ASL perfusion signal in areas where treatments were effective. Another area of future research is the added value of quantification of the cerebral blood flow in regions of interest of the tumor compared with a qualitative assessment of the perfusion signal in the brain tumor region.

Furthermore, on the technical side, ASL comparison studies have to be performed for further improvements in the methods to enhance ASL perfusion measurements. Although the pseudocontinuous ASL is currently most often used because of its high signal/noise ratio, it is possible that the signal/noise ratio may further increase based on optimization of the best possible readout strategy. Furthermore, especially in patients after surgery, surgical material (clips) may cause artifacts, which could be reduced with readout strategies that are less sensitive for MR field distortions.

## Other Advanced MR Imaging Sequences

### Susceptibility-weighted imaging

SWI is a 3D fast low-angle shot (FLASH) MR imaging technique that is extremely sensitive

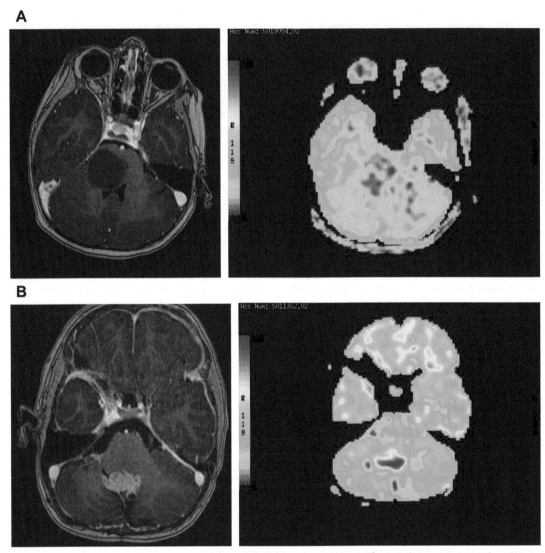

**Fig. 17.** ASL perfusion signal in 2 patients with a medulloblastoma. Patient A has a primary tumor, patient B was a local recurrence (*A, B*). In patient A, ASL perfusion images show low perfusion signal (*A*) and, in patient B, ASL shows high perfusion signal in the tumor (*B*).

to susceptibility changes. Various paramagnetic, ferromagnetic, or diamagnetic substances, such as air/tissue or air/bone interfaces, can cause these susceptibility changes. Compared with T2*-weighted (ie, gradient-echo) images (**Fig. 18**), SWI uses not only the magnitude of the signal loss but also the phase information to reveal anatomic and physiologic information about brain tissue and venous vasculature. The underlying contrast mechanism is primarily associated with the magnetic susceptibility difference between oxygenated and deoxygenated hemoglobin, leading to a phase difference between regions containing deoxygenated blood and surrounding tissues, resulting in signal cancellation. Therefore, SWI is sensitive for calcifications and blood products, like T2*-weighted images, but is also sensitive in visualization of venous vessel because of its deoxyhemoglobin concentration (**Fig. 19**). However, SWI contrast is also affected by other factors like hematocrit, red blood cell integrity, clot structure, molecular diffusion, pH, temperature, field strength, voxel size, previous contrast material use, blood flow, and vessel orientation.

Because of its magnetic susceptibility effects, SWI is extremely sensitive to small changes within brain tissues that are likely not visible

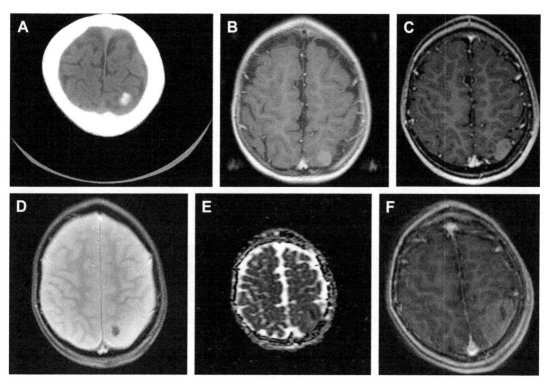

Fig. 18. A 3-year-old boy presents with an incidental finding on a trauma screening computed tomography scan (*A*). A calcification is seen in the left parietal lobe. Eight years later the child had an insult. MR shows the calcified lesion on the susceptibility-weighted image (*D*) and enhancement of the surrounding tissue (*B*, *C*). Two months later the lesion increased in size (*E*, *F*). On histology the lesion was an anaplastic ependymoma.

with conventional MR techniques. Thus, SWI can be used to identify even small alterations in hemorrhage, calcifications, and new vessel growth. SWI can be used to detect calcifications in brain tumors, suggesting a low-grade tumor. Also hemorrhage, often seen in rapidly growing tumors, is easily detected, suggesting a high-grade tumor. In addition, SWI can show areas of neovascularization in the tumor, which may help guiding tumor biopsy. Besides detection of small tumor vessels, SWI can also assess contrast agent uptake and oxygenation of the brain tumor.[23,24]

## Functional MR imaging

fMR imaging uses regional changes in cerebral blood flow and metabolism that are induced by brain activation. During neuronal activation, there is a change in blood oxygenation levels, which results in minor magnetic susceptibility differences. The blood oxygenation level–dependent (BOLD) contrast depends on the differences between the amount of deoxygenated and oxygenated blood present in the brain region being activated. With this technique,

radiologists can noninvasively identify important cortical areas, controlling language, motor, and memory functions. This ability could be essential for the decision to undertake neurosurgery or choose another treatment option. If neurosurgery is the best option, fMR imaging can help in presurgical planning, assisting in the decision of the best surgical approach as well as helping to determine the possible extent of the resection (Fig. 20). In addition, fMR imaging may help to select the patients who need an intraoperative cortical stimulation procedure, in cases in which the eloquent cortical areas are adjacent to or within the tumor. A disadvantage is that this procedure can only be performed in cooperative children. An important consideration concerning brain activation with fMR imaging is that it is easier to map the motor cortex using motor tasks than to map language areas (Broca and Wernicke) in children.

To overcome many of the limitations of task-dependent fMR imaging, resting state fMR imaging has been introduced. Several studies show that this method in combination with connectivity analysis is useful in the presurgical

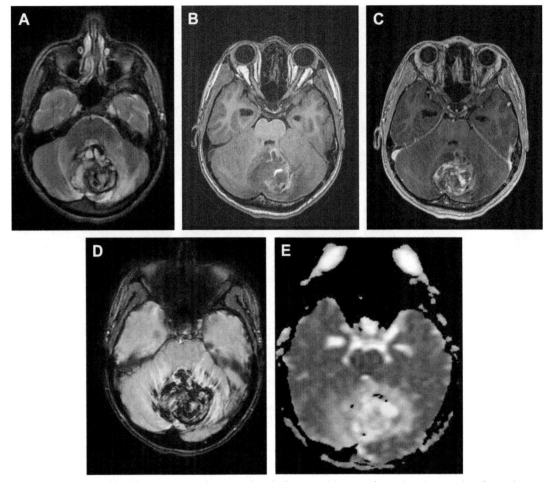

**Fig. 19.** A 16-year-old girl presents with acute headache, vomiting, and ataxia. Conventional MR images (*A–C*) show a midline tumor with intratumoral bleeding best visible on SWI (*D*). ADC map (*E*) does not show diffusion restriction but is unreliable because of hemorrhage in the lesion. Histology was pilocytic astrocytoma.

evaluation of pediatric patients with brain tumors. Moreover, it may improve postoperative outcomes.

Recently, fMR imaging has been integrated with electroencephalography (EEG) to optimize the information on brain function around the brain tumor. The advantage of this combination is the high temporal resolution of EEG and high spatial resolution of fMR imaging. The EEG changes produced by the tumor depend primarily on lesion size, rate of growth, distance to the cortical surface, and specific structures involved. To date, experience has only been gathered in adult patients.

## Future Perspectives

As stated earlier, extensive progress is being made in pediatric neuroradiology. Recent discoveries about the genomic characteristics of brain tumors have changed the understanding of tumor genesis and biology, which may have a great impact on the diagnostic power of the conventional and advanced MR methods discussed earlier. Also epigenetic factors, like histone mutations in pediatric high-grade gliomas, add another layer of complexity. However, all these new insights may clarify the previously poor understanding of biological and imaging phenotype features and variations, such as location, prognosis, and therapeutic response.

Future advances in molecular biology will alter neuroradiologic concepts and thinking and add information to that obtained from conventional and advanced MR imaging techniques, which will benefit pediatric patients with brain tumors.

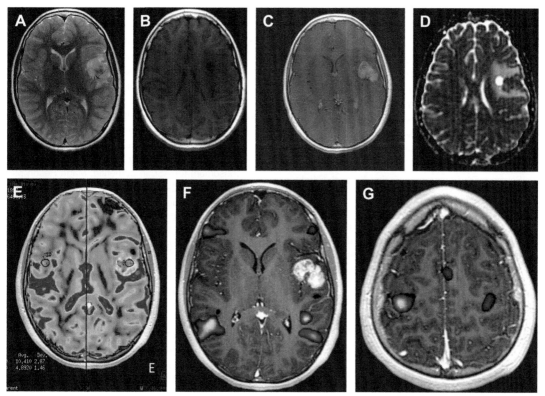

**Fig. 20.** In this 14-year-old girl, a total brain tumor work-up is done. The conventional MR sequences show a heterogeneous tumor in the left frontal lobe (A–C). ADC map (D) shows diffusion restriction. DSC study (E) shows hyperperfusion compared with the contralateral brain parenchyma. fMR imaging was performed to localize speech and language areas (F) as well as the motor strip (G). These areas were not involved by the tumor. Also, fMR imaging showed that the tumor was more than 2 cm from the activated areas, which implies good prognosis concerning surgical resection. Histology of the resected tumor was consistent with an anaplastic ependymoma.

## REFERENCES

1. Plaza MJ, Borja MJ, Altman N, et al. Conventional and advanced MRI features of pediatric intracranial tumors: posterior fossa and suprasellar tumors. AJR Am J Roentgenol 2013;200(5):1115–24.
2. Borja MJ, Plaza MJ, Altman N, et al. Conventional and advanced MRI features of pediatric intracranial tumors: supratentorial tumors. AJR Am J Roentgenol 2013;200(5):W483–503.
3. Brandão LA, Poussaint TY. Pediatric brain tumors. Neuroimaging Clin N Am 2013;23(3):499–525.
4. Poretti A, Meoded A, Cohen KJ, et al. Apparent diffusion coefficient of pediatric cerebellar tumors: a biomarker of tumor grade? Pediatr Blood Cancer 2013;60(12):2036–41.
5. Lee WJ, Choi SH, Park CK, et al. Diffusion-weighted MR imaging for the differentiation of true progression from pseudoprogression following concomitant radiotherapy with temozolomide in patients with newly diagnosed high-grade gliomas. Acad Radiol 2012;19(11):1353–61.
6. Mong S, Ellingson BM, Nghiemphu PL, et al. Persistent diffusion-restricted lesions in bevacizumab-treated malignant gliomas are associated with improved survival compared with matched controls. AJNR Am J Neuroradiol 2012;33(9):1763–70.
7. Nowosielski M, Recheis W, Goebel G, et al. ADC histograms predict response to anti-angiogenic therapy in patients with recurrent high-grade glioma. Neuroradiology 2011;53(4):291–302.
8. Park JE, Kim HS, Goh MJ, et al. Pseudoprogression in patients with glioblastoma: assessment by using volume-weighted voxel-based multiparametric clustering of MR imaging data in an independent test set. Radiology 2015;275(3):792–802.
9. Hoisak JD, Jaffray DA. A method for assessing voxel correspondence in longitudinal tumor imaging. Med Phys 2011;38(5):2742–53.
10. Van Cauter S, Veraart J, Sijbers J, et al. Gliomas: diffusion kurtosis MR imaging in grading. Radiology 2012;263(2):492–501.
11. Seo HS, Chang KH, Na DG, et al. High b-value diffusion (b = 3000 s/mm²) MR imaging in cerebral

gliomas at 3T: visual and quantitative comparisons with b = 1000 s/mm². AJNR Am J Neuroradiol 2008;29(3):458–63.

12. Tzika AA, Vigneron DB, Dunn RS, et al. Intracranial tumors in children: small single-voxel proton MR spectroscopy using short and long-echo sequences. Neuroradiology 1996;38:254–6.

13. Kovanlikaya A, Panigrahy A, Krieger MD, et al. Untreated pediatric primitive neuroectodermal tumor in vivo: quantitation of taurine with MR spectroscopy. Radiology 2005;236(3):1020–5.

14. Seymour ZA, Panigrahy A, Finlay JL, et al. Citrate in pediatric CNS tumors? AJNR Am J Neuroradiol 2008;29(5):1006–11.

15. Huang RY, Neagu MR, Reardon DA, et al. Pitfalls in the neuroimaging of glioblastoma in the era of antiangiogenic and immuno/targeted therapy – detecting illusive disease, defining response. Front Neurol 2015;6:33.

16. Griffith B, Jain R. Perfusion imaging in neurooncology: basic techniques and clinical applications. Radiol Clin North Am 2015;53(3):497–511.

17. Pal D, Bhattacharyya A, Husain M, et al. In vivo proton MR spectroscopy evaluation of pyogenic brain abscesses: a report of 194 cases. AJNR Am J Neuroradiol 2010;31(2):360–6.

18. Richards TL. Proton MR spectroscopy in multiple sclerosis: value in establishing diagnosis, monitoring progression, and evaluating therapy. AJR Am J Roentgenol 1991;157(5):1073–8.

19. Ho CY, Cardinal JS, Kamer AP, et al. Relative cerebral blood volume from dynamic susceptibility contrast perfusion in the grading of pediatric primary brain tumors. Neuroradiology 2015;57(3): 299–306.

20. Alsop DC, Detre JA, Golay X, et al. Recommended implementation of arterial spin-labeled perfusion MRI for clinical applications: a consensus of the ISMRM perfusion study group and the European consortium for ASL in dementia. Magn Reson Med 2015;73(1):102–16.

21. Boudes E, Gilbert G, Leppert IR, et al. Measurement of brain perfusion in newborns: pulsed arterial spin labeling (PASL) versus pseudo-continuous arterial spin labeling (pCASL). Neuroimage Clin 2014;6: 126–33.

22. Yeom KW, Mitchell LA, Lober RM, et al. Arterial spin-labeled perfusion of pediatric brain tumors. AJNR Am J Neuroradiol 2014;35(2):395–401.

23. Wagner MW, Poretti A, Huisman TA, et al. Conventional and advanced (DTI/SWI) neuroimaging findings in pediatric oligodendroglioma. Childs Nerv Syst 2015;31(6):885–91.

24. Tong KA, Ashwal S, Obenaus A, et al. Susceptibility-weighted MR imaging: a review of clinical applications in children. AJNR Am J Neuroradiol 2008; 29(1):9–17.

# Index

Neuroimag Clin N Am 27 (2017) 191–193
http://dx.doi.org/10.1016/S1052-5149(16)30110-1
1052-5149/17

# Moving?

## Make sure your subscription moves with you!

To notify us of your new address, find your **Clinics Account Number** (located on your mailing label above your name), and contact customer service at:

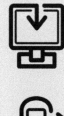

**Email: journalscustomerservice-usa@elsevier.com**

**800-654-2452** (subscribers in the U.S. & Canada)
**314-447-8871** (subscribers outside of the U.S. & Canada)

**Fax number: 314-447-8029**

**Elsevier Health Sciences Division
Subscription Customer Service
3251 Riverport Lane
Maryland Heights, MO 63043**

*To ensure uninterrupted delivery of your subscription, please notify us at least 4 weeks in advance of move.

Printed and bound by CPI Group (UK) Ltd, Croydon, CR0 4YY

03/10/2024

01040384-0019